PHYSICIANS PRAISE *The End of Heart Disease*

"*The End of Heart Disease* is the most comprehensive and valuable resource ever created for patients with heart disease. Dr. Fuhrman's extensive review of the research and rich clinical career lay the foundation for true informed consent and empower people to choose the best treatment pathway to prevent, suspend, and reverse the root causes of their heart disease. If you have heart disease this book is a must-read!"

 —Scott Stoll, M.D.
 Author, Speaker, Olympian
 Co-Founder Plantrician Project

"Outside of emergency lifesaving surgery, I have never seen any intervention come close to the breadth and depth of benefits that a nutrient-dense diet comprised of plant foods provides. The comprehensive information supplied by this book will empower patients and physicians to make healthier lifestyle choices. *The End of Heart Disease* may just save your life."

 —Robert Ostfeld, M.D., MSc., FACC
 Director, Preventive Cardiology
 Associate Professor of Clinical Medicine
 Montefiore Medical Center

"What distinguishes the excellent medical opinion from the mediocre is the synthesis of an accurate analysis of the scientific literature with sound clinical judgment. Science alone is not enough. Regardless of their field of expertise, a great doctor can separate the proverbial 'wheat from the chaff' when it comes to application of the continual barrage of medical research to the clinical setting. Dr. Fuhrman is one of those unique clinicians. The gift Dr. Fuhrman has shared with all of us, with the publication of this great work, is not only his brilliant evaluation of the medical literature but also descriptions of the seminal clinical work that have helped him, and now us, understand which nutritional approaches actually work to decrease the risk of heart disease."

 —Gregory S. Weinstein, M.D.
 Professor and Vice Chair
 Director, Division of Head and Neck Surgery
 Co-Director, The Center for Head
 The Department of Oto   Surgery
 The University of Penns

"*The End of Heart Disease* means exactly what it says. This empowering plan will protect and strengthen your heart and transform your overall health. Dr. Fuhrman draws on a wealth of experience to present everything you need to know and answers your questions along the way. I have often relied on Dr. Fuhrman's wisdom, and now you can too."

    —Neal D. Barnard, M.D., FACC
        Associate Professor of Medicine, George Washington University
        School of Medicine
        President, Physicians Committee for Responsible Medicine

"For more than a quarter century I have battled heart disease in the cath lab, watching young people suffer and even die. No more! *The End of Heart Disease* lays out the science and steps to prevent and reverse the epidemic of heart disease. This must-read book will be required for every one of my patients and family. *The End of Heart Disease* has taken a giant leap forward with the plan."

    —Joel Kahn, M.D.
        Kahn Center for Cardiac Longevity
        Professor of Medicine
        Author of *The Whole Heart Solution*

"*The End of Heart Disease* explains the downsides of conventional medical approaches in treating heart disease and evaluates the most effective diets designed to promote heart health. This well-crafted book uses evidence-based science to clear some of the misconception that media generates about nutrition, and to describe easy-to-do lifestyle changes that everyone should make to regain a healthy heart as well as adding longer and better-quality years of life."

    —Naila Khalaf, M.D., Ph.D., M.P.H., M.Arch,
        Kaiser Permanente, Los Angeles Medical Center

"Today's standard diet has resulted in an epidemic of coronary artery disease, obesity, and hypertension. Medications do not address the root cause of these diseases. Dr. Fuhrman's Nutritarian diet-style is a natural human diet that leads to health optimization and reversal of many diseases. In his latest book Dr. Fuhrman demonstrates an evidence-based approach, demonstrating the multiple cardiovascular benefits of this whole-food, high-nutrient, plant-rich diet. If one day this becomes the mainstream way of eating, society will become way healthier, happier, safer, and more productive!"

    —Aram Shahparaki, M.D., FRCPC
        Internal Medicine

"A well-aimed shot across the medical bow of a system that swallows up 84 percent of our national medical budget mostly on managing the symptoms of our common chronic disease with pills and procedures without effecting a cure. It's a shot that needs to be heard around the world, to empower people everywhere to better understand Dr. Fuhrman's NDPR (Nutrient-Dense, Plant-Rich) diet, largely consisting of 'foods as grown' as a safe and proven reversal strategy for heart disease and other lifestyle-related chronic diseases, where benefits often begin to show up within weeks, as published in peer-reviewed medical journals."

    —Hans Diehl, Dr.H.Sc., M.P.H., FACN
       Bestselling Author
       Founder of the CHIP program and the Lifestyle Medicine Institute
       Clinical Professor of Preventative Medicine, Loma Linda School
         of Medicine

"*The End of Heart Disease* is a must-read for all physicians and medical students as well as for anyone with a heart who wants it to continue beating! Fuhrman shares the extensive knowledge he has gained via thorough research and more than twenty-five years of helping patients reverse their disease processes. It's brilliant!"

    —Amanda McKinney, M.D., CPE
       Fellow ACOG, Director of Lifestyle Medicine, Beatrice Community
         Hospital

"On page one, Dr. Fuhrman makes the bold claim that this nutritional program can make it almost impossible for you to have a heart attack. He then backs that claim with science. The facts are there; the choice is yours. A must-read for anyone interested in their heart health."

    —Larry Antonucci, M.D., M.B.A.
       Chief Operating Officer, Lee Memorial Health System

"This book by Dr. Fuhrman is probably his best iteration and I see it as a game changer. I cannot overstate the importance of following his recommendations to the letter. Besides my experience using Dr. Fuhrman's methods on myself and with my patients, I have been reading hundreds of books by experts on the topic, but every time I read one of Dr. Fuhrman's books I find myself in awe and blown away once again by his honesty on one hand and his perseverance to leave a Fuhrmanian legacy that lingers on and on for generations to come. Spare yourself the platitudes of many other nutrition books and read the real thing!"

—Basim Ayoub, M.D.
Hospitalist CMC–Union NC
Stroke Department Program Co-Director

"Dr. Fuhrman's book discusses a powerful, scientifically documented approach for both preventing and reversing heart disease and diabetes. This book is a must-read for both doctors and the public since Dr. Fuhrman gives hope, twenty-five years of clinical proof, and scientific validity. This inspiring book can save lives!"

—Roopa Chari, M.D.
Medical Director, Chari Center of Health

"Are you truly committed to the most effective dietary change to lower your cholesterol, blood pressure and reduce your risk from heart disease? Dr. Fuhrman's carefully researched book can serve as a guidepost to a natural (nutritional) lifestyle to help achieve your goal."

—Austin "Ken" Kutscher, M.D., Fellow of the American College
of Cardiology
Associate Clinical Professor
Department of Internal Medicine
Robert Wood Johnson University of Medicine

"I am honored to support Dr. Fuhrman's latest teachings and his expertise in the area of heart disease, which focuses on prevention as well as a treatment approach that encourages patients and health care providers alike with the knowledge that heart disease IS reversible. His focus on eating (the right foods) to live a healthy life is spot on! As the title of his latest book states, we should *plan to prevent* heart disease; and when the disease does occur, Dr. Fuhrman's "Nutritarian" approach to healthy eating helps each individual reverse his or her disease and look forward to a more functional and fulfilling future. I discuss Dr. Fuhrman's medical approach to heart disease with my patients and also with many other physicians knowing that laypeople and health care providers also need more education in the area of nutrition. The information in Dr. Fuhrman's series of books develops a nutritional foundational and a practical way to deal with the number one killer in the USA. Dr. Fuhrman gives us hope that we can (and will) win the war against heart disease. Thank you, Dr. Fuhrman, for being a champion for healthy living!"

—Sal Lacagnina, D.O.
Fort Myers, Florida

"Once again, Joel Fuhrman has hit the mark. His 'Nutritarian' diet is supported by clinical evidence and illustrated with clear charts, graphs, and recipes. Many people could reduce their risk of both systemic and eye diseases by adhering to this diet."

—Joshua L. Dunaief, M.D., Ph.D.
Adele Niessen Professor of Ophthalmology
Perelman School of Medicine, University of Pennsylvania

"Dr. Fuhrman's latest text advises us on a program to achieve recovery for even those with advanced heart disease. He reviews the complete body of science that supports his twenty-five years of clinical achievements demonstrated by those following his nutritional protocol. He logically evaluates the most common nutritional recommendations to prevent and reverse heart disease and clearly and comprehensively addresses proper exercise, weight reduction, impact of alcohol, tobacco, and medications such as statins, anticoagulants, and anti-hypertensives. A key conclusion is that: 'Every step in the right direction will reduce risk and bear health dividends.' Even for those reluctant to be a convert to the 'Nutritarian' standard of living, reflection on his accomplishments to date may induce beneficial changes in how a reader lives."

—Eli A. Friedman, M.D., M.A.C.P., F.R.C.P.
Distinguished Teaching Professor of Medicine
SUNY, Downstate Medical Center

"The single biggest killer across the globe, heart disease, is almost 100 percent preventable and very often reversible. In the *End of Heart Disease,* Dr. Fuhrman lays out the science of ending and reversing heart disease using the most powerful drug on the planet: food. A whole foods, predominately plant based diet works faster, better, and is cheaper than any currently available treatments to prevent and reverse heart disease. Dr. Fuhrman cuts through the noise and provides a clear path to health for millions. If you have a heart, read this book!"

—Mark Hyman, M.D.
Director, Cleveland Clinic Center for Functional Medicine
Author of the *New York Times* bestseller *Eat Fat Get Thin*

"It's not if, it's when . . . when your heart disease will reverse is quite simply whenever you start this diet!"

—Alona Pulde, M.D., and Matthew Lederman, M.D.
Transition To Health Medical & Wellness Center

"Another brilliant book by Dr. Fuhrman calling patients and doctors alike to end heart disease by following a Nutritarian diet. He identifies the biochemical mechanisms by which plants in their whole form can reverse heart disease and how animal saturated fat and protein promote inflammation and vascular disease. This is a great read for all those wishing to promote health in themselves and their patients. Thank you, Dr. Fuhrman."

—Jaimela Dulaney, M.D., FACC
Cardiologist and Nutritional Educator

"As an orthopedic surgeon, I look for evidence-based treatments, results that can stand up to the scrutiny of research. I also know that replacing a joint or fixing tears and strains is only half the equation. Healthy people make healthy patients. Dr. Fuhrman's nutrient-rich diet and lifestyle approach changes lives, something I have witnessed time and again in my practice as well as in the health and well-being of my family and friends. His program is solid science and should be a mainstay of preventative care for the young and old."

—George Tischenko, M.D.
Muir Orthopaedic Specialists

"Dr. Fuhrman has written a Magnum Opus about nutrition and the heart!! Reading this book and following the dietary recommendations with delicious recipes he prescribes may save your life!!"

—Jill R. Baron, M.D.
Integrative and Functional Medicine Physician

"Dr. Fuhrman's twenty-five years of clinical experience, extensive research, and knowledge of nutrition has resulted in this book, which outlines an eating plan that will make patients not just survive, but thrive. Side effects of this diet include reduction/elimination of medication, cancer prevention, loss of excess weight, improved immunity, more stable blood sugars, and increased brainpower.

"What drug can claim this? Dr. Fuhrman includes his tastiest and time-tested recipes that will make anyone want to try this way of eating. Dr. Fuhrman has published multiple peer-reviewed articles in medicine journals, and this book is a synthesis of his research findings. This approach will be useful not only for heart disease, but for any medical condition for which lifestyle changes are helpful. The book is not only scattered with real clinical anecdotes that can inspire people, but also heavily referenced with the latest studies to back up all his advice and satisfy any health professional or scientist."

—Ashwani Garg, M.D.
Family Physician and Lifestyle Medicine Specialist

"A MUST-read for everyone wanting to be truly informed of their options to not only treat but to REVERSE heart disease and its risk factors. Dr. Fuhrman has no ulterior motive—he simply summarizes the evidence in a thorough yet easy-to-read fashion. At the same time, he dispels many of the mistruths about healthy eating. This book is a game changer!"

—Arvinpal Singh, M.D.
Medical Director, Emory Bariatric Center–Atlanta, GA
Diplomate, American Board of Obesity Medicine

"When it comes to protecting your heart and melting away plaque in your arteries, you will not find better guidance than *The End of Heart Disease*. With solid science, clear explanations, and inspiring real-life case studies, Dr. Fuhrman cuts through nutritional (and medical) nonsense to reveal a practical plan for avoiding heart attacks, stents, and bypasses, naturally and forever. 'Let food be your medicine' was never more effectively (and deliciously!) presented than in *The End of Heart Disease*—Hippocrates would be proud!"

—Michael Klaper, M.D.
Physician, True North Health Center, Santa Rosa, CA

"Easy to read. Clearly explains why and how to implement this health-saving strategy. Being open to this simpler lifestyle has allowed my patients and me to decrease medication dependence."

—Romeo A. Caballes Jr., M.D.
Internal Medicine

"Dr. Fuhrman is able to shine a light on the true role of food in our lives, which is to sustain us, keep us healthy, and not to promote disease. He puts into perspective the role of vegetarian diets, fats, and meats, and how to best nourish ourselves to optimal health. His diet program is about achieving success and balance and, in doing so, finding the best way to prevent the incidence of heart disease. Simply said, food is medicine, and in this book, Dr. Fuhrman provides us with a perfect prescription."

—Suzanne Steinbaum, D.O., Fellow of the American College
of Cardiology
Director, Women's Heart Health
Heart and Vascular Institute, Lenox Hill Hospital

"Dr. Fuhrman has done it Again! Years ago, when I first heard of him and his book *Eat to Live,* I assumed he was a quack because most diet and nutrition books were fluff and full of inaccuracies. With my scientific background, I read that book very critically and looked up multiple sources referenced by it in order to evaluate whether he had correctly interpreted the original studies. I fully expected to 'bust him' as inaccurate and was pleasantly surprised by his astounding ability to take very complex scientific studies and interpret them down into layman's terms without oversimplifying, and without losing the real meaning behind the findings. Once again, Dr. Fuhrman has taken a huge amount of scientific information and made it accessible to the layperson, and done it in such a way that they can apply this knowledge (including recipes) and make monumental improvements in their overall health and, more specifically, in most cases actually reverse coronary artery disease and ischemic heart disease, the #1 killer in America and around the world!"

—David Bullock, MSW, D.O., BCIM
President, Life Enhancement Medicine and Rehabilitation
Physical Medicine and Rehabilitation Specialist

"Finally, a scientific compilation of studies proving that food is medicine as well as an excellent alternative. I have already enjoyed the success of several of my patients cutting their LDL cholesterol in half and being able to stop all medications pertaining to cholesterol and hypertension, because eating as a Nutritarian makes sense. In fact, just to be sure this eating plan was doable, I tried it myself and my LDL cholesterol went from 120 to 65 in six months."

—Connie Hahn, D.O.
Family Physician

"Dr. Fuhrman propels the science of healthy eating well past vegan and even whole-food plant-based nutrition by focusing on the healthiest nutrient-dense foods. He clearly lays out how a healthy enough diet can not only be cheaper and safer than pills and procedures for heart disease and high blood pressure but, critically, *more effective.*"

—Michael Greger, M.D., FACLM
Founder of NutritionFacts.org

"As a physician who specializes in heart attack and stroke prevention via nutrition and lifestyle medicine, having such a thoroughly researched, well-organized, and user-friendly guide for my clients will be truly invaluable. My only criticism is having had to wait this long for it to be written! Nothing will help you prevent or reverse cardiovascular disease more powerfully than the ideas and recommendations in this book. Thank you, Dr. Fuhrman. You just made my job a whole lot easier!!"

—Daniel Chong, ND

"Lifestyle medicine is the most important and fastest-growing trend in health care today. In this important book, Dr. Joel Fuhrman describes why."

—Dean Ornish, M.D.
Founder and President, Preventive Medicine Research Institute
Clinical Professor of Medicine, UCSF
Author of *Dr. Dean Ornish's Program for Reversing Heart Disease* and *The Spectrum*

"In *The End of Heart Disease,* Dr. Fuhrman points us toward a solid, scientific path for dealing with heart disease by treating its cause with nutritional excellence. In the light of current science, the old approach focused on pills and procedures is not only outrageously expensive for little benefit for most, but antiquated, and now constitutes malpractice. It is my hope that many will experience a much more vibrant and longer life through availing themselves of this more rational and practical way of dealing with heart disease."

—Marc Braman, M.D., M.P.H., FACLM, FACPM
President, Lifestyle Medicine Foundation
Former President, The American College of Lifestyle Medicine

THE END OF HEART DISEASE

THE END OF HEART DISEASE

The Eat to Live Plan to Prevent and Reverse Heart Disease

Joel Fuhrman, M.D.

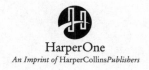

HarperOne
An Imprint of HarperCollinsPublishers

HarperOne

HarperCollins books may be purchased for educational, business, or sales promotional use. For information please e-mail the Special Markets Department at SPsales@harpercollins.com.

HarperCollins website: http://www.harpercollins.com

FIRST EDITION

Interior design by Laura Lind Design

Library of Congress Cataloging-in-Publication Data
Fuhrman, Joel, author.
The end of heart disease : the eat to live plan to prevent and reverse heart disease / Joel Fuhrman, M.D.
First edition. / New York, NY : HarperOne, 2016.
Includes index.
ISBN 978–0–06–224935–7 (hardback)
ISBN 978–0–06–224937–1 (e-book)
ISBN 978–0–06–237240–6 (audio)
1. Heart—Diseases—Prevention—Popular works. 2. Heart—Diseases—Diet therapy—Popular works. 3. Heart—Diseases—Nutritional aspects—Popular works.

16 17 18 19 20   RRD(H)   10 9 8 7 6 5 4 3 2 1

The results of any diet or medical intervention can vary from person to person. Some people have a medical history and/or condition that may warrant individualized recommendations and, in some cases, drugs and even surgery. Do not start, stop, or change medication without professional medical advice, and do not change your diet if you are ill or on medication except under the supervision of a competent physician. Neither this nor any other book is intended to take the place of personalized medical care or treatment.

A CAUTION TO THE READER

If you are taking any medication, especially medication for diabetes or high blood pressure, do not make dietary changes without the assistance of a physician, as your medication will need adjustment to prevent excessive lowering of your blood pressure and blood sugar levels. Very low blood glucose levels (hypoglycemia) and low blood pressure (hypotension) from using too much medication can be dangerous. This dietary program is very effective at lowering both, so any medication you are on for either of these conditions will need to be adjusted and, with time, maybe discontinued.

Hypoglycemia and hypotension can cause weakness and fainting, which can lead to a fall or a motor vehicle accident. The overuse of blood pressure medication can even damage your kidneys. Because this nutritional program is so effective at reversing heart disease, dropping body weight, and reversing diabetes, it is even more important to consult with a knowledgeable physician who is familiar with reducing medication as a result of aggressive dietary modifications. Do not underestimate the effectiveness of this program.

Many physicians, not realizing how effective this diet-style is, may be hesitant to taper medications sufficiently. Make sure you warn your physician about this and follow your blood pressure and blood sugar levels more carefully, especially over the first few weeks after you begin this plan.

I discuss medications in more detail and give more guidance for their reduction for you and your physician later in this book. However, you must be aware that a book cannot take the place of individualized counseling from a physician who knows your medical condition. It is your responsibility to work with your physician to assure that your blood sugar and blood pressure readings are neither too high nor too low.

Note: The cases in this book are all real, but some of the names have been modified or omitted for privacy purposes.

I dedicate this book to physicians who utilize Lifestyle Medicine, showing they care by spending the extra time to communicate and motivate their patients to take control of their health, despite the challenges and resistance of society and even their peers. Millions of human life years have been saved by their dedication.

Contents

The Heart of
the Matter

Heart disease is the leading cause of death for both men and women in the United States. In fact, cardiovascular diseases claim more lives than all forms of cancer combined. About half of these needless deaths are caused by sudden cardiac death. This means a person dies immediately after symptoms begin, or within a short time afterward. The cause of sudden cardiac death can vary from an obstructive clot to a fatal arrhythmia. Another common cause is enlargement of the heart, specifically, left ventricular hypertrophy caused by many years of high blood pressure. Fifty-five percent of the men and 68 percent of the women who die of sudden cardiac death have no prior warning of significant heart disease. Heart disease kills many people many years prematurely, and most of them do not even make it to the hospital alive.

I am reasonably certain that the nutritional program in these pages can make it almost impossible for you to have a heart attack or to experience sudden cardiac death. Not only that, this program is effective even if you presently have advanced heart disease. It can radically lower your cholesterol and blood pressure, and it can reverse obstructive coronary artery disease (CAD) so effectively that it obliterates the need for angioplasty and bypass surgery. Unless you are one of the fewer than 1 percent of people who has advanced valve damage, a genetic defect, or electrical pathway disease, you should be able to reverse any heart disease you now have.

In other words, you will not merely lower your cholesterol, but you will also remedy other risk factors. By following this nutritional plan, you will

- Lower and normalize your blood pressure

- Lower your low-density lipoprotein (LDL) cholesterol

- Lower your weight, body fat, and waist measurements

- Lower your fasting glucose levels and resolve diabetes (type 2)

- Restore normal bowel function

- Improve your immune function, lowering the risk of infection

- Maintain your youthful vigor as you age, and age more slowly

This approach is the most effective and safest way to lower your blood pressure and cholesterol. But more importantly, I give you information that will assure you that you most likely will never have a heart attack. This is potentially lifesaving information. When you lower your cholesterol and blood pressure through superior nutrition, you lower your risk of heart disease much more radically than by using cholesterol-lowering drugs and blood pressure medication alone.

Other nutritional programs have demonstrated, in clinical practice and research trials, effective protection against and reversal of heart disease. As one would expect, those programs are similar to this one. Effective nutritional interventions must have significant similarities, or they would not be effective.

But the information presented in this book takes this science a step further. Based on my twenty-five years of clinical experience reversing heart disease in thousands of patients through nutritional excellence, this book provides the clinical protocols, the medical management, and the detailed application information not merely to prevent and reverse heart disease, but also to prevent sudden cardiac death, stroke, and dementia. My experience with thousands of patients has also given me invaluable insight so that I can give you the information that allows you to tailor the protocol to your individual needs. What you learn here will help you overcome obstacles to effective dietary

change, especially since dietary change can be challenging and unhealthy foods are highly addictive.

Existing heart ailments, obstructive atherosclerosis, and CAD can
improve and eventually resolve. In addition, you can gradually reduce
and eventually eliminate your need for medications that treat high
cholesterol, high blood pressure, and type 2 diabetes. This book delivers the most effective method to lose weight, lower cholesterol and
high blood pressure, and reverse heart disease, and it makes most
medical care and medical interventions for heart disease obsolete.
Plus, the results happen quickly in most cases, immediately lowering
risk and within a few months *entirely removing the risk* of ever having
a heart attack.

Over the past twenty-five years, I have counseled thousands of patients who've had advanced heart disease, many of whom experienced
angina (chest pain) or were told they needed urgent bypass surgery or
angioplasty. Not one of the individuals who followed my nutritional
recommendations ever had a heart attack or died from heart disease.

I do believe that the risk goes down gradually, over time, when a
person follows such a heart-protective diet-style. I do not think the first
week, or even the first month, will offer total protection against heart
attacks, but as months pass, I am certain that a heart attack would be
an incredibly rare occurrence.

In my opinion, this lifesaving book should be distributed to every
heart patient in the United States because conventional care, with its
usual poor outcome, is bad medicine. Cardiac patients typically worsen
and usually die of heart disease despite the finest medical management. Every physician caring for people presenting with heart disease
should offer them the information found in this book. Not informing
patients about this simple advice—advice that could make the difference between life and death—should be considered malpractice.

Patients are not given the information they need to make a definitive decision to *not* have a heart attack. Many may choose to eat the
heart disease–causing Standard American Diet (SAD) and sprinkle a
few drugs on top to try to lessen the risk a bit. That's their choice. But
others—and I hope this is *you*—will do more. They will say "No!" to

angina and heart attack. They will learn that superior nutrition can reverse and prevent heart disease, and save them from getting some other diseases as well.

If what I am saying is true, and if what I call a Nutritarian diet-style is this effective, then the foundation of traditional cardiology is subpar, even negligent. If a patient with heart disease is not told about effective dietary interventions and instead is offered only drugs; invasive, interventional procedures; and surgeries, then that person is denied informed consent. That patient has effectively been corralled into risky interventions that are expensive and high-tech—and mostly do not work.

I hope that with a careful review of the information and scientific references in this book, you, working with your doctor, will help modify the way medicine is practiced. This book provides comprehensive, informed consent. That means every person on high blood pressure medication, or offered cholesterol-lowering drugs by their physicians, should be advised to read this information first.

In addition, it is critical that any patient with known atherosclerosis who is considering an intervention such as angioplasty or bypass surgery should be told that this dietary approach is a safer and more effective option. (Of course, this does not include people who are in unstable or emergency situations, such as those in an emergency room having a heart attack or with unstable angina and a heart attack looming shortly.)

The following case history makes an important point, showing the dramatic effectiveness of this approach for heart disease. It demonstrates what I have seen routinely occur and the time frame in which individuals typically see results.

Barry's Story: Dramatic Change
in Twelve Weeks

I went to Fort Wayne, Indiana, to give a lecture to a large church group of more than seven hundred people. Gaby Henderson coordinated this event. She had lost more than 100 pounds following my advice and had kept the weight off for more than four years. She was excited about sharing my Nutritarian approach with her community.

She had mentioned to me in a prior e-mail correspondence that her husband, Barry, age 53, was experiencing increasing chest pressure and shortness of breath with exertion. It had slowly worsened in intensity, to the point where he could no longer run or even walk uphill. He called his diet "Fuhrman-light" because he still ate out almost every day, in addition to eating the healthy food Gaby prepared for them in the evening. There was Barry, sitting right in the front row of the church, ready to listen to my lecture.

While we were waiting for people to arrive, I asked him how he was feeling, and he told me that recently the pain had become significantly worse. He had been experiencing continuous chest pain, even at rest, since the previous day. In fact, he was having chest pressure and significant discomfort sitting right there in his chair. Wow, I thought to myself. He had really waited too long to get "on board."

I told him that he was now in a potentially life-threatening position called "unstable angina," since his condition had advanced to the point that he felt chest pressure even at rest that worsened with activity. He needed to go the emergency room immediately; he could even have been experiencing a heart attack at that very moment.

I don't know whether it was because of his religious beliefs or his fear of medical care, but he refused. Barry said he would rather die than go to the hospital and be treated for heart disease, and he asked me whether I would still help him.

So I told him that he and his family needed to be aware that he could have a fatal heart attack at any time, because his condition was unstable, and he was placing himself at extremely high risk.

I was concerned that a heart attack was imminent. Certainly, I did not want Barry to die, and I did not want to be held responsible if something bad happened. But he adamantly refused medical care. Instead, he agreed to let me totally control what he put into his mouth.

I told him that he should not make *any* decisions about what to eat or not eat. I would make those decisions for him, and I would also talk to Gaby about his dietary and supplemental regimen so that she could help him, too.

When he began the Nutritarian diet program, Barry, who was 5 feet 10 inches tall, weighed 183 pounds and had an average blood pressure of 160/108 mmHg. Within three months, he lost 30 pounds and his angina symptoms faded away. The sensation of chest pressure lightened in a few days, and within a week he no longer experienced chest pain at rest. His blood pressure came down to 130/80 during that first week. After two to three weeks, he was able to walk a few blocks without experiencing chest pain. After eight weeks, he was able to jog without symptoms. And after twelve weeks, he was able to do any amount of physical activity, even run fast, without any signs of angina. After one year on the program, his weight was down to 154 pounds, his blood pressure averaged 112/75 mmHg, and he continued to live in excellent health without any angina symptoms.

In twelve weeks, Barry went from being a cardiac cripple, unable to walk without pain and hovering close to death's door, to feeling normal—all without a stress test, cardiac catheterization, stent placement, or bypass surgery. He would still have been recovering and rehabbing from bypass surgery at that twelve-week point if he had gone to the emergency room, yet in the same time frame, after a different choice, he was essentially cured.

Barry never should have waited until his condition was so precarious to seek help. But even with the most severely obstructed patients, this life-threatening condition can completely resolve quickly with dietary intervention alone. Of course, Barry's atherosclerosis was not entirely gone within those twelve weeks, but it will continue to lessen as he stays on the program. Most importantly, his vulnerable (most dangerous) plaque transformed and became nonvulnerable and nonobstructing.

This simple, illustrative case makes an important point and is an excellent teaching tool, especially when you recognize that bypass surgery and angioplasty do not prevent future cardiac events or extend life span in heart patients. These procedures just relieve symptoms temporarily, like a Band-Aid, while the disease process remains and advances throughout the coronary vasculature.[1] In Barry's case, his reversal reflected a true reduction of risk, not a temporary fix like one gets from drugs and surgical interventions.

Where Is the Evidence?

As you read this book, it is helpful to be aware of the hundreds of references, and the large body of knowledge, that lead to the inescapable conclusions reported here. It is not only my experience, case histories, and recorded and published medical journal data that lend evidence to the effectiveness of this approach. Many other physicians, scientists, and researchers have evaluated and contributed to these conclusions as well.

As more scientific studies and corroborating evidence become available in the future, the information will encourage more physicians and health professionals to embrace this approach with enthusiasm. But the truth is, it has been happening already. The results keep coming in that a nutrient-dense, plant-rich (NDPR) Nutritarian diet is extremely effective in protecting against and reversing heart disease.

A recently published case series and survey study evaluating more than one thousand individuals following my dietary recommendations to various degrees offered compelling results documenting the effectiveness of this approach in the general population.[2] It is important to note that the results reported on the group of participants 80 percent or more compliant with my recommendations. Numerous individual cases demonstrating reversal of even advanced heart disease were presented in this study. Of the 443 individuals with high blood pressure, the average drop in systolic blood pressure after a Nutritarian diet was followed for at least one year was 26 mmHg. In contrast, standard blood pressure medications lower systolic blood pressure on average about 10 mmHg.[3] The drop for the Nutritarian patients in diastolic blood pressure was about 15 mmHg. These results dwarf what can be achieved with routine blood pressure medications—and they are achieved without the risks of side effects. Similar dramatic benefits were seen for lowering cholesterol and body weight reduction, and I discuss the details of this study in Chapter 3.

There will always be those who insist that the evidence presented and the results reported are not sufficient. But take a moment to consider, what is their motivation for doubting the consistent lifesaving outcomes resulting from using this nutritional method? I chose the cases highlighted in this book for their severity and teaching points. But thousands more people have experienced lifesaving results from following my guidance.

I am not the only physician using the methods described within these pages. I communicate regularly with many doctors specializing in lifestyle medicine who use this program with what have to be considered phenomenal results, by anyone's standard. Many of my patients have described what has happened to them as "a medical miracle." I've heard these words time and time again, and they demonstrate that heart disease is not the inevitable consequence of aging—instead, our food is killing us.

Certainly, much more scientific investigation is needed for this information to fully permeate society and the medical industry. Some of those additional studies are being performed right now. I am devoting much of my time, effort, and resources to making such studies happen. But make no mistake: Although this additional data may be needed to persuade the skeptics, it is not needed for you to benefit from this information today.

Implementing this lifesaving strategy today can save your life. It has happened already—not hundreds, but thousands of times, to people all across our country and many around the world who have used this approach to reverse their heart disease.

This year, more than seventeen million people will die from heart disease. More die of heart disease than AIDS and all cancers combined. Not only does sudden cardiac death, in most cases, give no warning—half of those victims are younger than age 65.

In 2011 the total cost of treating cardiovascular disease in the United States was $320 billion; in comparison, the estimated total cost of treating cancer in 2009 was $217 billion.[4] But that is only the beginning: How do we measure the pain, suffering, and emotional distress thrust on individuals and families as a result of the staggering epidemic of broken hearts? It is even more tragic when you contemplate that all this suffering and premature death does not have to happen. And yet it continues, despite modern medical facilities and some of the best medical care available in the world.

Every hour across the United States, patients go to their physicians with high blood pressure, high cholesterol, and glucose intolerance, or diabetes. They are put on medications, and (generally) they are never told that changing their diets could rid them of their problems, and even save their lives.

Very often, doctors believe that dietary modifications this effective are simply too difficult for most people to follow and stick with. They rationalize this belief by telling themselves that, since patients won't do it anyway, what's the use in taking the time to educate them?

This is an opinion that I heard in medical school, and I still hear it now from some cardiologists and endocrinologists. The general consensus is: "Oh yeah, I know it can work, but I tried that and nobody would listen. It's just a waste of time. People want a pill; they aren't going to radically change their habits and their diets." They recognize that the conventional approach is not ideal, but they rationalize their treatment choice.

Some doctors have given up because they believe they can't make enough money if they change their practice, and/or they don't want to practice differently from their peers. They just continue what they were taught, even though it doesn't work.

Fortunately, I see that this status quo is changing rapidly. The American College of Lifestyle Medicine has been growing by leaps and bounds. More and more doctors are recommending that patients embrace significant dietary change. Leading hospitals and research institutions are setting up centers of lifestyle medicine and utilizing and testing nutritional approaches. Top physicians and scientists are recognizing that this information is sorely needed to help our suffering population—and many of them are eating this way themselves.

Many doctors today realize that patients suffer and die needlessly when they do not give those patients the information they need to save their lives. That is why this book is so important. A little bit of knowledge does not work very well. People need *all* the right information to make the right decisions for their lives.

What I call "standard" medical care is ending. *Doctors can no longer effectively—or ethically—treat patients with medications without discussing the power and absolute necessity of nutritional interventions.*

I am not limiting my definition of "standard" medical care to the use of coronary angioplasty and bypass surgery. I am referring to the uses and abuses of the prescription pad as well.

Imagine that a physician notes that her elderly patient has high blood pressure and writes a prescription. In many cases, the doctor will soon get a phone call telling her that the patient fell, fractured a hip, and is now in the hospital. As surprising as this sounds, it is not an unusual event. In fact, in people 66 years and older, the likelihood of hip fracture increases almost 50 percent during the first six weeks of starting blood pressure medication.[5]

This "prescription pad" approach to medicine raises a great many questions: Was this patient told that there was a safer option to lowering blood pressure? Was this patient informed of the increased risk of hip fracture with the use of medication? Was this patient told of studies that demonstrate a 50 percent increased risk of breast cancer for people taking certain blood pressure medications? What if a statin drug caused liver failure, requiring hospitalization? What if the patient died or suffered brain damage while undergoing angioplasty or bypass surgery? It all comes down to one critically important question: *Why wasn't the patient informed that there was a safer, more effective option?*

Things are changing because the way medicine has been typically practiced has resulted in needless suffering and the needless death of patients. Patients may choose not to comply with dietary recommendations, but that should be *their* decision, not the doctor's. All people who visit a family doctor, internist, endocrinologist, or cardiologist have a right to know that they have the potential to get well without being exposed to the risks that medical care can create. This is especially true when so many medical procedures and medications have been adequately demonstrated to have negative consequences.

Since heart disease and stroke are now the leading causes of death worldwide, I think every adult should be aware of the superior power of nutritional excellence to treat and eliminate heart disease, compared with the unimpressive results associated with standard cardiovascular medicine. This information is of vital importance and impacts every man, woman, and child. It should be taught in our schools.

Certainly, all doctors caring for adults should be making an effort to inform their clients of this information. Any doctor who fails to do so is violating the physician's oath—"First, do no harm"—and is breaking the rule of informed consent.

If your physician is recommending or making this information available to you, then you are working with an enlightened individual. Providing you with the tools to recover your health demonstrates your doctor's goodwill toward you. The hope that you can get well is a form of care of the highest magnitude. The role of doctor-as-teacher is the most valuable part of health care because correct information saves lives.

I have cared for thousands of patients with cardiovascular disease, and thousands of individuals whom I have never met have read my books, received guidance via my website, and followed my advice. Of the more than ten thousand individuals whom I have counseled over the years, most were seriously ill and often at a phase in their disease evolution that was extremely serious. The results of following this nutritional protocol have been consistent and dramatic. Even people with the most advanced disease were able to see dramatic improvements in their conditions, with the vast majority achieving complete recovery and becoming able to discontinue all medications.

Of course, no dietary approach to heart disease and diabetes will succeed without attention to other risk factors. It is critically important to alter a sedentary lifestyle, to stop smoking, and to get enough sleep. The road to wellness involves making a commitment to a healthy lifestyle.

When they started this dietary approach, many of these individuals were not able to exercise—some could hardly even walk. But the inability to exercise did not prevent them from obtaining dramatic benefits. In fact, most often, those who adopt this approach regain the ability to be active and in time learn to enjoy exercising after they have already made a significant recovery. Exercise and activity are helpful; however, being unable to exercise much, or at all, at the beginning will not prevent this approach from working for you.

What is so disappointing is seeing so many people suffer and die needlessly—especially the millions of people who were never told that they did not have to die prematurely; they had the opportunity to recover. I am writing this book with the hope that it can reach a vast number of people. I hope that it will prove useful to both patients and physicians in evaluating the risks and benefits of medical care versus nutritional excellence, and in delineating the precise nutritional recommendations for optimal protection and recovery.

Having or not having heart disease is merely a decision, because ultimately, it is all up to you. Your doctor cannot force you to do anything; he or she can only present the options. It is *your* life—and you get only one chance to live it. I hope you choose to make this life a healthy, joyful, and long one.

My sincere wish is that you and your doctor receive tremendous joy and satisfaction from monitoring your recovery and taking part in your healing. Thank you for giving me the opportunity to play a role in helping you achieve better health. I applaud all physicians who re-educate themselves and buck the medical establishment to give their patients a better quality of care.

I have taken every effort to make sure that all the data and scientific evidence quoted, discussed, and referenced in this book are accurate. If any scientist, physician, or researcher finds an error, I would appreciate that it be brought to my immediate attention, so it can be remedied. Even though the information is not yet the "standard of care" in medicine in the United States, I invite scientific and medical readers who investigate this evidence to see whether they disagree with the conclusions drawn from logic, experience, and conservative sensibility.

CHAPTER ONE

Food Can Either
Kill or Heal,
the Choice Is Yours

The standard American diet (SAD) is heartbreaking—in the most literal sense of the word. It damages the heart in almost every single person who eats it. Heart disease and strokes kill about half of all Americans, and that does not mean that atherosclerosis (blood vessel hardening and plaque deposition) develops in only half of the people in this country. The only reason cardiovascular disease doesn't kill most of the other half is because cancer or some other diet-related disease kills them first. The diet-style of most Americans is overwhelmingly unhealthy and causes atherosclerosis in everyone who eats convention-ally. The result is that almost all Americans develop heart disease, re-gardless of genetics. Autopsy studies on adult Americans of all ages who die in car accidents show that more than 90 percent of them have some degree of atherosclerotic heart disease.[1]

It is a simple fact that certain foods lead to superior health and other foods lead to ill health. It is impossible to not gradually damage blood vessels when you regularly consume disease-causing foods. And it is also almost impossible to escape from the biological laws of cause and effect even if you are taking medicine to offset the symptoms; the negative effects of the modern eating style in most of the modern world are too powerful to overcome. The SAD is deadly; that is why I often call it the DAD, or deadly American diet. And, this way of eating has permeated much of the world today.

CASE HISTORY: PROOF FROM A PATIENT

I was always overweight and battling it with every fad diet there was, without success. So I gave up trying to lose weight. For over a decade I had nasal polyps and was frequently on steroids and antibiotics. In August 2013, at age 35, I was trying to get medically cleared to have surgery on my nose. At the cardiologist's office, I weighed 303 pounds. Several nurses took my blood pressure and then brought in the doctor, who told me that my blood pressure was 265 over 140. He said that I couldn't leave his office unless I went straight to the emergency room. He even suggested I take an ambulance there. I thought they were crazy.

Eventually, I was pumped full of pills until I vomited. I wound up taking as much medication as my stomach could tolerate, and my blood pressure was still high. I was only 35, my wife was pregnant, and I was going to die of a heart attack. To make matters worse, my mother died of a heart attack at age 38, when I was just 5 years old. That I could leave my wife and child in the same awful circumstances my mother left me in was a wake-up call.

I tried dieting, controlling portions, and working out. I also did four cycles of hCG hormone shots. I was given injections for diabetes, too. And with all this effort I lost 26 pounds in eighteen months, and I still was no better. I thought I just was a "big guy" and I'd lost my opportunity to get healthy and improve my life.

Then my diet coach introduced me to the Fuhrman plan. In three months, I lost 74 pounds. I am now down to 203 pounds and my blood pressure is great and I don't need medications anymore. My polyps shrank and most disappeared. I can do push-ups and chin-ups and run like I never could before. The number of benefits I have felt in all aspects of my life are amazing and outweigh a hundred times needing junk food, meat, or cheese on my plate. I am also enjoying new delicious foods I never knew tasted so good.

David Montanaro

Atherosclerosis starts in childhood, even in infancy for those infants whose mothers eat the SAD during pregnancy. Atherosclerotic plaque develops over decades, with sickness and death mostly occurring later in life. With the growing waistlines of our population and the increased consumption of processed foods and fast foods over the past few decades, we are observing more diabetes, more strokes, and more serious diseases in younger people. In men older than 50 and women older than 60, the rate of atherosclerosis accelerates and the vessels become stiffer and less flexible, increasing the risks associated with blood vessel disease.

Certainly, some acquired and genetic defects are not caused by diet, but those are the rare exceptions. We are often told that high blood pressure, high cholesterol, diabetes, and heart disease are consequences of aging and genetics and that all we can do to mitigate them is take the medications prescribed. Our "numbers" may look better, but the underlying disease process worsens each year. But these issues are not predominantly the direct result of genetics and need not be the expected outcome of aging. Superior nutrition can prevent high blood pressure and CAD from ever occurring at all stages of life.

Some authors and advice-givers claim that eating meat and fat is the culprit; others claim that you can eat all the meat and fat you want and that the culprit is sugar. The reality is that both excess simple sugars and excess animal products promote atherosclerosis and heart disease. This has been well documented and will be discussed in detail later. In order for you to really have the tools and motivation to prevent and reverse heart disease, you need to have a degree of expertise in nutritional science. This requires knowing what is wrong with the way people are eating today, as well as understanding the therapeutic value of certain foods.

I divide food into four main categories:

- Produce
- Whole grains
- Refined or highly processed foods
- Animal products

In the typical American diet about 30 percent of calories come from animal foods such as dairy, meat, eggs, and chicken, and about 55 percent of calories come from processed foods such as pasta, bread, soda, oils, sugar, puffed cereals, pretzels, and other adulterated products. This means that only about 15 percent of calories come from a combination of whole grains and produce. Cancer and heart disease are the inevitable consequences. It is essential for your health and survival to reduce both processed foods and animal products in your diet and replace those calories with more vegetables, fruits, whole grains, beans, nuts, and seeds. This can improve the health of people in modern countries the world over, as well as dramatically reduce health-care costs.

The Deadly American Diet

The SAD, or the deadly American diet (DAD), includes only a small amount of produce, particularly greens, mushrooms, onions, seeds, and colorful vegetables and fruits. This leads to an overall deficiency in micronutrients, especially in the antioxidants and phytochemicals necessary for normal health, cellular repair, and immune function. These nourishing unrefined plant foods are rich in fiber and nutrients that help prevent cancer and protect blood vessels, yet Americans eat very little of them. Almost every nutritional scientist in the world

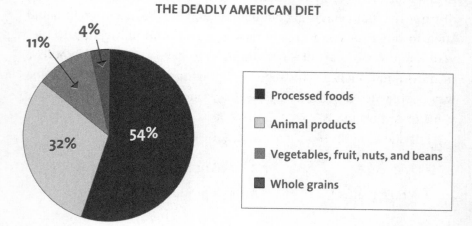

THE DEADLY AMERICAN DIET

11% 4% 32% 54%

- Processed foods
- Animal products
- Vegetables, fruit, nuts, and beans
- Whole grains

agrees that we need to eat more vegetables, beans, seeds, and nuts and less processed foods.

There is one thing that all powerful, long-term, and large epidemiological studies have in common, and that is the demonstrated benefits from eating more vegetables, beans, nuts, and seeds. This common denominator of more plant foods and less animal products is also seen in all the so-called Blue Zones of the world, that is, where the people who have the longest life expectancy live. The population with the longest documented life expectancy in the world doesn't eat any meat at all: the subset of the Seventh-Day Adventists in Loma Linda, California, who are vegetarians and regularly eat nuts and seeds.

When the Mediterranean diet was evaluated in the large PREDI-MED study, the data corroborated that the more produce and the less animal products consumed, the greater the longevity enhancement. This pattern held to a consistent dose-dependent relationship, meaning that each serving of plants extended life span more and each serving of animal products decreased it accordingly. The benefits were dramatic: Cutting back on animal products by two-thirds, to one serving a day instead of three, reduced deaths by more than 40 percent.[2]

Other large-scale studies have confirmed the same thing. Of particular interest is the 2012 article "Low-Carbohydrate, High-Protein Diet and Incidence of Cardiovascular Diseases in Swedish Women: Prospective Cohort Study."[3] The researchers followed more than forty-three thousand women, 30 to 49 years old, for more than fifteen years. The study was notable for the large number of participants and the care taken to access the degree of dietary adherence to the high-protein, low-carbohydrate diet protocol. The researchers gave the subjects a diet score from 1 to 20 based on how closely they followed the low-carb, high-protein dietary pattern. Those with the lowest diet score were eating the least amount of animal products, and those who were eating the most were scored as 20.

The researchers tracked cardiovascular events for years and found a dose-dependent increase in risk: a 5 percent increase in risk of cardiovascular events per 2-point increase in the low-carb, high-protein diet adherence score. Overall, a 60 percent increased risk of cardiovascular events was seen in women adhering to a low-carb, high-protein diet (diet score greater than 16). The results also showed a gradual and consistent increased risk of experiencing cardiovascular disease and cardiovascular death with a higher consumption of animal products and reduction in plant food. The researchers compared these results with those from at least four other studies that examined the same issue and found that their results were consistent with those from these earlier, smaller studies. These results collectively offer conclusive, indisputable evidence that diets low in protective plant foods and high in animal products are dangerous.

It is not merely the fat in animal products that can promote atherosclerosis, but also the high concentration of biological protein. It has been demonstrated in animal studies for decades that saturated fat and cholesterol alone do not account for all the increased atherosclerosis seen with increases in animal protein over plant protein.[4] When you eat more animal products, you develop more heart disease, and not merely because of the fat or type of fat they contain. One thing we know for sure: animal products do not contain the longevity-promoting antioxidants and phytochemicals that plants have, but modern science is uncovering other important reasons accounting for these findings.

Study data in humans show a strong association in various countries between the amount of animal protein eaten and heart disease deaths.[5] In 2004, scientists looking at the Iowa Women's Health Study, which followed twenty-nine thousand women for more than fifteen years, addressed this issue head-on.[6] Instead of comparing which of the potential negatives was worse, animal products or processed carbohydrates, researchers isolated the effects of animal protein and compared protein derived from animals with protein derived from plants.

They found a 40 percent lower risk of heart disease deaths in women whose eating pattern was higher in vegetable protein and lower in animal protein. These benefits were not seen from eating more whitish plant foods, such as bread, rice, and potatoes, but only with vegetables, beans, seeds, and nuts, which are higher in plant protein. There was a 30 percent decrease in heart disease deaths with the highest intake of vegetables, along with a lower intake of animal protein. When the foods were studied individually, it was found that meat and dairy increased risk, while nuts, vegetables, and beans decreased risk significantly.

In short, we have lots of conclusive evidence to support the need to eat more vegetables and less animal products in general.

Research studies funded by various commercial concerns have sought to deny this relationship and protect their favored foods by demonstrating conflicting findings. You can always show that a food is good, rather than bad, when you use it in place of something worse. What is typically done to achieve results showing that animal products are not harmful is to reduce animal products somewhat and replace them with more refined, high-glycemic carbohydrates. This can demonstrate an even worse outcome, thus exonerating the animal product in question. These conflicting studies that attempt to vindicate animal products prove nothing because when refined products are replaced with vegetables, nuts, seeds, and beans, disease rates *always* go down; and when animal products are replaced with vegetables, nuts, seeds, and beans, disease rates *always* go down too.

What Is a Nutritarian Diet?

I recommend a diet rich in vegetables. This plant-rich diet also contains beans, fresh fruit, nuts and seeds, and whole grains. Animal products are permitted, but in smaller quantities than are usually consumed. I call it a *Nutritarian diet.* It has also been called the nutrient-dense, plant-rich diet, or *NDPR diet.* It is a dietary style that is rich in the nutrients that humans need to maintain good health.

A Nutritarian diet has no fundamental philosophical, ethical, social, or environmental objectives. Its primary objective is to enable individuals to enjoy a diet-style that is the most longevity-promoting and the most therapeutically effective for the prevention and treatment of common chronic diseases. Its foundation is designed from an unbiased and comprehensive evaluation of the preponderance of scientific evidence on the subject.

A Nutritarian diet can be *flexitarian* (that is, containing a limited amount of animal products) or be *vegan* (no animal products at all), depending on personal preferences and individual needs. A Nutritarian diet-style, designed to maximally support health and longevity in a diverse population base, has four distinguishing characteristics:

1. *It is nutrient dense.* The Nutritarian diet-style strives to be high in micronutrients per calorie. It achieves this with increased consumption of nutrient-rich plants, such as greens, berries, seeds, and other colored produce.

2. *It is hormonally favorable.* The Nutritarian diet-style strives to avoid excess hormones, especially excess insulin and insulin-like growth factor-1 (IGF-1) (read more below), that can promote fat storage, premature aging, and cancer.

3. *It is comprehensively adequate.* The Nutritarian diet-style strives to be nutritionally adequate in a comprehensive fashion, using supplements (when deemed necessary on the basis of dietary history and available blood work) to assure optimal levels of vitamins D and B12, iodine, zinc, eicosapentaenoic acid (EPA), and docosahexaenoic acid (DHA).

4. *It avoids toxins.* The Nutritarian diet-style strives to avoid foods containing toxins, carcinogens, infectious agents, and other contaminants that can contribute to food-related morbidity and mortality.

Scientific advancements have enabled researchers to measure parameters of aging and markers of disease. It is well established that modest micronutrient insufficiency is ubiquitous and can lead to DNA damage, mitochondrial decay, and telomere decay—all factors that can significantly shorten life span. In addition to vitamins and minerals, adequate phytochemical intake also enables cells to slow the progression of these indicators of aging. I classify phytochemicals as a form of micronutrient because of their positive relationship to immune function, protection against disease, and longevity. Considering the functional importance of micronutrients, we must classify almost all

Americans, both vegetarians and meatatarians, as being deficient in micronutrients, and especially deficient in those longevity-promoting nutrients derived from green vegetables.[7]

Eating healthy is all about eating healthful foods. This isn't a brilliant or original idea, but nobody seems to understand which foods are truly healthy. Lots of people think a diet designed around pasta, chicken, and olive oil is healthy, but are these actually healthy foods? It is this confusion and the promulgation of misinformation about nutrition that is at the core of why so many people suffer with cardiovascular disease and cancer.

The healthiest foods are those with the highest ratio of nutrients to calories. To achieve optimal health we must know which foods naturally contain a significant concentration and broad array of nutrients that we need, and then eat more of those foods. But in addition to eating nutrient-rich food, we must take care not to consume more calories than we require. Nutritional adequacy without caloric excess is the only thing that has been "proven" to significantly extend life span in hundreds of corroborating scientific studies.

Vitamins, minerals, fiber, antioxidants, bioflavonoids, and phytochemicals are all necessary for normal body function—they are not optional. So we must design a diet-style that gives us an adequate amount of all these protective nutrients, leaving none missing, without providing too many calories. An added benefit is that when we receive optimal levels of a broad spectrum of human-required nutrients, we don't experience unhealthy food cravings and overeating anymore. After we achieve an adequate level of micronutrients, our brains get the appropriate signals that our nutritional needs are met and we stop eating.[8] Cravings and excess hunger diminish when our nutrient requirements are met.

Essential Nutrients

An *essential nutrient* is one that we must get from our diet because our bodies cannot make it in sufficient quantity to meet our needs. Categories of essential nutrients include vitamins, dietary minerals, essential fatty acids, and essential amino acids. *Micronutrients* refer to essential nutrients we need in relatively small amounts throughout life. These include vitamins and minerals as well as thousands of plant-derived phytochemicals. We need *macronutrients* too—water, protein, carbohydrates, and fats—but the major origin of dietary-induced disease is an excess of macronutrients from eating calorically dense foods that contain insufficient levels of micronutrients.

Much of the modern world today suffers from *high-calorie malnutrition.* This means we are eating foods that are rich in calories but contain insufficient micronutrients. It is important to note that only colorful plant foods contain *phytochemicals,* which have antioxidant and anti-inflammatory effects. Animal products do not contain phytochemicals and are very low in other antioxidants. In contrast, natural plants contain thousands of healthful, life span–enhancing phytochemical compounds.

High-nutrient foods ⟶ vegetables, beans, seeds, and fruits

Low-nutrient foods ⟶ processed foods, white flour products, sweets, oils, and animal products

Would you expect to achieve excellent health consuming a diet consisting of cotton candy and a daily multivitamin? Of course not! But most people eat a diet that has such a low nutrient density that the body cannot be expected to function normally. Bread, pasta, cold cereals, oil, and animal products are all low-nutrient foods that are cornerstones of the SAD. Why should we expect a normal lipid profile or adequate defenses against cancer and heart disease to result from a diet so low in antioxidant nutrients and phytochemicals? Remember, thousands of phytochemicals in plant foods do not inhabit the inside of a vitamin pill.

A food is good or not so good on the basis of the amount of fiber, phytochemicals, antioxidants, minerals, vitamins, and other (yet to be discovered) nutrients it contains in proportion to its number of calories. When we eat low-nutrient foods, we cannot be expected to achieve the disease-free life that our bodies are capable of. Consuming nutrient-rich foods is the critical secret explained in this book that will help you lower your cholesterol and protect yourself from heart disease.

The Health Equation and ANDI Scores

The information presented here is well supported by today's science, and I and some of my physician-colleagues have applied it clinically for many years. Thousands of my patients have experienced phenomenal results. The secret lies in simply understanding my health equation, which will change your life forever.

$$H = N / C$$
Health = Nutrients / Calories

This equation means that how long you are going to live—whether you are resistant to infection, whether you are prone to dementia, and whether you are at risk of heart disease—can be predicted by the nutrient-per-calorie density of your diet over your lifetime. Putting this equation into action means that we want to consume lots of valuable health-preserving nutrients as we seek our caloric needs, because when we don't, disease can result. This equation, $H = N / C$, represents the basic principle that to maximize healthy life expectancy (H) we have to eat a diet rich in micronutrients (N) per calorie (C).

The *Aggregate Nutrient Density Index* (ANDI) ranks the nutrient value of many common foods on the basis of how many nutrients they deliver to your body for each calorie consumed. Unlike food labels, which list only a few nutrients, ANDI scores are based on thirty-five important nutritional parameters. Foods are ranked on a scale of 1 to 1,000, with the most nutrient-dense cruciferous leafy green vegetables (such as kale) scoring at 1,000. Because phytochemicals are largely unnamed and unmeasured, these ANDI rankings may underestimate the healthful properties of colorful, natural plant foods, so the nutrient density of natural whole foods may be even higher than ANDI scores indicate.

The ANDI is a useful tool to help you visualize the high concentration of micronutrients in green and other colored produce compared with micronutrients in animal products and processed foods. This scoring tool has been demonstrated to be remarkably effective at Whole Foods Market to increase the sales and consumption of nutrient-rich produce across the country. This can have a major effect on the health of our society, since green vegetables are the foods most powerfully linked to a reduction in both cardiovascular disease and cancer. On the basis of this nutrient-per-calorie (N/C) criterion, you can grade food quality, construct menus, and make food choices that support excellent health. Once you know which foods have the highest nutrient density, you will know more about nutrition and weight loss. It is that simple.

However, this is not all you need to know to devise a diet with maximal health benefits, because some foods with only a moderate nutrient density have salient features that make them valuable for disease resistance. For example, mushrooms and flaxseeds contain powerful anti–breast cancer components that are not reflected in their ANDI scores. These important foods will be discussed later.

ANDI SCORES AND HOW THEY ARE DETERMINED

To determine ANDI scores, an equal-calorie serving of each food was evaluated. The following nutrients were included in the evaluation: fiber, calcium, iron, magnesium, phosphorus, potassium, zinc, copper, manganese, selenium, vitamin A, beta-carotene, alpha-carotene, lycopene, lutein and zeaxanthin, vitamin E, vitamin C, thiamin, riboflavin, niacin, pantothenic acid, vitamin B6, folate, vitamin B12, choline, vitamin K, phytosterols, glucosinolates, angiogenesis inhibitors, organosulfides, aromatase inhibitors, resistant starch, and resveratrol plus ORAC score (oxygen radical absorbance capacity, a measure of the antioxidant or radical scavenging capacity of a food). For consistency, nutrient quantities were converted from their typical measurement conventions (milligrams, micrograms, and international units) to a percentage of their dietary reference intake (DRI). For nutrients that have no DRI, goals were established based on available research and current understanding of the benefits of these factors. To ease the comparison of foods, the raw point totals were converted (multiplied by the same number) so that the highest-ranking foods received a score of 1,000 and the other foods received lower scores accordingly. (A more comprehensive list of ANDI scores can be found in my book *Nutritarian Handbook and ANDI Food Scoring Guide.*)

ANDI Scores

FOOD	SCORE	FOOD	SCORE
Collard greens	1,000	Grapes	119
Kale	1,000	Pomegranates	119
Mustard greens	1,000	Garlic	118
Watercress	1,000	Cantaloupes	118
Swiss chard	895	Onions	109
Bok choy	865	Snow peas	106
Spinach	707	Plums	106
Arugula	604	Flaxseeds	103
Romaine lettuce	510	Edamame	98
Radishes	502	Oranges	98
Brussels sprouts	490	Black rice	96
Carrots	458	Yellow squash	92
Cabbage	434	Cucumbers	87
Broccoli	340	Pinto beans	86
Cauliflower	315	Tofu	82
Radicchio	271	Beets	80
Bell peppers	265	Chia seeds	77
Pumpkin	249	Apricots, fresh	75
Butternut squash	241	Sesame seeds	74
Mushrooms	238	Lentils	72
Asparagus	205	Watermelon	71
Tomatoes	186	Tempeh	66
Strawberries	182	Hemp seeds	65
Sweet potatoes	181	Peaches	65
Blackberries	171	Kiwi	61
Zucchini	164	Kidney beans	64
Artichokes	145	Sunflower seeds	64
Raspberries	133	Green peas	63
Blueberries	132	Black beans	61
Iceberg lettuce	127	Figs, fresh	56

FOOD	SCORE	FOOD	SCORE
Wild rice	56	Plain yogurt (low fat)	28
Chickpeas	55	White potatoes	28
Cherries	55	Cashews	27
Pineapples	54	Tilapia	27
Persimmons	54	Apricots, dried	26
Apples	53	Chicken breasts	24
Mangoes	53	Pork, loin	23
Peanut butter	51	Beef, ground (85 percent lean)	21
Corn	45	Figs, dried	21
Spaghetti squash	44	Feta cheese	20
Acorn squash	44	Beef, top sirloin	20
Split peas	43	Frozen yogurt, vanilla	18
Pears	40	Dates	17
Pumpkin seeds	39	Raisins	15
Nectarines	39	French fries	12
Pistachio nuts	37	Cheese pizza	12
Oats, old fashioned	36	Apple juice	11
Shrimp	36	Cheddar cheese	11
Salmon	34	White pasta (unfortified)	11
Eggplant	31	Fast food chicken sandwich	11
Honeydew melon	31	Olive oil	10
Milk (1 percent)	31	Fast food hamburger	9
Eggs	31	White bread (unfortified)	9
Bananas	30	Vanilla ice cream	9
Walnuts	30	Granola bar, chocolate chip	9
Whole wheat bread	30	White rice (unfortified)	8
Almonds	28	Corn chips	7
Avocados	28	Bagel (unfortified)	5
Pine nuts	28	Apple pie	4
Quinoa	28	Cola	1
Brown rice	28		

FEATURES OF A NUTRITARIAN DIET

- Large green salads with seed/nut-based dressings

- Bean soups with carrot/tomato juice and cruciferous vegetables

- Green vegetables, onions, and mushrooms steamed or cooked in a wok

- Animal products limited to no more than three small servings per week

- No dairy, white flour, and white rice

- No processed foods, cold cereals, and sweets

- No sweeteners, except fruit and limited unsulfured dried fruit

- Carbohydrates with high nutritional quality such as beans, peas, squashes, lentils, and intact whole grains

- Protective foods such as walnuts, mushrooms, onions, berries, and seeds

Issues with the SAD

Now that I have shared the dietary basics of the Nutritarian diet for maximizing disease protection and heart health, let's examine some of the common issues with the SAD. The key to remember is this: The choice about what to eat is yours to make. The right foods have remarkable health-giving properties that can protect against disease and reverse existing conditions. The wrong foods are the very thing that has put your health at risk. Food-related disease inevitably worsens while being treated with medications, invasive procedures, and surgeries; such medical care cannot do what nutritional excellence can. The choice in front of you should be clear.

Let's look at some of the specific ways our diet choices affect our health.

Glycemic Load

Refined grain products—such as white bread, pasta, bagels, white rice, most breakfast cereals, and other denatured and processed grains—are almost as nutrient-deficient as sugar. The nutritional value of these "foods" falls very low on the scale compared with healthful, whole plant foods. As these low-fiber, refined carbohydrate foods are digested, they are converted to, and absorbed as, simple sugar. This spikes the glucose level in the bloodstream in the same way as if you had consumed a cube of sugar. At this point in the history of nutritional science, the evidence is overwhelming that high glucose levels appearing frequently or sustained in the bloodstream promote heart disease and cancer.

Glycemic index and glycemic load consider the rate at which glucose builds up in the bloodstream over time. The more rapid and concentrated the elevation of glucose in the blood, the higher the glycemic index or glycemic load of a particular food and the more significant the risks of developing heart disease. The same can be said of fat entering the blood quickly. In other words, there is an advantage to fat calories being more gently eased into the bloodstream. Oils and even concentrated animal fats can enter the bloodstream rapidly, but the fat content of seeds and nuts is absorbed over several hours, allowing the calories to be burned for energy, rather than stored as fat. This slow entry of calories into the blood can delay hunger and more effectively reduce the body's demand for calories.

Greens, mushrooms, onions, tomatoes, beans, nuts, and seeds have lower glycemic loads, and eating them instead of lower-quality carbohydrates results in a dramatic lowering of diabetic and cardiovascular parameters. For example, in a trial of 117 diabetic individuals randomized to eat an equal caloric amount of nuts or muffins or both daily, the nut group showed dramatic improvement in both glycemic control and serum lipid levels, including improvement in LDL cholesterol.[9]

The modern world has been bombarded with nutrient-deficient, high-calorie foods, often called *empty-calorie foods*. Nutrient-poor fake food is spreading all over the globe, and in recent years obesity, diabetes, and heart disease have become the leading causes of death almost everywhere. These foods are poor sources of nutrients, and their consumption is linked directly to heart disease, strokes, and many cancers—diseases that kill more than 85 percent of all Americans.

In fact, diabetes and heart disease are exploding in China, even though Chinese people are not yet as overweight as Americans. Vegetable consumption has decreased there, and soda and sugar consumption has increased, along with the consumption of animal products and oils. In other words, when you already have lots of high-glycemic white rice in the diet and then add more sweets, meat, and oil, health effects worsen. That combination of high-glycemic-load carbohydrates and more animal products and fewer vegetables promotes chronic disease very effectively.[10]

Diabetes is not a lightweight problem; it is the fourth leading cause of death by disease in the United States, and the number of people developing it worldwide is soaring. White flour, white rice, and other refined grains such as sweetened breakfast cereals, soft drinks, and even fruit juices can cause weight gain and lead to diabetes. Heightened levels of glucose in the bloodstream can raise triglyceride, cholesterol, and C-reactive protein levels, as well as dramatically increase pro-inflammatory cytokines, leading to blood vessel inflammation and synergistically increasing the risk of heart attack.[11]

The more rapid and concentrated the elevation of glucose in the blood, the higher the glycemic load and its associated risks. So the

FAST FOOD VERSUS SLOW FOOD

Fast Food
(oil and white flour)

Slow Food
(beans and nuts)

Calories in
bloodstream

Hours   1   2   3

glycemic load of your diet, or the amount of high-glycemic carbohy-drates you eat, is directly proportional to your risk of having a heart attack, whether you have diabetes already or not. For example, in an in-teresting and well-designed study with a Chinese population, remov-ing one serving of rice or noodles a day and substituting one serving of vegetables reduced the risk of heart disease by 24 percent.[12] And that was after just one switch a day!

Some Foods Are Like Candy

You may love your bread, bagels, crackers, pizza, and pasta, but these foods can affect your body like candy. When you take a whole wheat berry and process it into white flour to make such foods, more than 90 percent of the fiber and vitamin E and more than 75 percent of the minerals are lost. Your body breaks down the carbohydrate into simple sugars, and the physiological response is not much different from what would happen if you had eaten cotton candy. White pasta, white rice, and white bread are just like sugar; because their fiber has been removed, the body absorbs these nutrient-deficient foods too rap-idly. This in turn raises glucose, triglyceride, and insulin levels in your blood. Even minimal amounts of refined grains are undesirable and can sabotage your weight-loss and cholesterol-lowering efforts.

All refined sweets—including sugar, honey, corn syrup, agave nectar, maple syrup, molasses, and corn sweeteners—are low in nutri-ents and fiber and are rapidly absorbed by the body. They all contain insignificant amounts of nutrients (per calorie) and no fiber. More and more studies offer evidence that the consumption of these sweets and white flour products contributes significantly to the development of obesity, diabetes, heart disease, and even cancer.[13]

Added sugars come in several forms other than table sugar, such as evaporated cane juice and high-fructose corn syrup. Calorie-containing sweeteners like maple syrup, honey, agave nectar, and coconut sugar are marketed as "natural" and are often touted as healthier alternatives to these types of added sugars. But the reality is that all concentrated sweeteners add substantial calories to the diet while contributing very little nutritional value.

COMPOSITION OF SWEETENERS

	FRUCTOSE (%)	GLUCOSE (%)	SUCROSE (%)	OTHERS (%)
White sugar, granulated			100	
Maple syrup	1	3	96	
Honey	50	45	1	4
Molasses	24	22	54	
Agave nectar	82	18		
Corn syrup, light	7	93		
High-fructose corn syrup	42	53		5
Brown rice syrup		100		
Coconut sugar	3–9	3–9	70–80	2–4

Even maple syrup and honey elevate blood glucose similarly to sugar (sucrose), leading to disease-causing glycemic effects in the body. Sucrose is half fructose and half glucose, as it is made up of one fructose molecule linked to one glucose molecule. Agave nectar is marketed as a low-glycemic sweetener because of its high fructose content (agave is approximately 80 percent fructose). Though high-fructose corn syrup and agave nectar may not have a high glycemic load compared with honey and white sugar, they are still just as bad, because the high fructose load can promote fat production in the body.

When fructose is absorbed, it is transported directly to the liver, where it is broken down to produce energy. Fructose itself does not stimulate the pancreas to secrete insulin; however, much of the fructose is metabolized and converted into glucose in the liver, so it does raise blood glucose levels somewhat. Fructose stimulates the liver to produce fat, which causes direct fat deposition and elevated blood triglyceride levels, a predictor of heart disease.[14] Concentrated ingestion of fructose also increases sugar cravings and hunger, leading to increased calorie intake at subsequent snacks and meals.[15] When you ingest any caloric sweetener, you get a mix of disease-promoting effects: the glucose-elevating effects of added glucose, and the triglyceride-raising and fat-building effects of added fructose.

All sweeteners (and fruits) contain some combination of glucose, fructose, and the two bound together as sucrose. Maple syrup contains 96 percent sucrose, so it is very similar to regular white sugar (see table above). Coconut sugar contains 70–80 percent sucrose, and honey contains about 50 percent fructose and 45 percent glucose. All caloric sweeteners have effects that promote weight gain, diabetes, and heart disease, regardless of their ratio of glucose to fructose or what type of plant they come from.

Whole fruits are different because they have the necessary fiber to regulate the entry of glucose/fructose into the body and buffer the effects with the polyphenols and other nutrients they contain.[16] Plus, the threshold of fructose is lower with fruits. Because they contain only a few grams of fructose per serving, whole fruits do not expose you to enough fructose to trigger fat storage, unless you consume lots of fruit juice or dried fruits.

The whiter the bread, the sooner you're dead.

Every time you eat processed foods you exclude not only the important known nutrients from your diet, but also hundreds of other undiscovered phytonutrients that are essential for normal human function. For instance, it is the outer portion of the wheat kernel (the part that is removed when white flour is made) that contains trace minerals, phytoestrogens, lignans, phytic acid, indoles, phenolic compounds, and other phytochemicals as well as all of the vitamin E. It is the amount and diversity of micronutrients, both known and unknown, that are necessary to ward off heart disease and cancer.

Additionally, when we eat baked goods, cold breakfast cereals, and snack foods such as pretzels, we are eating heart disease–promoting *trans* fats, along with a high dose of acrylamides. *Acrylamides* are toxic, cancer-promoting compounds produced when foods are baked or fried at high temperatures. Chips, pretzels, cold breakfast cereals, roasted soy nuts, browned foods, crusted foods, and fried foods contain high levels of these toxic compounds that are formed when carbohydrates are exposed to high dry heat. These harmful compounds are not formed when foods are water cooked, such as when you steam vegetables or make soups. These carcinogens in overly cooked carbohydrates cause intravascular inflammation and heart disease, too.[17]

On the other hand, low-glycemic carbohydrates have the opposite effect. Almost all vegetables are low glycemic, and vegetables that are raw, boiled, steamed, or cooked in a wok are associated with a lower risk of heart disease. If you eat enough vegetables in your diet, you will not develop heart disease. And if you have developed heart disease from prior poor eating habits, it is reversible.

Elevated insulin levels do not merely increase the risk of diabetes and heart disease, they also have pro-angiogenic and cancer-promoting effects.[18]

Glossary

Angiogenesis—the growth of new blood vessels from existing vessels. Angiogenesis is a fundamental step in permitting the growth of fat cells on the body and also in the transition of tumors or dysplastic cells to malignancy.

For example, in a meta-analysis of thirty-nine studies, a high glycemic load was associated with an increased risk of colorectal and endometrial cancers,[19] and a meta-analysis of ten prospective studies demonstrated a link between higher glycemic load and breast cancer.[20] Another study demonstrated that for every 100 grams of white rice consumed per day, breast cancer risk increased 19 percent, whereas the same amount of whole grain, brown rice, or beans had almost the direct opposite effect.[21]

Recent research suggests that high-glycemic processed foods promote heart disease even more powerfully than saturated fats from animal products. This is a chilling concern, considering all the white bread, white rice, and white potato products that people around the world consume.[22]

GLYCEMIC LOAD OF COMMON FOODS[23]

White potato	29	Apples	9
White rice	26	Kiwi	8
White pasta	21	Green peas	8
Chocolate cake	20	Butternut squash	8
Corn	18	Kidney beans	6
Sweet potato	14	Black beans	6
Grapes	14	Watermelon	6
Rolled oats	13	Oranges	4
Whole wheat	11	Cashews	2
Mango	11	Strawberries	1
Lentils	9		

The white potato is an example of a high-glycemic carbohydrate with a favorable caloric density, because one potato contains only about 120–160 calories. The Nurses' Health Study demonstrated an 18 percent increased risk of diabetes for each potato eaten daily by overweight women. Notably, it was the glycemic load of potatoes, rather than the added or associated butter or oil, that was implicated.[24] Ominously, data from the North Carolina Colon Cancer Study, which looked at more than one thousand cases of colon cancer compared with one thousand controls, demonstrated a more than 50 percent increased risk of rectal cancer in participants eating three potatoes a week compared with one, and more than an 80 percent increase comparing 5.6 servings a week with one.[25] These are shocking findings, but note that these heightened risks were observed only for refined grains and potatoes, and not for any added fats, suggesting that the association is demonstrating significant glycemic risk for the food itself and not merely an association with a dietary pattern of adding fatty toppings.

It has also been observed that the association of white potatoes with increased disease risk becomes more pronounced as a person's body weight and insulin resistance increase, thus specifically identifying the potato's glycemic effect as the culprit. High-glycemic foods become a more significant stimulator of excess insulin release as a person's body weight increases. The more fat on the body, the more insulin resistance, and the more the pancreas responds by pumping out larger insulin loads in response to foods that stimulate insulin release.

And because of the fat-promoting effects of insulin, high-glycemic foods can make it more difficult for an overweight person to lose weight.[26]

Overall, it is not the inclusion or exclusion of a whole plant food like a potato that will make a diet good or bad. However, you should take care to eat only a limited amount of white potato and to eat it with greens, beans, nuts, and seeds. Even then, eat only half of a medium potato or one small potato. Starches such as turnips, rutabaga, butternut and acorn squash, chestnuts, parsnips, carrots, peas, corn, and intact whole grains are better choices.

Certainly, there are lots of worse foods you can eat than white potatoes and white rice. However, when you eat these foods, especially while consuming oils, meats, and cheeses, the body can store fat even more effectively than it can if you eat just the meat alone with greens or the potato and rice alone with greens. Nevertheless, though it is not as bad as sugar and white flour, a white potato is still not a favorable high-starch vegetable to choose, and white rice is not a preferred form of grain to use.

Virtually everyone interested in nutrition knows that products made with white flour are not healthful carbohydrate sources for a longevity-enhancing or disease-reversing diet. This can be understood by comparing the nutritional profile of white flour products with those of more healthful carbohydrate sources such as peas, corn, or beans. We can do the same with white potatoes, comparing them to peas, corn, or beans.

When comparing the nutritional profiles of high-carbohydrate plant foods, we must consider

- Fiber content

- Percentage of slowly digestible starch

- Percentage of resistant starch

- Micronutrient content

- Caloric density

- Glycemic index/load

- Beneficial qualities of other foods that may be displaced to allow room in the diet for this food

We can classify carbohydrate-rich foods on a hierarchal scale based on their nutrient levels, fiber content, and amount of resistant starch. As the amount of fiber and resistant starch increase (see table below), more dramatic benefits for people who are overweight and/or diabetic are noted. Resistant starch is counted as calories on labels and charts, but during digestion, 90 percent of resistant starch calories are lost, thus acting more like a type of fiber. I generally emphasize beans, starchy vegetables, intact grains, and other nutritious, high-carbohydrate natural foods most heavily in my recommendations because of these criteria.

Resistant starch is present in all foods that contain natural carbohydrates. Other starches are broken down by digestive enzymes, converted into simple sugars, and absorbed in the small intestine. Resistant starch, on the other hand, is more like a fiber because it resists enzymatic digestive degradation in the small intestine and travels to the colon for degradation by bacterial action, so only a small percentage of its calories become absorbed and utilized for energy. Public health authorities in recent years have accepted the food value of resistant starch because of its benefits in helping prevent diabetes and promote weight loss. A committee of the United Nations and World Health Organization stated that the discovery of resistant starch has been "one of the major developments in our understanding of the importance of carbohydrates for health in the past twenty years."[27]

Not only is resistant starch satiating and calorically barren, it also promotes health and weight loss by other mechanisms:

- It encourages the growth of beneficial bacteria, reducing intestinal pH and the production of bile acids and ammonia.

- Its breakdown by bacteria produces short-chain fatty acids, which have beneficial effects on fat metabolism and fat storage in the body.

- Its intake reduces the glycemic effect of other foods, even those eaten at separate meals.

By considering the hierarchal scale of carbohydrate quality, which includes not just the information in the table below but also the amount of slowly digestible starch and the level of nutrient density, we can devise a dietary protocol that reduces exposure to the highest-glycemic carbohydrates and incorporates more beans. Beans run away with the prize for the healthiest carbohydrate choice. And when you eat more beans in your diet, along with more raw and cooked greens, other low-glycemic vegetables, and more nuts and seeds, you achieve dramatic glucose-favorable benefits that are especially helpful if you are diabetic, prediabetic, or have metabolic syndrome.

RESISTANT STARCH AND FIBER CONTENT[28]

FOOD	RESISTANT STARCH (%)	RESISTANT STARCH (%) + FIBER (%)
Black beans	27	70
Navy beans	26	62
Lentils	25	59
Split peas	25	58
Corn	25	45
Brown rice	15	20
Rolled oats	7	17
Whole wheat flour	2	14
Pasta	3	9
Potato	3	5

As an example, a two-group controlled trial had one group increase legume intake by 1 cup a day and the other group increase whole grain intake by the same amount. A clear benefit was seen for the group adding more whole grains, but more dramatic benefits occurred for the bean group, as shown in the table below from an individual baseline.[29]

PARAMETER	WHOLE GRAIN GROUP	BEAN GROUP
Fiber increase (g/1,000 cal)	1.9	10
Glycemic load reduction	−5	−48
HbA1c (%)	−0.3	−0.5
Body weight (lbs)	−4.4	−5.7
Fasting glucose (mg/dl)	−7	−9
Triglycerides (mg/dl)	−9	−21
Cholesterol (mg/dl)	−2	−9
Systolic blood pressure (mmHg)	0	−4
Diastolic blood pressure (mmHg)	0	−3

Beans are not merely glycemically favorable themselves, but their fermentation and probiotic effects also lower the glucose absorption from other foods in the diet. These glucose-lowering benefits occur not merely in the meal that includes beans, but in later meals as well, even if they don't include beans—something that has been called the "second-meal effect."[30] Beans have multiple benefits for favorable glycemic response, weight reduction, and protection against cancer.

Across five different regions and ethnicities, legumes were found to be the most consistent and reliable predictor of longevity. A 7 to 8 percent reduction in death rate was reported for every 20 grams (2 tablespoons) of beans eaten daily.[31] Beans, nuts, and seeds have numerous anticancer compounds, including phytic acid and inositol pentakisphosphate (IP-5), which has been shown in animal studies to inhibit tumor growth, migration, and invasion and to augment NK (natural killer) cell activity.[32] Eating more beans as a replacement for other foods aids in all metabolic parameters that enhance cardiovascular health.[33]

Animal Protein and the Dangers of IGF-1

Insulin-like growth factor–1 (IGF-1), a human growth hormone, is one of the body's most important growth promoters during fetal and childhood growth. However, later in life, higher levels of IGF-1 are not a good thing. They promote cellular replication and growth that can accelerate the aging process and promote cancer. IGF-1 is primarily produced in the liver, and its production is stimulated by pituitary-derived growth hormone.

Diets high in animal products and animal protein promote not only heart disease, but also cancer—predominantly by increasing the body's production of IGF-1. In adults, higher blood levels of IGF-1 have been shown to promote the growth, proliferation, and spread of cancer cells. Elevated IGF-1 levels are linked to increased risk of all major cancers, including colon cancer, breast cancer, and prostate cancer.[34]

IGF-1 stimulates mitosis (cell division) and inhibits apoptosis (a process leading to cell death). That means it not only promotes the spread of cancer cells, but also inhibits the immune system's ability to identify and kill abnormal cells before they become cancerous (apoptosis). As we age, high circulating IGF-1 levels stimulate the replication of injured cells that would not have otherwise progressed to malignancy.

Heightened IGF-1 signals are involved with numerous processes promoting the growth, proliferation, survival, adhesion, migration, and invasion of tumor cells, as well as angiogenesis (increased blood vessel growth) and metastatic growth.[35] Reduced IGF-1 levels in adulthood are associated with reduced oxidative stress, decreased inflammation, enhanced insulin sensitivity, and longer life span.[36]

Unquestionably, IGF-1 is a major player in the development of breast cancer. The European Prospective Investigation into Cancer and Nutrition (EPIC) found that elevated IGF-1 levels were associated with a 40 percent increased risk of developing breast cancer for women older than 50.[37] In the Nurses' Health Study, high IGF-1 levels were associated with a doubling in risk in premenopausal women.[38] Additional human studies, reviews of the literature, and five meta-analyses have also associated elevated IGF-1 levels with breast cancer.[39] In other words, it is broadly supported and accepted in the scientific literature that higher IGF-1 levels promote this common cancer.

The principle dietary factor that determines IGF-1 levels is animal protein, so the excessive meat, fowl, seafood, and dairy intake common in our society is responsible for high circulating IGF-1. Interestingly, when we were children we were taught that animal products were important in our diets because of their biologically complete protein that was essential for good health. Now, research in the past ten years has resulted in accumulating evidence that the increased amounts of high biological protein is the most damaging feature of animal products, which makes limiting their use so important.[40] When we get our protein from plant foods, we support our health without supporting the growth of cancer.

Milk products likely raise IGF-1 more than other animal products. This is likely due to other bioactive growth-promoting compounds, along with milk's protein content; but meat, fish, and poultry also increase IGF-1 considerably. Ten different observational studies and several interventional studies have confirmed a positive correlation between milk and heightened IGF-1 levels.[41]

Prostate cancer seems to be particularly sensitive to IGF-1 levels, and its incidence increases sharply in countries that have high consumption of dairy and meat.[42] Researchers tracked 21,660 men in the Physicians' Health Study for twenty-eight years, and those who had one serving of milk a day had double the risk of dying from prostate cancer compared with men who rarely drank milk.[43] Meat consumption was also a risk factor, shown to raise IGF-1 levels and risk of prostate cancer death in this study. Meat, poultry, and fish have been confirmed to raise IGF-1 in multiple studies.[44]

The link between IGF-1 and cancer is the big story here, because legions of dieters have jumped on the high-protein bandwagon, thinking they are aiding their health by eating egg whites, fish, and lean meats. In fact, this thinking may be fueling an explosion of cancer. A Nutritarian diet-style, on the other hand, is specifically designed to maximize cancer-protective nutrients and minimize cancer-promoting ones. However, some questions here are still unanswered.

IGF-1 and Heart Disease

The link between IGF-1 and heart disease was examined in a 2009 study published in the *European Journal of Endocrinology*. Researchers followed individuals aged 50 to 89 years (mean age, 68 years) for an average of five years and determined that higher levels of IGF-1 were linked to higher all-cause mortality. They also noted a significant increase in deaths due to congestive heart failure in the group with the highest IGF-1.[45] They did not see a relationship between higher IGF-1 and heart attack deaths. Apparently, with the frailty of aging, IGF-1 can drop too low as a sign of advancing illness, confusing some of the data linking higher IGF-1 with ischemic heart disease. Most research today confirms that both excessively low and high IGF-1 are associated with higher cardiovascular mortality.[46]

A larger and longer-term study published in 2014 helped clarify these findings. This important study compared low-glycemic diets that were high in animal protein and low in sugar with diets that were low in animal products and low in added sugars. Researchers followed more than six thousand people for more than eighteen years. In the 50–65 age range, researchers found a fourfold increase in cancer death risk in the group consuming more animal protein compared with the group consuming lower animal protein as well as a 75 percent increase in overall mortality over the eighteen years.[47]

There were three study groups: a high-protein group (20 percent or more of calories from protein), a moderate protein group (10–19 percent from protein), and a low-protein group (less than 10 percent from protein). The researchers isolated the negative effects of the high-protein intake and found that the damage was solely related to animal protein; higher-protein plant foods did not increase disease risk. Also of interest was the threefold higher risk of cancer deaths even for those in the moderate protein group; so animal products, consumed even moderately, were strongly cancer-promoting.

It is important to note that the highest-protein group was consuming the average amount (or less) of protein that most Americans consume, and certainly less animal protein. Many popular diets encourage the consumption of much higher amounts of animal products. For example, some advocates of the Paleo diet suggest that 50–75 percent of calories come from animal products, which may be drastically more dangerous than was reported here. In this study, the lowest-protein group, which had the greatest longevity, consumed less than 10 percent of calories from protein (more than half of which was likely animal protein), which is less than a third of what Americans currently consume.

Note that these research scientists found a seventy-three-fold increased risk of developing diabetes in the higher-protein group and a twenty-three-fold increased risk in the moderate-protein group compared with the lower-protein group. This increased risk of diabetes with higher protein intake was consistent across all ages, including the most elderly. Researchers were careful to emphasize that this increased risk of diabetes and death held only for intake of animal proteins, not for plant proteins.

In contrast, in the oldest cohort of this study (average age older than 70), the study demonstrated an increased cancer death rate for those in the lowest-protein, lowest IGF-1 group over the next eighteen years. So eating less animal protein is beneficial until later in life, when health may be deteriorating and weight is dropping excessively. The researchers hypothesized from the data, and from other studies and their work in animal models, that after age 75 some adults develop a reduced ability to assimilate nutrients and experience weight loss and increasing frailty that could require more protein in their diets (and higher IGF-1) to maintain adequate muscle mass and immune function. They advised that 10 percent of calories from total protein be the lower limit after age 75.

In other words, eating sufficient protein (using higher-protein plant foods such as hemp seeds, sunflower seeds, and beans), even including animal products (if necessary), may be important late in life if digestive capacity and increasing frailty are issues. Premature aging and frailty with advancing years is a more realistic scenario for a person who has been eating the SAD and much less likely for a person who has eaten a longevity-promoting Nutritarian diet for many years.

Studies investigating IGF-1 in the elderly are still conflicting and uncertain, complicated by the use of foods to raise IGF-1 and the effect of those foods. For example, more fish in the diet in the elderly may raise IGF-1, but any benefits observed may be from the anticlotting effects of fish fat. Some evidence even exists that higher IGF-1 protects against plaque instability in the frail elderly and aids in insulin sensitivity, contributing to extended life span.[48] This complicated subject is actively being investigated by researchers today. But right now, we know that lower IGF-1 is beneficial through most of a person's adult life and that toward the end of life, it is most likely best if IGF-1 is not too low or too high.

At this point we can conclude that increasing protein intake during the last ten years of a projected life span—that is, after age 85 in a healthy eater and after age 70 in an unhealthy eater—may be indicated. However, the need to include some animal products for extra protein would best be made on an individual basis and not by some rote formula based on age. Even when individual requirements indicate that it is beneficial to use animal products in a person's diet, their use should still be held to low amounts to achieve the desired benefits with minimal risk. It is life span–beneficial to rely on protein-rich plants such as greens, seeds, and beans, not animal foods, for the majority of our protein requirements even toward the end of life.

If you want to be a centenarian, the road to get there is clear. Centenarians have low levels of IGF-1 and high levels of anti-inflammatory molecules from nutrient-dense plant foods. The combined effect of a reduction in IGF-1 and a high-phytochemical diet, resulting in lower levels of oxidative stress, is the secret to maximizing longevity and cancer protection.[49] The amount of animal products that can safely be added to a longevity-promoting diet is not clearly defined and may differ from person to person. As a reasonable estimate, averaging more than 7 ounces a week for a woman and 10 ounces a week for a man may be risky because the IGF-1 curve starts to increase considerably above this level.[50] This certainly is an area of evolving science, but this estimate offers a reasonable guideline based on the information available today.

Who Should You Believe?

I make a considerable effort to present the research findings and clinical evidence without predetermined bias or any environmental, ethical, or philosophical agenda. There may be other excellent reasons why someone might recommend or support a certain diet-style, but my efforts and twenty-five years of expertise are narrowly focused on devising the gold standard of nutritional therapy. You can be confident that this information is the most effective because the evidence is overwhelming, the logic is clear, and the results are consistently effective.

When I began my medical practice as a specialist in nutrition, I focused my attention on individuals who were looking for nutritional intervention in order to reverse their medical conditions and avoid medication and invasive surgery. The consistent outcome then and now shows that people committed to superior health through nutritional excellence are able to reduce and eventually stop their dependence on medications for controlling high blood pressure, diabetes, high cholesterol, and a host of other conditions. Spectacular disease reversals are the norm, not the exception.

My twenty-five years of experience with thousands of patients have confirmed that when people eat a diet composed of the most nutritious and powerful anticancer plant foods, their cholesterol levels drop more dramatically than they can with the use of standard cholesterol-lowering medication. Their heart conditions and angina symptoms disappear, and they get well within weeks to months, not years. Their diabetes also goes away. I am confident when I say to them: "Let's not just treat your diabetes and control it. Let's get rid of it and make you nondiabetic."

Over the years my focus has never been on calorie restriction; rather, it has been on eating more high-nutrient foods, and as a result, eating less of everything that is not a high-nutrient food. Besides reversing chronic disease and preventing heart disease and cancer, I have found that my patients are able to reach their ideal weights with ease—with no calorie counting, no complicated formulas, no pills or unfulfilled promises. The basic plan is simple: Just take the healthiest foods, make them taste great, and then eat as much as desired. My patients have dropped the weight they could not lose before, with associated health benefits, and they have achieved these results relatively quickly.

There is an often-repeated cliché about weight loss: If you lose weight too rapidly, the loss won't stick and you will gain all the weight back. I have never advocated that people be in a race to lose their excess weight. I see no reason to eat unhealthy foods or to eat when you are not hungry under some notion that losing weight more slowly is better. The reality with the Nutritarian diet is that your body drops its unhealthy weight quickly and naturally while you eat well and sufficiently.

For many people who were at high risk of heart attack and death, their adoption of the Nutritarian program without compromise has saved their lives. Very often, moderate improvements toward dietary excellence provide little or sometimes even no benefits, but a complete commitment to excellence begets spectacular results.

Over time, people find that they prefer a Nutritarian diet-style—they like the way they feel, they like the way the food tastes (as their taste buds adjust), and they love being freed from the fear of chronic disease that makes life miserable for so many Americans.

The Nutritarian diet-style supplies outstanding results in the weight-loss arena that are sustainable because once people become nutritional experts and experience the results, they want to eat this way forever. The secret to success is to be educated and gain the knowledge first. The more you learn, the easier it becomes to eat this way for the rest of your life, especially knowing that other people are committing suicide with food all around you.

Many people think they are already eating a healthy diet; but they are not. These people are following a misguided notion of a "balanced" diet. Under this formula, when they want to lose weight, they try to eat less. But this almost never works in the long run. It is very hard to cut portion size and not feel hungry, and it is even more difficult to feel hungry and not eat. People continue to drastically cut portion sizes, follow popular fads, and go on and off diets. Through all of this, they still don't eat enough healthy, nutrient-dense food, and they still consume low levels of crucial nutrients.

Traditional calorie-restriction dieting is unhealthy in the long run and cannot be sustained for many reasons. The traditional view of dieting, which entails watching portion sizes and calories, has already been shown to fail more than 90 percent of the time because as dieters' nutrient levels go down, they develop cravings and feel poorly. We will never permanently succeed at weight loss until we care about our long-term health and decide to consume a better quality diet that contains lots of nutrient-rich foods. Then, as a consequence of eating a high-nutrient diet and getting fueled with antioxidants and phytochemicals, we will gradually and naturally lose our desire to overeat.

What makes the Nutritarian program for lowering cholesterol, improving health, and losing weight work so effectively is the large volume of healthy food I ask you to eat. By eating so much of the "good stuff," you will naturally desire less food that is not rich in nutrients. You will also find it easy and fulfilling to make the necessary changes to achieve the results you have been looking for. Gradually your taste and food preferences will change, and you will find that healthy dishes and foods are what you prefer and enjoy the most.

Why do I personally eat this way? Because I enjoy eating as much food as I want. I like eating great-tasting food. I like the fact that I can maintain my ideal weight without any effort or dieting. I value the fact that I can be emotionally and intellectually secure in feeling that I am totally protected from heart disease and stroke. I feel great and am able to maintain my youthful stamina and strength. For me, eating healthfully is not a sacrifice, nor does it require a will of iron. It is the way I enjoy eating so I can live life to the fullest. It is a blessing.

Losing Weight Becomes Effortless
Getting thinner is extremely important to maximally lower your cholesterol and protect yourself from heart disease and cancer. It is well established in the scientific literature that your heart disease risk increases as your percentage of body fat gets higher.[51]

Visceral fat (intra-abdominal fat and the central deposition of fat around the organs) is particularly and independently related to heart attack risk.[52] This means that visceral fat has heart disease–promoting effects that are in addition to, and separate from, high cholesterol, high blood sugar levels, and high blood pressure.[53] In other words, controlling risk factors is not sufficient; you have to get rid of the dangerous fat in your body too.

Body fat drops quickly with a Nutritarian diet, but you do not have to worry about dropping weight too fast because you are flooding your body with health-supporting micronutrients. As you get closer to your ideal weight, your weight loss will gradually slow down and then stop. Your body is a very intelligent machine, and when you eat correctly, it will achieve its ideal weight and you will lose both *subcutaneous fat* (the pinchable fat under the skin) and visceral fat.

If you consume a diet rich in nutrient-dense foods, you can disease-proof your body. Superior nutrition has such a powerful effect on the body's ability to defend itself against illness that it can force genetics to take a secondary role. This means that our genetic weaknesses can remain at bay. However, if you have already developed serious disease, you cannot merely dabble in healthy eating—every mouthful of food counts toward making you better. With a diet-style that is perfected to maximize disease reversal, you can earn back your health. You can do what drugs and surgeries cannot do. Only nutritional excellence gives you the ability to adequately protect yourself and recover from your dietary-induced medical conditions.

If you want to throw away your medications and recover from high blood pressure, diabetes, asthma, fatigue, allergies, or arthritis (to name just a few), you can put this information into action and bring about a predictable improvement in your health. The Nutritarian program can even reverse the amount of obstructive plaque and fatty deposits in your blood vessels, restoring normal blood flow to the heart. With the help of your doctor, this program can help you to slowly reduce—and to eventually cease—your dependence on drugs. It may enable you to avoid open-heart surgery and other invasive procedures. It has saved the lives of countless others, and it could save your life too.

CHAPTER TWO

Bypassing Angioplasty

When it comes to treating heart disease, modern medical technology, including surgical intervention and drug therapy, is expensive, invasive, and largely ineffective.

Traditional medical approaches, such as angioplasty with stent placement and coronary artery bypass grafting (CABG), pose serious risks and, studies show, do not benefit stable patients. What is most alarming is that these treatments target stable plaque that is not in danger of rupturing to form a clot and ignore the dangerous, unstable plaque that doesn't show up in tests. In contrast to the traditional approach, a Nutritarian diet approach, which emphasizes a diet rich in nutrient-dense plant foods, can resolve and even reverse cardiovascular disease and rejuvenate the blood vessels.

You ate the SAD for most of your life. You developed heart disease. And now, your cardiologist is telling you that you need angioplasty or CABG, also called bypass surgery. Faced with the evidence of a 95 percent obstruction in a major coronary vessel, you require treatment to open up the occluded blood vessel so the blood can flow into your heart—or, you are told, you could die. Is that true? What should you do?

Certainly, these modern medical technologies, surgical techniques, billions of dollars of procedures, and hospital real estate would not exist unless they were useful and could extend your life, right? These procedures have to work, or your doctor would not be insisting on them, right?

Wrong! On both counts.

A careful review of medical studies on this issue demonstrates that even if you have advanced cardiovascular disease, these procedures likely *shorten* your life, not lengthen it. But before you can understand why traditional medical care is futile and in most cases harmful, you need to understand some basics about the heart and heart disease.

What Is Heart Disease?

Your heart is a powerful muscle that pumps 3,000 gallons of blood through your body each day. Like other muscles, it requires a continuous supply of energy and oxygen. But because it is always working, the heart is a large utilizer of oxygen in the body. The heart gets the oxygen

CASE HISTORY: PROOF FROM A PATIENT

A 47-year-old, 240-pound man with high blood pressure and high cholesterol was evaluated with Doppler ultrasound of his carotid arteries and found to have an 80 percent obstructed carotid artery on the left side. His physician warned him that he was at high risk of having a stroke and suggested he have a carotid endarterectomy to remove the obstructive plaque. He read my book *Eat to Live*, changed his diet, and lost 80 pounds in one year. His high blood pressure resolved, but most surprisingly his LDL cholesterol levels dropped exactly 80 points too. A repeat ultrasound of his carotid artery demonstrated only a 40 percent obstruction, meaning that half had melted away. Two years after he began my dietary recommendations, no plaque was detectable on ultrasound.

His results from changing to a Nutritarian diet:

• 80 pounds lost

• 80-point reduction in LDL cholesterol

• 80 percent obstruction gone

and nutrients it needs from the coronary arteries, which supply it with blood. Most heart disease is *coronary artery disease (CAD)*.

Glossary

Coronary artery disease (CAD) is the narrowing or obstruction to blood flow that develops inside the lumen (interior) of the coronary vessels, usually caused by *atherosclerosis,* or hardening of the arteries. Narrowing can also be caused by *stenosis,* or a type of scarring that occurs after a medical procedure.

Atherosclerosis is the buildup of cholesterol-laden fatty plaque in the interior of blood vessels. Over time, as plaque builds up, inflammatory products and calcium stick to the fatty streaks and softer plaque in the wall, and it develops a harder, calcified cap over the softer fatty (lipid) base.

When enough obstruction and resistance to blood flow occurs, the heart muscle experiences a restriction in blood flow, or *ischemia,* which can result in chest pain, or *angina.* Ischemia causes a shortage of the oxygen and glucose needed for cellular metabolism and healthy tissues. If the blood flow in that vessel is suddenly and completely cut off, the death of that section of heart muscle can occur. This results in a heart attack, or *myocardial infarction.*

Most heart attacks are caused by a clot that forms within the blood vessel and enlarges to the extent that it obstructs the flow of blood. Clots are prone to form in areas where there is plaque with a thin, calcified cap that is most vulnerable to cracking or rupture. If the hard surface of the plaque cracks or tears, the soft fat inside is exposed, spilling into the *lumen* (open center) of the artery and releasing inflammatory cytokines that attract platelets to the site of the injury. When these platelet cells clump together, they can form a clot large enough to block the artery.

For years, doctors thought that the main cause of heart attacks was the buildup of fatty plaque. They believed that over time the vessel would become so narrow that flow would be compromised, and eventually the vessels would close up or be clogged.

Now we know that the facts are much different. Most of the large clots that create heart attacks occur in parts of the heart where the arteries are *not* severely narrowed. Instead, they occur in areas where the plaque is soft and has a thinner cap, sitting on an unstable, cholesterol-laden base. The propensity of plaque to rupture and create a complication or infarct depends on two other important criteria: the tensile stress (destabilizing pressure) on the fibrous cap, and the amount of inflammatory white blood cells (leukocytes) that have infiltrated the lipid segment.

Older, more stable plaques, whose inflammatory reaction has cooled, have been infiltrated by more smooth muscle and more fibrotic (scar) tissue and have thicker, calcified caps. The bases of these older plaques are also under less stress than the stress at the periphery of non-obstructing, eccentric plaques of varying density and consistency. The older, more stable plaques, though more uniform, are larger and more likely to obstruct blood flow, leading to angina. Those are the plaques typically treated with angioplasty and stenting, yet they are *not* vulnerable plaques and *not* likely to initiate a clot that can cause an infarction.

Now we know that a certain type of plaque and a certain type of biochemical event most often trigger a heart attack. These plaques are often not visible to conventional cardiac testing, such as stress tests and angiograms, because they do not obstruct blood flow, or impinge on the vessel lumen sufficiently to be visualized by such tests.

The important takeaway message here is how important it is to be able to understand what distinguishes risky coronary plaque from stable coronary plaque. It is important to recognize that

> *Plaque can become stable with dietary excellence,* and it can become unstable relatively quickly with dangerous eating. It is the more recently deposited, and more recently modified, plaque, resulting from eating dangerously, that can create vulnerable plaque and make semi-vulnerable plaque more vulnerable, precipitating a cardiac event.

> *Angioplasty and bypass surgery do not address or fix the vulnerable plaque* in a person's coronary circulation. These procedures

mostly address the least dangerous (old) plaque and therefore have no effect on reducing the risk of future cardiac events. However, eating carefully, in the manner I prescribe, can immediately make plaque less vulnerable by reducing inflammatory cells, reducing soft plaque, and reducing tensile stress. Superior nutrition stabilizes both the base of the plaque, to keep it from rupturing, and the cap of the plaque, to keep it from cracking.

AVOID THE "HOLIDAY HEART ATTACK"

For many years, researchers have been intrigued by a disturbing pattern: The number of deadly heart attacks increases during the winter holiday season, with distinct spikes around Christmas and New Year's Day. The cardiologist Philip Ettinger coined the term "holiday heart syndrome" in 1978 in a study of twenty-four patients who drank heavily and regularly but also had a holiday or weekend binge before the study.[1] He demonstrated the toxic effects of alcohol on the heart and the rhythm disturbance it promoted.

In a 2004 study researchers examined fifty-three million U.S. death certificates from 1973 to 2001. They noted that "the number of cardiac deaths is higher on Dec. 25 than on any other day of the year, second highest on Dec. 26, and third highest on Jan. 1."[2]

These findings of holiday heart attacks, or the "Merry Christmas Coronary" and "Happy Hanukkah Heart Attack," shoot up consistently across the country. They hold true even in balmy climates such as Los Angeles, where the winter weather stays mild and no one ever wields a snow shovel. During the holidays, legions of Americans eat and drink too much. They eat out at gatherings of family and friends, they receive food as gifts, and they take in more salt. To put it simply, they just get full of food—and much of it is unhealthy food, too. Add increased caffeine and alcohol consumption to the mix, and you have the perfect ingredients for cardiac problems, such as atrial fibrillation and stroke.

The point is this: Celebrations that include excess eating and drinking and that focus on dangerous foods cause many people to die needlessly.

The rapid weight gain associated with holidays, and vacations, doesn't just increase fat on your waist—it also enhances visceral deposits of fat, including soft lipid accumulation in plaque. Then the increased inflammation from sugar and alcohol immediately affects the *endothelium* (the interior

CHARACTERISTICS OF DANGEROUS (MOST VULNERABLE) PLAQUE

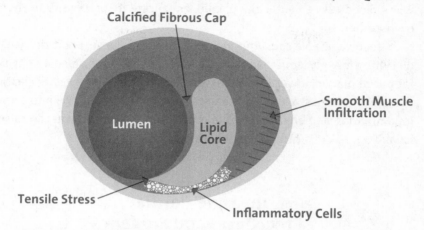

- The lipid segment of the plaque is more substantial.
- The lipid segment is infiltrated with many inflammatory cells (especially macrophages).
- The fibrous cap is thin.
- There is significant tensile stress at the edge of the plaque.

CHARACTERISTICS OF LEAST DANGEROUS (LEAST VULNERABLE) PLAQUE

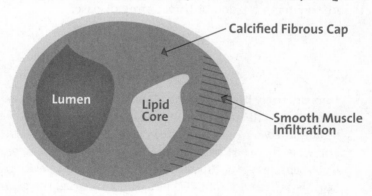

- The smooth muscle segment of the atheroma (fatty buildup) is more substantial.
- There are few inflammatory cells.
- The fibrous cap is thick.
- There is less tensile stress on the plaque.

lining of the blood vessels) by increasing microvessels, or pores. This allows white blood cells to enter the plaque, enhancing its propensity to rupture even further.

Green vegetable consumption and a nutrient-dense, plant-rich (NDPR) diet with a low-glycemic load work in the opposite way. You lose weight, suck fat out of plaque, lower blood pressure, and restore blood vessel elasticity (lessening tensile stress). Antioxidants and phytochemicals help to prevent inflammation and enhance plaque repair. In other words, you can raise or lower your risk of a cardiac event within days.

Invasive Cardiac Procedures and Surgeries Are Not Effective

Do you think that being evaluated by a cardiologist or radiologist to determine whether you have significant coronary blockage will enable an intervention at an early enough point to save your life? If you do, I have some bad news for you: That kind of thinking is dead wrong. Angioplasty and stents, as well as cardiac surgery, treat symptoms and ignore the major burden of threatening disease.

Glossary

Coronary artery bypass grafting (CABG), commonly known as *heart bypass surgery,* is the most common heart surgery in the United States. A healthy artery or vein is connected (grafted) to the obstructed coronary artery, creating a new path for the blood to flow to the heart muscle. The blood bypasses the obstructed vessel, with a resulting relief in angina.

The serious risks of CABG include an increased risk of stroke and overall death rate compared with percutaneous coronary intervention (see below), loss of mental function in the elderly, atrial fibrillation, and other more unusual events, such as failure of the sternum to close properly after surgery.

Percutaneous coronary intervention (PCI) (or angioplasty with stent placement) is a nonsurgical procedure during which the physician feeds a thin flexible tube, or catheter, from the groin or arm into the heart. The catheter has a deflated balloon on the end, and when the tube reaches the blockage, it is forced though. The balloon is then inflated to open the artery, allowing blood to flow better. Then a stent, or short metal wire tube, is placed to prevent the stretched vessel from closing up again quickly.

The most serious risks of PCI include death, heart attack, stroke, ventricular fibrillation (nonsustained ventricular tachycardia is common), and aortic dissection. Heart attacks induced by heart muscle injury occur in 3–5 percent of patients, and one study showed that 1.2 patients out of every 100 died in the hospital undergoing PCI.[3] Restenosis (the growing back of scar tissue and plaque around the stent) still occurs in about 20 percent of people who undergo angioplasty and stenting.

When more extensive disease is present or the obstructed vessels are not amenable to stenting, CABG is preferred over PCI.

During **cardiac catheterization** a catheter is put into a blood vessel in the arm, groin (upper thigh), or neck and threaded to the heart. Through the catheter, a doctor can perform diagnostic tests and treatments.

During **coronary angiography** or **coronary angiogram** a special type of dye is injected into the catheter; it then flows through your bloodstream to your heart and makes the interior lumen of your coronary arteries visible on radiographs.

Since atherosclerotic plaque blankets many parts of the numerous vessels in the heart, bypassing or removing the most obstructive portion still does not address all the shallow and nonobstructive lipid deposits that are more vulnerable and thus more prone to cause heart attack. The major burden of disease is left intact, and therefore the potential for a deadly heart attack is largely unaffected.

The tactic of using surgical and high-tech interventions as a substitute for a healthy diet is doomed to fail. Whenever CAD is present and surgical intervention occurs, the vast bulk of plaque is still left untreated. Atherosclerosis is a dietary-induced disease that spreads throughout the heart, not only in those areas visualized by angiograms. The vast majority of patients who undergo these interventions do not have fewer new heart attacks or live longer.[4]

The procedures themselves expose patients to more risk of new heart attacks, strokes, infection, encephalopathy (disease in the brain), and death. Angioplasty, with or without stenting, also damages the treated blood vessel. It increases inflammation in the treated vessel and raises levels of C-reactive protein, which creates restenosis and increases the risk of recurrent coronary events.[5] Restenosis, which occurs in 30–50 percent of angioplasty-treated patients,[6] is more resistant to regression with nutritional approaches than native atherosclerosis.

Once an individual has a stent placed, that foreign body in the vessel wall increases inflammation at the edge of the stent. This can enhance the potential for the treated area to generate a clot, leading to a future heart attack. It is routine to combine aspirin with another anticlotting drug to help lessen this risk. Patients are typically kept on these medications for years, increasing their risk of gastrointestinal bleed or hemorrhagic stroke (bleeding into the brain).

To accommodate the increased risk of the stent, patients have no option but to increase their future risk of bleeding to death. I suppose this might be acceptable if patients had no other option, but they *do* have one—and it's much more effective than stenting. That option is to adopt a Nutritarian NDPR diet-style that has a low glycemic load.

Stenting represents not only a risky and flawed medical procedure, but also a serious economic burden on society. It is costly, and when it fails, further treatment strategies include even more expensive approaches. Even the temporary relief of angina (symptomatic benefits) from angioplasty and subsequent interventions erode with time.

In the United States alone, the total cost for the diagnosis and treatment of heart disease with angioplasty and coronary bypass surgery now exceeds $100 billion annually, despite the limited effectiveness of these procedures. Almost all of these costly and invasive procedures represent what I call "uninformed malpractice." In other words, these invasive procedures are most often done without patients being truly informed about their limited benefit and their significant risks. In addition, patients most likely are not told of the effectiveness and safety of nutritional excellence, as shown by numerous studies available today.

Without this critical information, how can patients compare the two approaches and give truly *informed* consent?

These medical interventions do not address the cause of the disease; they treat only the symptoms—an approach that lessens pain for a limited period of time. So it is not surprising that patients undergoing bypass surgery and angioplasty experience disease progression, graft shutdown, restenosis, and more procedures as their heart disease continues to advance. This nearly ubiquitous advancement of pathology is inevitable, because *these treatments simply do not work.* Most patients who undergo these procedures needlessly die prematurely from heart disease because their disease remains essentially untreated.[7]

When we combine these medical interventions, which are ineffective or at best only marginally effective, with the incorrect dietary advice that most doctors and dietitians provide (specifically, to reduce fat and cholesterol intake and eat less red meat and more chicken and fish), we get predictable future cardiac tragedies. Numerous studies have demonstrated that following the typical dietary recommendations of the American Heart Association to hold cholesterol to less than 200 mg/day and to reduce dietary fat to less than 30 percent just doesn't work.[8] These "politically correct" diets fail to recognize that the nutritional cause of heart disease is not simply a question of eating less fat. Moderation kills, because heart disease still advances.

Getting Tested and Treated for Coronary Obstructive Disease Won't Help

> Everyone who eats the traditional SAD, is overweight, and has high blood pressure and high cholesterol is at risk.

Even a small coating of vulnerable plaque, invisible to standard cardiac testing, can cause a heart attack—and typically does. The important point to remember is this: Individuals *without* major blockages of their great vessels, who might have only 30–50 percent narrowing of the vessels, are just as likely to have a fatal cardiac event as those with more significant blockages. And yet, stress tests and angiography don't even show these individuals as having heart disease.

Stress tests identify only those blockages that obstruct more than 85 percent of the vessel lumen. A "normal" stress test *does not* mean that you do not have significant heart disease, do not have lots of dangerous plaque, or will not shortly have a heart attack.

When lipid-filled atheromas first develop on the wall of a blood vessel, the walls remodel outward, preserving the lumen. These are the most vulnerable or lethal plaques, and they do not obstruct or encroach on the blood flow. Even coronary catheterization (angiography) does not identify these smaller, non-occluding atherosclerotic deposits. Therefore, interventional strategies do not treat patients with shallower lesions, despite the fact that these are the people who suffer the most heart attacks.[9]

If the plaque deposit does not impinge significantly on blood flow or compromise the lumen by 30 percent or more, the plaque is typically not even seen on coronary angiography. And since you now know that it is not the *extent* of the blockage that determines risk but rather the *vulnerability* of the plaque, or its propensity to rupture, you can understand why 70–80 percent of all myocardial infarctions are caused by plaque that is not obstructive or visible on angiography or stress tests.

What Do Authorities Recommend?

The majority of cardiologists today recommend cardiac catheterization followed by a revascularization procedure to improve blood flow, or bypass surgery for individuals with abnormal stress tests and subsequent angiogram for those experiencing heart-related chest pain with activity. But this is not the current standard of practice recommended by the American Heart Association or the American College of Cardiology. These organizations now realize that no high-quality scientific data suggest that patients with stable CAD should even be evaluated with angiography, let alone treated with angioplasty and stenting or CABG. "Stable CAD" means disease that is not rapidly worsening, thereby being suggestive of older, obstructive plaque.

These newest guidelines, intended to advise cardiologists and other physicians on the most updated scientific investigations, recognize that cardiac catheterization procedures have significant risk and that little is gained by identifying and treating stable CAD.[10]

The studies on this subject show that, even compared with something as ineffective as what is known as optimized medical therapy, which is essentially just giving patients cholesterol-lowering drugs and treating high blood pressure, an invasive evaluation with cardiac imaging and revascularization treatment does nothing to prevent future cardiac events and hospitalizations or to extend life.[11] And of course, such therapy does not include optimal *nutritional* therapy, which is the missing piece of this puzzle.

These official guidelines recognize that invasive diagnostic procedures have significant complications. Reported complications of angioplasty include death, stroke, heart attack, bleeding, infection, allergic or anaphylactic reactions, vascular damage, kidney damage, arrhythmias, and sometimes even the need for emergency surgery. And these complications are more likely to occur in people who are older than 70. The guidelines state further that "the concept of informed consent requires that risks and benefits of and alternatives to coronary angiography be explicitly discussed with the patient before the procedure is undertaken."

The guidelines also clearly advise that angiography and subsequent interventions are appropriate only if it is determined beforehand that a patient is amenable to percutaneous or surgical evaluation. I can't imagine that anyone who has been adequately informed (such as those of you reading the information within these pages) would choose an invasive, expensive, and potentially dangerous procedure— and one that probably won't even help—over changing the way he or she eats.

Given the recent advances in and findings on the reversibility of even severe and advanced CAD with nutritional intervention, it is vital that doctors inform their patients about this nutritional option before those patients are corralled into expensive, dangerous, and usually needless medical evaluations and treatments.

Unless doctors tell heart patients about the
documented effectiveness of superior nutrition,
those patients are not getting complete information
and therefore are not giving proper, informed
consent for any coronary revascularization
procedures they may undergo.

The American Heart Association and the American College of Cardiology supplied conventional guidelines on when revascularization would be appropriate in patients with very severe CAD. These guidelines are based on the assumption that revascularization offers a survival benefit in these cases—something that is still unlikely compared with a change to a healthy, nutrient-dense diet. These organizations concluded that revascularization is appropriate in the following cases:

1. When severe CAD is suspected to be the cause of depressed left ventricular ejection fraction or transient heart failure. A low ejection fraction can be determined with an ultrasound of the heart, which is a safe test that does not involve using contrast dye, breaking the skin, and performing radiation and associated risks.

2. When severe CAD is suspected as the cause of severe ventricular arrhythmias.

I understand that in these cases evaluation and revascularization can benefit patients. But even under these relatively unusual conditions, we do not know whether revascularization would beat nutritional intervention in a head-to-head trial. My guess is that it would not. I base my opinion on the reasons discussed above: first, on the failure of the revascularization procedure to generally benefit the average patient; and second, on the effectiveness of the Nutritarian diet in bringing about relatively quick and dramatic improvements in blood flow to all areas of the heart, not just the areas addressed by medical intervention.

Of course the above discussion is referring to the *stable* patient, not one who is undergoing a heart attack and needs urgent care. When that is happening, every minute counts, and reestablishing circulation with angioplasty or clot-busting drugs can be lifesaving. Unstable angina or increasing pain, even at rest, is another legitimate indication for acting urgently to establish blood flow, as it could be suggestive of clot development, leading to a heart attack. *All acute coronary syndromes require emergency evaluation and treatment.*

Glossary

Stable angina is chest pain of cardiac origin resulting from decreased blood flow through the coronary vessels supplying the muscle (myocardium) of the heart. Stable angina increases with activity and exercise and improves with rest.

Unstable angina could be a new symptom or a change from prior symptoms, but its persistent hallmark is that the chest discomfort and other symptoms of angina occur when a person is at rest, not just during exertion. Unstable angina is significant for increased risk of heart attack and should be treated appropriately as a medical emergency. It may be the only appropriate indication for coronary artery angioplasty and stenting other than those procedures done while a person is experiencing a heart attack.

Acute coronary syndromes include both heart attacks and unstable angina usually associated with a defect or rupture in the plaque and partial or complete clot formation of a coronary artery (thrombosis). All acute coronary syndromes require emergency evaluation and treatment.

So what do I recommend if you have CAD? How do my recommendations differ from those you might get from a typical cardiologist? If you "just" have high blood pressure and high cholesterol and are overweight or diabetic, I recommend aggressive nutritional intervention and an exercise program customized to your fitness level and tolerance.

If you have symptoms suggestive of angina with exertion, then I recommend you also use aggressive nutritional intervention to reduce the plaque burden and stabilize the plaque so that it doesn't form a clot. You should monitor your blood pressure and undergo blood tests. I also recommend that you get a noninvasive test to monitor heart output and wall motion, such as a cardiac ultrasound along with a carotid ultrasound, which can include (if possible in your area) measurement of the intima-media thickness, as well as an accurate determination of body fat to monitor the lowering direction of plaque burden and body fat stores.

Even if someone has chest pain with light exertion, with documented left main disease (disease in the left main coronary artery) with a reduction in ejection fraction, I still recommend nutrition as the primary treatment in a stable patient. This is because my experience (and that of my physician colleagues using this method) has shown that in two or three months, ejection fraction can improve dramatically and angina can already be significantly improved. I do not recommend angiography and stenting or bypass unless acute coronary syndrome is present, worsening ejection fraction on repeat ultrasounds is demonstrated, or ventricular arrhythmias are severe or worsening.

The exciting news is that even in very advanced cases of CAD, a slow and steady reversal of the disease is possible through a committed change to a Nutritarian diet. It is exceedingly rare that a person will not see heart disease resolve with this program. I include an emergency diet approach in Chapter 8 that starts patients with serious disease on an aggressive dietary intervention for maximizing results (see "Radical Weight Reduction Menu" on page 247).

The Good News

All of the symptoms of heart disease, as well as blockages, can melt away with superior nutrition—without any cardiac intervention. The risks and complications of cardiac interventions and bypass surgeries are simply not necessary when people adopt an effective nutritional strategy. Instead of prescribing drugs and recommending expensive and invasive medical procedures, doctors need to educate themselves and then educate and motivate patients to take charge of their own health.

People are committing suicide in daily increments, using their knives and forks. When they experience the warning signs of cardiovascular disease, they turn to doctors, expecting to be saved. Unfortunately, it is almost impossible to escape from the biological laws of cause and effect. Good health can't be bought. Doctors can't give it to you and health insurance can't provide it. Good health has to be *earned.*

Compelling data from numerous population and interventional studies show that a natural plant-based diet will prevent, arrest, and even reverse heart disease. We look at this more thoroughly in the next chapter. Only via superior nutrition can you remove and resolve the invisible but potentially dangerous plaque throughout your coronary arteries.

Unlike surgery and angioplasty, the Nutritarian dietary approach presented in this book does not merely treat your heart, but rejuvenates all your blood vessels and protects your entire body against heart attack, stroke, pulmonary embolism, venous thrombosis, peripheral vascular disease, and vascular dementia. A Nutritarian diet-style is your most valuable insurance policy to secure a longer life free of medical tragedy.

CHAPTER THREE

Nutritional Excellence, Not Drugs

The standard of modern medical care is to medicate rather than educate people suffering from cardiovascular disease, high blood pressure, and a host of problems that can be improved and even reversed through nutritional excellence. In most cases, aggressive drug treatment and surgery offer limited benefits in terms of life span enhancement, although they can give the illusion of safety. In contrast, the Nutritarian diet, with its emphasis on nutrient-dense foods that are high in phytochemicals, is designed to give the body the tools it needs to heal itself. Combined with exercise, the Nutritarian diet-style is the best defense against the ravages of disease caused by the SAD. Remember, your health is truly in your hands—primarily the one that holds your fork.

Think about this for a minute: Heart attack rates vary widely on the basis of where you live and the typical eating and exercise habits of the people in your region. We know some countries have much more heart disease than other countries, but did you know that right here in the United States, heart attack rates vary tremendously from region to region?

For example, according to data from the Centers for Disease Control and Prevention (CDC) the southern states of Alabama, Arkansas, Louisiana, and Mississippi have about four times the number of heart attacks per thousand compared with Arizona, Colorado, New Mexico, and Utah.[1] This implies that the dietary habits of people in those southern states are exceedingly dangerous.

More than one and a half million people will have a heart attack or stroke this year in the United States, with about one million deaths caused by heart disease. In practical terms, this amounts to a needless death every thirty seconds. In 2011, the direct medical costs attributed to cardiovascular disease came to $320 billion—more than any other medical condition, including strokes, peripheral artery disease, and high blood pressure.[2]

Here are some heart-stopping statistics:

- More than one in three—or eighty-three million—U.S. adults currently live with one or more types of cardiovascular disease.

- Nearly sixty-eight million U.S. adults have high blood pressure, and about half of them do not have this condition under control.

- An estimated seventy-one million U.S. adults have high cholesterol.

Drugs, medical procedures, and surgery are the recommended approaches for dealing with heart disease in the United States. As a result, the demand for high-tech, expensive, but largely ineffective medical care is high, causing already high medical costs and insurance rates to skyrocket. The lifetime medical costs accrued for each patient with heart disease now averages more than $750,000 and can approach $1 million in those with CAD.[3]

The medical answer to heart disease is both financially devastating and futile. An entire medical industry, with exploding costs, has developed to attempt to deal with the dangers of disease-causing food. Patients need to be told that there is another option that is more effective—one that can reverse heart disease and protect their lives with certainty. If all patients had access to this information, then they could choose which road was right for them.

My goal is for all patients to know that they can get well and be safe—and avoid expensive, invasive, and futile medical care. I want to make sure people know that they have a safer, noninvasive, and more effective choice, and that they can effectively prevent a needless, premature death.

CASE HISTORY: PROOF FROM A PATIENT

A 72-year-old man with a history of CAD sought nutritional management of his angina. He had complained of chest pain radiating to his arms while walking. A thallium stress test showed multivessel CAD, and a cardiac catheterization showed a 95 percent stenosis of his left anterior descending artery. He refused angioplasty and bypass surgery, instead requesting aggressive nutritional management. The man was taking diltiazem and aspirin daily and sublingual nitroglycerin as needed.

On his own, he had started a grain-based vegan diet before visiting his doctor's office, which resulted in his losing 14 pounds (from 180 to 166 pounds); his total cholesterol lowered from 240 to 218 md/dl, with an LDL concentration of 146 mg/dl. His angina was also starting to improve.

Two months after starting the Nutritarian diet-style, the man lost an additional 14 pounds, and his blood pressure averaged 120/70 mmHg on diltiazem (from a previous average of 136/64). Over time, the diltiazem was discontinued gradually, and his blood pressure remained favorable at future visits. In a short time, his chest pain resolved, and he did not need any further sublingual nitroglycerin. His lipid profile also dramatically improved, with a total cholesterol of 177 mg/dl and LDL concentration of 107 mg/dl. His cardiologist supported his decision at this time to continue with nutritional management instead of undergoing angioplasty.

At the age of 78 he had a repeat exercise stress test that showed increased exercise tolerance, improved heart rate and blood pressure, and regression of disease when compared with the previous stress test results. His lipid profile continued to decrease, with a total cholesterol concentration of 189 mg/dl and LDL concentration of 81 mg/dl. Now in his 90s, he has continued to be free of high cholesterol, high blood pressure, and angina and has remained medication-free and in good health.

What's More Effective—Food or Drugs?

Why bother with exercise, eating right, or losing weight, if we can just pop some pills? Because the pills don't do such a good job in guarding against cardiovascular disease.

The INTERHEART study showed that for men and women, old and young, and in all areas of the world, nine potentially modifiable factors such as diet, exercise, and smoking accounted for greater than 90 percent of the risk of having a heart attack.[4] A recent analysis of data from the Nurses' Health Study showed almost the same thing: that 92 percent of heart attacks could be prevented by adherence to healthy lifestyle habits.[5]

The point is that conventional physicians, who do not use an optimized dietary approach to disease prevention, have to recognize that even moderately healthier choices, such as exercising, eating fruits and vegetables, maintaining a favorable weight, and not smoking, can reduce the incidence of heart disease, stroke, and diabetes by 80–90 percent.[6] Even hereditary hypercholesterolemia (very high cholesterol) is rare enough that more than 99 percent of people can protect themselves without the use of cholesterol-lowering drugs if they adopt a Nutritarian diet. It is important to note that common (and ubiquitous) atherosclerotic heart disease is acquired by eating an unhealthy diet; it is not genetic.

Pharmacological therapies, on the other hand, including cholesterol-lowering and blood pressure–lowering drugs, reduce cardiovascular disease risk by only 20–30 percent—and even these low figures are questioned by many researchers who are skeptical of the clinical trial results reported by industry-sponsored scientists. So even among patients taking these drugs, 70–90 percent of heart attacks still occur, depending on which studies you consider.

The first step to applying this lifesaving information is to understand that traditional medical care is risky and largely ineffective, as we just saw in Chapter 2. An aggressive nutritional approach is substantially more effective, even for people with advanced CAD. But in order for patients to make the right choice, they need to understand the futility and risks of conventional medical management. If you fully knew the risks and dangers of the medications prescribed for high blood pressure, diabetes, and high cholesterol—and understood how relatively ineffective they are—you would be more likely and more willing to change the way you eat.

The fact is that *medical care can kill you*. And your loved ones have no legal recourse when it does, because your doctor practiced the current "standard of care." In other words, your doctor did what other doctors mostly do.

The decision is yours: Choose a favorable diet-style and lifestyle that can effectively protect your health, or rely on drugs and surgical procedures, which cannot.

Reversing CAD via nutritional excellence is now an accepted and proven fact. Doctors do their patients a disservice if they do not advocate superior nutrition and insist on its implementation. Physicians must fight aggressively for patient compliance with nutritional excellence and dispense dietary advice that offers patients the opportunity for a complete recovery. As I've already said, and say again, anything less should be considered malpractice.

Physicians rely on medications for lowering high blood pressure and cholesterol (and blood sugar, for diabetics) in an attempt to limit the damage caused by eating the SAD (or DAD—deadly American diet). Then, when that fails and angina develops, they recommend angioplasty with stenting or coronary artery bypass surgery.

This raises a series of questions: Are these medicines effective? Are they safe? Do they significantly extend human life span? Let's first review typical medical interventions used for high blood pressure and lowering cholesterol, along with some of the known risks and how effective those interventions are at offering protection.

High Blood Pressure

> High blood pressure (or hypertension) is typically
> the first sign of heart attack risk.

High blood pressure is a strong risk factor for developing heart disease and kidney failure, strokes, and death. Letting your blood pressure run dangerously high is not wise.

Hypertension is often called "the silent killer" because it usually has no symptoms until the body is already damaged and a deadly heart attack or stroke occurs. Blood pressure is made up of two numbers: systolic blood pressure and diastolic blood pressure. According to the U.S. National Institutes of Health, systolic pressure is considered normal when it is 120 mmHg or lower, and diastolic should be less than 80 mmHg: that is, 120/80 mmHg.

About 95 percent of hypertension is *essential hypertension,* which means that the high blood pressure is not the secondary effect of some other condition such as a tumor or kidney disease.

Essential hypertension is caused mostly by enhanced peripheral resistance from blood vessels that have lost their elasticity due to atherosclerosis or hardening of the arteries. Another important contributor is the increased activity of the sympathetic nervous system. This is a more complicated issue but arises often as a result of many years of consuming excess sodium. The SAD also takes its toll, inducing chronic low-grade inflammation to the interior lining of the arteries (endothelium) with all its low-nutrient, processed, high-glycemic-load foods and animal products. The body-wide stress or inflammation from a poor diet is often called *oxidative stress,* because it reflects the increased presence of free radicals.

So in summary, three main causes of high blood pressure are

- Atherosclerosis (stiffened and narrowed blood vessels)

- Chronic high salt intake, leading to increased sympathetic and vascular tone

- Chronic inflammation damaging the endothelial lining, causing constriction and decreased elasticity

Right now, most people older than 65, and 27 percent of our entire population, are taking blood pressure–lowering medications, making them the most commonly prescribed class of drugs in the United States.[7] There are six classes of drugs used to lower blood pressure:

- Diuretics

- Beta-blockers

- Calcium channel blockers and direct vasodilators

- Angiotensin-converting enzyme (ACE) inhibitors and angiotensin II receptor blockers (ARBs)

- Alpha-blockers

- Nervous system inhibitors

The current consensus among physicians and medical authorities is that once established, high blood pressure is a lifelong condition, is largely irreversible, and requires medication for the rest of a person's life. My contrary position is that *high blood pressure is reversible in most cases* through dietary excellence, which is substantially more effective than medical management of high blood pressure. Dietary excellence is also effective in reducing morbidity and premature mortality, whereas medications usually are not.

Case Studies

I now turn to some results from my case series and medical journal study evaluating more than one thousand individuals following my dietary recommendations to various degrees for more than a year. The group of participants were 80 percent or more compliant with my recommendations. Of the 443 individuals with high blood pressure, the average drop in systolic blood pressure was 26 mmHg. In contrast, standard blood pressure medications lower systolic blood pressure on average about 10 mmHg.[8] The drop for the Nutritarian patients in diastolic blood pressure was about 15 mmHg. These results are far superior than the changes seen with standard blood pressure medications, with the added benefits of zero side effects.

BLOOD PRESSURE REDUCTION COMPARISON

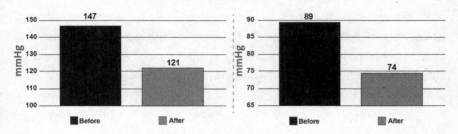

For the 328 individuals who reported high cholesterol but were not taking any medications, LDL cholesterol dropped an average of 42 mg/dl. For the 166 individuals who had high triglycerides, those levels dropped an average of 80 points. Seventy-five individuals whose starting body mass index (BMI) was above 30 kg/m² and whose data we had for at least three years, lost an average of 50 pounds by the end of year one; the average weight lost was greater each consecutive year. All these results would have been even more spectacular if the study had evaluated only those people who were 100 percent compliant with my dietary recommendations.

A sampling of patients with advanced disease who used this approach was also published. Looking at some of these published case studies sheds light on the impact of applying this nutritional approach and gives you an idea of its potential benefits.

Reducing blood pressure, body weight, oxidative stress, cholesterol, blood sugar, and other metabolic markers synergistically restores health to vessels in the heart, brain, and peripheral circulation. The dramatic effects seen for a reduction in blood pressure parallel the benefits seen for lowering cholesterol, and the resultant reduction and eventual resolution of atherosclerosis.

Case #1

This 48-year-old man had a past medical history of obesity, alcohol abuse, and CAD. At 6 feet tall, his starting weight was at least 300 pounds (his home weight scale went up to only 300 pounds, so he likely weighed more), putting him in the morbidly obese category, with a BMI of 40.

After having CABG on four vessels in September 2005, he resumed his poor diet, along with smoking two to three packs of cigarettes per day and occasionally binge drinking. In July 2008, he awoke with rest angina, which subsequently resulted in the placement of three cardiac stents in one of the coronary arteries that had not been bypassed. Shortly after the procedure, he continued having severe angina, experienced at the slightest exertion, and was unable to work. His medication list included metoprolol succinate, 200 mg; irbesartan, 300 mg; atorvastatin, 20 mg; clopidogrel bisulfate, 75 mg; and aspirin, 325 mg. He had a poor prognosis and was forced to be sedentary because of angina even with minimal walking.

CASE #1

PARAMETER	JULY 2008	JULY 2009
Weight (lbs)	300+	160
Blood pressure (mmHg)	161/110, on irbesartan, 300 mg / metoprolol, 200 mg	110/68, off medications
Total cholesterol	270, on atorvastatin, 20 mg	120, off medication
LDL	148	75
Triglycerides	300+	63
Fasting glucose	100–120	80–90

Realizing he had no other options, this man adopted a Nutritarian diet-style, which he learned about via an Internet search. He also quit smoking. He received further guidance via website forums and discussion groups. He lost 35 pounds in the first month, and 47 pounds in nine weeks. At this point, his angina improved dramatically, but he still had morning angina symptoms with mild exertion that resolved during the day. After six months, he had lost 100 pounds and had no further angina symptoms, even with exercise. At that time, he had stopped all medications other than 81 mg aspirin daily. After one year, his weight, lipid panel, glucose, and blood pressure were dramatically lower.

He can now exercise without angina or irregular palpitations. He also stopped his smoking and binge drinking. Now, more than five years later, he maintains his superior health without any medications and without any further cardiac symptoms.

Case #2

A 60-year-old man with no significant past medical history was following a diet-style for ten years that avoided red and processed meats and included vegetables, fruits, whole grains, olive and flax oil, butter, salmon, and chicken. At 5 feet 7 inches tall with a weight of 155 pounds, he had a BMI of 24, placing him in the "normal weight" category.

CASE #2

PARAMETER	JUNE 2006	JUNE 2007
Weight (lbs)	155	135
Waistline (in)	35	30.5
Blood pressure (mmHg)	130/90	96/60
Resting heart rate (bpm)	72	55
LDL	126	63
HDL	39	47
Triglycerides	80	50
Lp(a)	144	72

In March 2006, he began a power walking exercise program and experienced exertional chest pain. A visit to a cardiologist revealed a normal physical exam, electrocardiogram, echocardiogram, and a lipid panel with LDL 126, high-density lipoprotein (HDL) 39, and triglycerides 80. In June 2006, the patient had a positive thallium exercise stress test and a computed tomography (CT) angiogram, which revealed multifocal disease in the left anterior descending artery with low-density obstructive plaque. He was started on aspirin and clopidogrel bisulfate but declined a statin medication. He started the Nutritarian diet-style in May 2006. By June, he stopped experiencing exertional angina. In January 2007, his primary physician discontinued all medications. The patient discontinued the aspirin on his own.

In June 2007, the patient had a repeat CT angiogram, revealing that the plaque in his left anterior descending artery was now nonobstructive and had changed from low density to mixed density. In August 2008, he had a magnetic resonance angiogram showing complete reversal of his coronary plaque, with no detectable disease, two years after he had begun the Nutritarian diet-style. Eight years later, he continued to be off all medications and free of angina.

Case #3

A 60-year-old man (5 feet 8 inches tall, 205 pounds, BMI 31) had a history of atrial fibrillation, hyperlipidemia, degenerative disc disease, and arthritis. He had chronic episodes of symptomatic atrial fibrillation during moderate exercise, with dizziness and fatigue. He complained of shortness of breath while climbing stairs and was unable to walk more than fifteen minutes because of pain. He had chronic indigestion requiring the use of antacids at bedtime for the previous twenty years. His medication list included metoprolol, atorvastatin, aspirin, warfarin, and fish oil.

In June 2012, the patient began a Nutritarian diet-style. After a few weeks, he was able to discontinue his antacids. He lost 15 pounds during the first seven weeks. By September 2012, he had lost 25 pounds. Two years later he weighed 168 pounds (BMI 25). His arthritis pains resolved. He could exercise without restrictions: run stairs, cycle for thirty minutes, and lift weights without fatigue or shortness of breath. The patient's episodes of symptomatic atrial fibrillation resolved. He was able to discontinue all medications. His lipid profile and blood pressure improved significantly.

Case #3

PARAMETER	DECEMBER 2009, ON MEDICATIONS	MARCH 2013, OFF MEDICATIONS
Total cholesterol	226	188
LDL	156	119
HDL	51	52
Triglycerides	96	83
Blood pressure	149/90	110/62

Critics may complain that these case studies, and the many others referenced in my published study and on my website, are carefully selected, best-case scenarios. These critics ask, "What about all the other people you did not record who did not do as well?" Some may even say case histories do not count.

The critics are right—to a degree. But remember, I have been using this approach on thousands of people in my medical practice for twenty-five years. I was in a busy private practice, seeing patients more than fifty hours a week. Those who dropped out and either didn't see great results or could not follow the diet-style are not included in these cases. But those who followed my nutritional guidelines to the letter have all had excellent results. I never claimed most people would be adherent to this approach in a randomized trial, I only claim those who do will get spectacular results. What the masses choose to do, has no bearing on whether there should be universal awareness of the effectiveness of superior nutrition on cardiovascular disease. However, full informed consent, such as offered by this book, is needed for individuals to be able to make an educated choice.

When you change to a Nutritarian diet-style, cut the salt out of your diet, exercise regularly, and lose weight, you remove inflammation, reduce atherosclerosis, and eliminate the inflammation of the endothelium. In other words, the causes of high blood pressure are eliminated, and the blood vessels begin to heal themselves.

Drugs, on the other hand, merely cover up the symptoms. This gives people a false sense of security, because even though the blood pressure *numbers* are better, the inflammation, thickening, hardening, and in-creased vascular tone are still problems. Most often, the condition slowly advances because people don't make adequate changes in their diet and lifestyle for the problem to be repaired. Prescription drugs encourage people to continue to make self-destructive eating choices. The drugs give them "permission" to continue to eat as they always have, because they mask the symptoms while allowing the causative pathologies to advance.

Modern Medical Care Is Heavily Biased

Modern medical care is based on scientific studies that evaluate drugs; however, these studies are heavily biased toward pharmacological in-terventions. The studies are funded, and results interpreted, by the pharmaceutical companies, or they are at least influenced by their funding sponsors.

Articles being published in the most prestigious medical journals are no longer composed of careful science; for decades they have been supported or conducted by pharmaceutical companies and as a result they are essentially drug advertisements. The information brought to and taught to the medical profession is shaped by its com-mercial value to drug companies. The fundamental purpose of most scientific research articles published today is how to improve corpo-rate profits.

Modern medical care has mostly evolved into a drug-distribution arm of the pharmaceutical industry, rather than being a profession pri-marily centered on improving people's health. A true health-care profes-sion that is concerned with maximizing patients' well-being would be focused on removing impediments to better health. The emphasis would be on the promotion of healthy habits, such as smoking cessation, exer-cise, and dietary improvement, as well as protection against exposure to chemicals, toxins, and other known causes of disease. Instead, prescrip-tion drugs, all of which have toxicities and dangers, have become the primary intervention for every dietary-induced health issue.

Contrary to public perception, doctors often do not review the potential negative consequences of medications when they prescribe them. As I have already pointed out, blood pressure–lowering medications are the most commonly prescribed class of medications in the United States, yet serious health risks associated with them are rarely discussed.

For example, *calcium-channel blockers (CCBs)*, a commonly prescribed class of blood pressure medication, have been linked to higher rates of cancer in women.[9] Longtime users of these drugs have been found to have more than double the risk for getting breast cancer, compared with women not using the medication. CCBs include amlodipine (Norvasc), diltiazem (Cardizem LA, Tiazac), isradipine (DynaCirc CR), nicardipine (Cardene SR), nifedipine (Procardia, Procardia XL, Adalat CC), nisoldipine (Sular), and verapamil (Calan, Verelan, Covera-HS).

The researchers found that taking CCBs for at least ten years was associated with increased risks of both ductal and lobular breast cancer, the most common types of breast cancer. Remember, cancer initiation and promotion must occur many years before cancer is eventually diagnosed—usually twenty to fifty years before diagnosis. So with only a ten-year follow-up, these data could be underestimating the cancer-promoting potential of these drugs.

It is common for pharmaceutical companies to claim that their drugs do not cause cancer by doing follow-up studies for only two to three years, when fifteen to twenty years would be needed to ascertain risk. Despite this major risk of cancer, physicians have not changed their prescribing habits, nor have they been advised to do so. The leading researcher reporting the results of this study wrote: "Despite the potential for concern raised by this study, the findings don't warrant any modifications of clinical practice. We need to see confirmation of these results before we make any recommendation for women to change what they are using." In other words: *Use drugs that are highly suspected to be unsafe first, and keep using them until we know the extent of risk with 100 percent certainty.* Doesn't this sound ridiculous?

Given the heavy use of these drugs in the United States, with more than 17 percent of women over the age of 65 taking them, the implication of a doubling of breast cancer risk is huge—and represents tremendous suffering and death. Wouldn't you expect, if there were a question of safety, that doctors would err on the side of caution? This practice is the opposite of "First, do no harm"—the Hippocratic oath that all physicians take.

But wait, it gets much worse. These women on CCBs are often also on statin cholesterol-lowering medications too, and those have been shown independently to double the risk of common types of breast cancer.[10] Imagine the cancer risk if studies looked at people on *a combination of* statins and CCBs. But scientific trials almost never consider or investigate the safety of drugs in combination.

In action, the Hippocratic oath has been interpreted to mean: Don't just stand there—prescribe medications, even if they are dangerous.

This pharma-centric attitude is even more distasteful when you consider the power and effectiveness of lifestyle medicine. Doctors could be highly persuasive in motivating their patients to adopt nutritional excellence as their path to superior health. But this would require them to be effectively trained and committed to doing so—and not to see drugs as their primary option.

Consider another blood pressure drug class, *beta-blockers*. In the large POISE trial, conducted in twenty-three countries, all 8,351 people enrolled had atherosclerosis or were at risk of heart disease. They had been admitted for noncardiac surgery and were randomized to take metoprolol (a common beta-blocker) or a placebo. After thirty days, more people died in the metoprolol group than in the placebo group (3.1 percent versus 2.3 percent), and the drug-treated group had almost double the incidence of stroke.[11]

Additional analyses did not identify any subgroup that benefited from metoprolol. The artificially lowered blood pressures had clear risks; the drugs caused more harm than good. They also can add more risk to eating the SAD, because beta-blockers cause weight gain and increase insulin resistance, predisposing patients to diabetes.

Generic names of beta-blockers include acebutolol, atenolol, bisoprolol, carvedilol, esmolol, labetalol, levatol, metoprolol, nadolol, propranolol, and timolol.

> Do not discontinue beta-blockers suddenly. Doing
> so can cause a rapid heart rate and increased
> cardiovascular risk. There is no definitive formula for
> weaning off the medication, and communication with
> and adjustment by your physician is necessary. Watch
> for a rapid increase in pulse or rebounding higher
> blood pressure. Depending on the medication used and
> the dose, doctors may prescribe five days of gradual
> decreasing dosage or they may cut the dose in half,
> and then, after one week, in half again. Your doctor
> should customize this to your needs and responses.

For decades, American physicians prescribed beta-blockers as a primary treatment for high blood pressure. More than one hundred million prescriptions were dispensed annually. Yet no data suggest that these drugs prevent heart attacks in healthy people with elevated blood pressures.

Despite the fact that beta-blockers had been used to treat hypertension for three decades, the authors of a 2007 paper noted that no study had shown that beta-blocker therapy reduces death in hypertensive patients, even when compared with placebo. The authors stated in their summary: "Given the increased risk of stroke, their 'pseudo-antihypertensive' efficacy (failure to lower central aortic pressure), lack of effect on regression of target end organ effects like left ventricular hypertrophy and endothelial dysfunction, and numerous adverse effects, the risk benefit ratio for beta-blockers is not acceptable" for patients with uncomplicated hypertension.[12]

The Cochrane Reviews, which are systematic reviews published by a global independent network of researchers, essentially found the same thing: Beta-blockers do not extend life span.[13]

Diuretics, which may be a safer choice for treating high blood pressure, have their own set of unique risks, including increased risk of developing gout. They can also increase the risk of diabetes, especially when combined with a statin drug used for lowering cholesterol.[14]

The liberal use of medications in an attempt to reduce the effects of our toxic diet-style has significant risks that counterbalance the supposed (mild) benefits. We pay a serious price for our eating habits, and then we pay an additional price from the risk of the medications—adding injury on top of injury, since almost every drug has potentially serious side effects.

All medications used to lower blood pressure can cause fatigue, lightheadedness, and loss of balance that can lead to falls and resultant hip fracture in the elderly. When the risk was investigated in people older than 70, it was found that antihypertensive medications were associated with a 30–40 percent increased risk of fall injuries, which was most severe in those with previous fall injuries.[15] This significant effect on functional loss and mortality was as severe as the heart problems these medications were supposed to protect against.

Lowering Diastolic Blood Pressure Can Be Dangerous

Systolic blood pressure is the first, higher number of your blood pressure reading. It represents the force of the heart pumping against the resistance offered by the blood vessel walls. *Diastolic blood pressure* is the second, lower number. It represents the pressure against the blood vessels during the relaxation and filling phase of the heartbeat. A healthy blood vessel is elastic, like a balloon; it spreads outward during systole and moves inward during diastole. The inward elastic movement (recoil) of our major blood vessels during diastole helps to continue the flow of blood back to refill the heart with blood during this relaxation phase of the heart pump.

Blood pressure: 120/80 = systolic/diastolic
Pulse pressure: The gap between systolic and
diastolic blood pressures
130/80: 130 minus 80 = 50 pulse pressure
140/70: 140 minus 70 = 70 pulse pressure

Perhaps the largest danger of blood pressure medications, in general, is the increased risk of death secondary to lowering diastolic blood pressure too far. Frequently, medications are prescribed in sufficient dose and in combination to adequately drop systolic pressure into a safe range. But in order to do that, these medications sometimes must lower the diastolic blood pressure too low, or widen pulse pressure, with grave results.

Low diastolic blood pressure and/or a widened pulse pressure is associated with increased risk of cardiac-related death.

When blood vessels stiffen with disease and aging, systolic pressure rises because the vessels do not expand during systole like they should, and the diastolic pressure falls, as the blood vessel walls no longer contract inward like they should. As physicians medicate to get the systolic number to a safe level, they can't stop the medication from also pushing the diastolic blood pressure down, too. This can be very unfavorable and even deadly, because with the loss of elasticity, and loss of diastolic pressure, the coronary blood vessels cannot fill adequately as they should during diastole. The heart muscle gets its supply of oxygenated blood primarily during diastole.

The excessive use of blood pressure medications that lower diastolic blood pressure too low has been shown also to increase the occurrence of atrial fibrillation and other serious rhythm disturbances of the heart, including deadly cardiac arrhythmias.[16]

In the elderly, moderately high blood pressure is not a risk factor for increased mortality, but the use of medication that brings the blood pressure below 140/70 mmHg is associated with excess mortality. The heightened risk and occurrence of death is found the more the drugs lower diastolic blood pressure. Because coronary artery filling occurs during diastole, people with CAD are at increased risk for coronary ischemic events (insufficient blood flow and oxygenation) when diastolic blood pressure falls below a certain level.

When international researchers studied twenty-two thousand patients in a fourteen-country study, they found a striking increase in heart attacks in those whose medications brought diastolic blood pressure below 84 mmHg. Those with a diastolic blood pressure below 60 had three times the occurrence of heart attacks compared with those with a diastolic above 80.[17] Even diastolic blood pressure medicated to be below 70 has been shown to almost double the risk of death.[18]

The only way to lower systolic blood pressure into a safe range without lowering diastolic too low is with diet and exercise, not drugs. Remember, this risk of death from excessive use of medication is observed in people with obstructive CAD who already have reduced blood flow and stiffened vessels. A low diastolic blood pressure is not a risk if it is not artificially medicated down and the systolic pressure is also favorable.

Plenty of healthy people of all ages, with healthy, elastic vessels, have blood pressures averaging 100/60 mmHg. In these cases, this low diastolic number is not a risk factor, as it would be in an older individual with systolic elevation and a drug-induced low diastolic reading.

What to Do If Your Blood Pressure Is High

To accurately know your blood pressure, you should take multiple readings at various times each day for a few days and take an average of the readings. Normal systolic blood pressure is below 120 mmHg, so if your average is at or below 120, congratulations! If your blood pressure is elevated, immediately take whatever steps are necessary to bring it down. These include the following:

- Eat an NDPR Nutritarian diet, which you will learn more about in following chapters.

- Do not add any salt to your food or eat any food or dish with added salt.

- Do some exercise every day, including interval training where you exert yourself for two to three minutes, sustaining a moderate elevation in heart rate at least ten times a week.

If you are taking medications for high blood pressure you will need to reduce the dose when you begin to follow the Nutritarian diet-style because it is so dramatically effective at lowering blood pressure. Even when medications are reduced at the onset of this diet program, further reductions and even discontinuation of all medications may be necessary after a few days, or your blood pressure may fall too low. *Remember: I recommend that blood pressure medications be slowly reduced as you follow this program. Do not stop them suddenly. Consult your physician.*

Whenever your systolic blood pressure starts to average below 130, it is time for your doctor to reduce your medication dose.

I have tapered the medications of thousands of my patients. Many of them were able to reduce from three medications to two within a few days, and then to one by the end of the first week. In other cases, patients reduced from two medications to one in the first few days and then—within a week—did not require any medications. However, depending on the medication and dosage used, lowering the dose rather than stopping the medication is often indicated. When a person is on only one medication, it is rare that it cannot be lowered at the onset and then stopped by the end of the first week of starting the Nutritarian diet-style. It is important to monitor your blood pressure at home during this period to make sure it does not get too high or too low and to keep your physician informed.

Remember that a medicated blood pressure is not the same as a nonmedicated blood pressure. Just because 120/80 mmHg and below are ideal readings in a healthy person does not mean that lowering blood pressure to that level with drugs will make a person live longer or reduce his or her risk of developing cardiovascular disease. Actually, if a person were to take drugs to achieve those readings, it would in fact *increase* their risk of heart attack, according to a 2013 trial.[19]

This relationship was confirmed in a recent study that investigated the outcome of 26,785 individuals followed for more than six years. It demonstrated that those taking more blood pressure medications had a 248 percent increased risk of stroke.[20] The more medications taken, the higher the risk of stroke, even if the treatment successfully lowered blood pressure into a favorable range.

In other words, compared with people who have normal blood pressure without medications, those who took three or more medications to lower their blood pressure had a stroke risk 2.5 times higher. Even the use of one medication to normalize blood pressure increased the risk of stroke 33 percent compared with those not taking medications. This information should make people wake up, realize that drugs are not the answer, and get serious about the need to change their diet.

Let's look at the most up-to-date recommendations from the Eighth Joint National Committee on the Prevention, Detection, Evaluation, and Treatment of High Blood Pressure (JNC 8), which consists of four hundred physicians and scientists studying this issue, to offer physicians prescriptive guidelines. Reviewing the existing evidence, JNC 8 reached the following conclusions:[21]

1. There is strong evidence that a benefit exists from treating people older than 60 with medications if their blood pressure is above 150/90 mmHg.

2. The goal of treatment is to get the average treated systolic blood pressure below 150 mmHg.

3. Evidence demonstrates that setting a drug-induced goal of systolic pressure lower than 140 mmHg in this age group provides no additional benefit compared with a higher goal of 140 to 150.

4. In younger individuals (ages 59 and below), there was insufficient evidence to treat elevations in systolic blood pressure with medication, but there was evidence to treat diastolic blood pressure above 90 mmHg.

This careful analysis from reputable physicians and scientists has relaxed recommendations and does not recommend treatment for high systolic blood pressure in the range of 130 to 150 mmHg. The reason for these more liberal recommendations is not because those readings are normal—they are not. It is because for most people the risks of using medications outweigh the benefits of using medications.

In other words, this means physicians should be using lifestyle modifications, not drugs, to lower the blood pressure of most of their patients. This does not mean a blood pressure of 145/88 should be ignored or that a blood pressure of 135/75 is ideal. These numbers should be aggressively treated, not with medications, but with a substantial change in diet, avoidance of salt, and daily exercise.

If doctors followed the updated guidelines of JNC 8, about six million U.S. adults could be taken off their blood pressure medications because their poorly controlled high blood pressure would be considered adequately managed. I am lobbying for much stronger and forceful recommendations to treat all ranges of systolic blood pressures above 125, and all diastolic blood pressures above 80, with effective lifestyle interventions, meaning a Nutritarian diet-style and exercise. (See Chapter 10 for exercise recommendations.)

Right before this book went to print, a news release went out publicizing the early outcome data of the Systolic Blood Pressure Intervention Trial (SPRINT).[22] This study randomized 9,361 individuals with known cardiovascular disease and/or kidney disease to determine whether adding more medication to aggressively lower the systolic blood pressure to 120 mmHg was better than 140. Scientists have still not fully analyzed the data at this time, and the official findings have not been published in a medical journal, however an early data review found significantly fewer heart attacks in the group more aggressively treated with medications. Why these results completely contradicted the earlier studies, including the ACCORD trial, published in 2010 is not totally clear yet.

The ACCORD study found that medicating diabetic patients to a systolic blood pressure below 120 did not result in a lower risk of cardiac events, and only resulted in more negative side effects.[23] One suggested reason for the contrary findings in SPRINT was that they studied a population that already had cardiovascular disease and almost a third of the participants had kidney disease. So they examined a different population who were at significantly higher risk. The evidence still indicates that for most people, not at imminent danger of a heart attack, staying on these medications for many years, and the drug-related risks associated with using multiple drugs in combination, would trump the potential benefits observed in the SPRINT study. Being overly aggressive with medications still has substantial risks. This one study does not erase all the other data we have from the earlier trials.

Though these new findings show a value in treating very high risk patients more aggressively, it does not change my guidelines stated here for the vast majority of people who have high blood pressure. Nor does it change the fact that drugs put you at needlessly heightened risks, and should only be considered after failure of aggressive dietary modification. Even in these high-risk and elderly patients, who require medication, dietary modifications are almost never optimized, and these are necessary and need to be strongly emphasized to all people considering and requiring medications. Plus, medicating the diastolic below 75 is still not ideal even in patients at high risk.

JENNIFER BARLOW'S PERSISTENCE PAID BIG DIVIDENDS

When I first met Jennifer Barlow, she was 54 years old and taking three medications to lower her blood pressure: a CCB (Norvasc, 10 mg), a beta-blocker (Inderal, 100 mg), and an ACE inhibitor (Prinivil, 20 mg). She was 5 feet 4 inches tall, weighed 180 pounds, and still had high blood pressure (165/80 mmHg), despite the three medications. I held off on adding any medications because I expected that my dietary recommendations would help her lose weight and lower her blood pressure rapidly.

During the first four months of her diet change, she lost 40 pounds, but her systolic blood pressure remained elevated: At two months her blood pressure was 150/80 and at four months it was 145/75. On the basis of these readings, which Ms. Barlow confirmed with her home blood pressure monitor, I kept her on all three medications throughout this period.

Although Ms. Barlow's experience was not typical, neither was it cause for alarm. Some people who develop high blood pressure at a relatively young age find it difficult to bring it down with diet and weight loss. I reassured her that, for many people, weight loss does not bring blood pressure down initially. The pressure comes down only after the weight drops below a certain threshold and the person has stayed off all salt for a year or longer.

Ms. Barlow persisted. Her health continued to improve, and she lost more weight. Eight months after her first visit, she weighed 135 pounds and her blood pressure was down to 130/75 mmHg. At that point, I started tapering the beta-blocker.

It was another twelve months before she was able to discontinue all of her medications, so in all it took her almost two years to get her weight below 130 pounds and to get her blood pressure in the normal range without any medications. Now, a few years later, she continues to have systolic blood pressure readings averaging between 110 and 120, with no medication.

The timetable for recovery through nutritional intervention is difficult to predict. Some people dramatically improve their diets, adopt an exercise program, lose weight, and still have high blood pressure for a period of time; while others see a rapid drop in one to four weeks. Whether the process is fast or slow, it is important to continue close monitoring of the blood pressure to prevent a problem that could arise from too much medication, excessive lowering of blood pressure, or both.

In Ms. Barlow's case, she learned that reversing a fifty-year history of unhealthful living could not be achieved in a few months. She also learned that persistence pays off: Not only did she lose weight and resolve her high blood pressure, but her dietary and lifestyle adjustments literally changed the structure and function of her body. The result? She restored the youthful elasticity to her blood vessels and removed blood vessel plaque. Medications never do this; they just cover up the gradually worsening pathology.

I hope you are convinced that taking blood pressure–lowering medications is not a great idea unless your blood pressure is high and the systolic reading does not come down below 140 mmHg after maximizing lifestyle improvements. If most people with high blood pressure learned the information in this book and took the right steps to protect their health, they would not have high blood pressure and they would not need medications.

The key point in this discussion of blood pressure is that for the greatest level of protection against heart disease, kidney disease, and brain disease later in life, it is vital to live in a manner that produces a favorable blood pressure *without* medications. If you require medications to lower your blood pressure, then you are at a higher risk of these diseases and you likely need to make further modifications to your lifestyle to improve the health of your cardiovascular system. You may need medication for now, and some people may have to remain on medication in the long term, but even if that is necessary, you should be working aggressively to fix the blood vessel damage, with the expectation that your blood pressure can improve and the dosage of medication can be reduced and eventually eliminated.

A Nutritarian diet dramatically lowers blood pressure.

For twenty-five years I have been observing that patients' blood pressures normalize when they follow my Nutritarian diet-style. Changes take longer for some people than they do for others, but it is rare that blood pressure does not normalize. The figure below shows additional data from 105 individuals on a Nutritarian diet for an average of two years. Note that even 80–90 percent compliance with my recommendations resulted in a 26 mmHg drop in systolic blood pressure. No medication is nearly that effective, safe, and lifesaving.

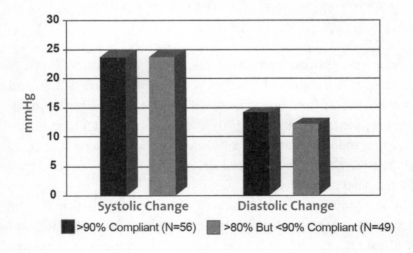

AVERAGE NUTRITARIAN BLOOD PRESSURE LOWERING

What About Cholesterol-Lowering Drugs?

Before you consider whether you need cholesterol-lowering medications or whether you should stay on such medications, there are some important points you should know about this subject.

First and foremost, your cholesterol level, in this case your *LDL (bad) cholesterol* level, is only one of many risk factors for heart disease. That means if your LDL concentration is considered elevated but you eat healthfully, are not overweight, are physically fit, and have good blood pressure, then you should not have a significant cardiovascular risk despite your elevated LDL levels. In other words, don't give LDL cholesterol more credit than it deserves as a risk factor. Also, when you eat healthfully, the inflammatory potential of the LDL particles changes—they get larger and fluffier, and the number of particles goes down. This renders the LDL safer, despite an elevated LDL cholesterol as shown on a blood test.[24]

LDL particle size and number provide independent measures of *atherogenicity* (the ability to form plaque, especially on the innermost layer of arterial walls) and are strong predictors of cardiovascular disease.[25] It is the oxidized version of LDL (ox-LDL) that is more actively negative, promoting inflammatory cells and plaque deposition. It is ox-LDL that primarily gets incorporated into vulnerable plaque and is most dangerous.

Oxidized LDL particles are more elevated in smokers, in people who are overweight, and in those eating unhealthy diets. They are not elevated in people who eat a diet rich in phytochemicals and antioxidants. Only relatively recently have blood tests been able to evaluate the ox-LDL number and other parameters that give a better indication of cardiac risk.

Unlike drugs, the Nutritarian dietary approach is spectacularly effective in decreasing multiple risk factors simultaneously. The degree of protection offered by the Nutritarian diet-style is not represented to its fullest extent if one considers only the decrease in LDL.

A Nutritarian diet lowers multiple risk factors simultaneously; the Nutritarian diet:

Lowers body weight and body fat

Lowers blood pressure[26]

Lowers intravascular inflammation[27]

Lowers blood glucose and triglyceride levels[28]

Lowers inflammatory markers, including C-reactive protein and white blood count[29]

Increases tissue antioxidant score[30]

Improves exercise tolerance and oxygen efficiency[31]

Enlarges the size of the LDL molecules and decreases particle number

Prevents LDL from becoming oxidized[32]

Lowers LDL cholesterol dramatically[*]

Of interest is that longtime Nutritarians run WBC (white blood cell counts) much lower than those following a standard diet. It is important to remember this so your doctor is not alarmed when your WBC comes back low, out of the conventional normal range. Scientific studies link lower WBC with less inflammation, lower risk of cancer, and a longer life. Levels between 2.5 and 5 are common among Nutritarians, whereas 5–10 is the conventional normal range.[34]

Not only does a Nutritarian diet significantly lower cholesterol in weeks, it also simultaneously lowers intravascular inflammation, body weight, and blood pressure and has beneficial effects on intravascular elasticity. This diet delivers benefits that protect the heart comprehensively, and almost immediately.

---

[*] A Nutritarian diet—which authors of a 2001 study called a "very high fiber, vegetable, fruit, and nut diet"[33]—is tremendously effective at lowering LDL, in addition to changing its functional parameters. Other dietary interventions have not been as effective or have been relatively ineffective at lowering cholesterol. Not only did LDL cholesterol drop a 33 percent average in just two weeks, but a favorable effect on triglycerides was also seen. The improvement is more significant than that seen with cholesterol-lowering drugs in clinical application.

> True protection from heart disease can be reached
> only when you achieve favorable blood pressure and
> cholesterol levels, *without* drugs.

In my medical practice, I recommend that my patients lower their cholesterol through natural methods whenever possible and use prescription drugs only when absolutely necessary, as most medications have potentially serious side effects, as we have seen. Almost all of my patients prefer this judicious and more effective approach, and it is very rare that they are not able to achieve protection from heart disease quickly.

For example, one day I had a medical student observing and taking notes as I saw patients in my office. At the end of the day, he alerted me to the fact that five of the patients seen that day had dropped their LDL cholesterol by more than 50 points from their last visit, without drugs. In fact, the range was 65 to 87 point reductions and they were all now near to or below 100 mg/dl, an impressive number. Don't forget, this was just *one day* in my medical practice.

Not only had all of these individuals suffered from dangerously high cholesterol levels two months earlier, but each had also reported additional health problems. Peggy suffered from chronic anemia. Eugene was tired all the time. Keith had chronic heartburn and allergies. Peter suffered from angina. Maria had become severely ill from a statin drug prescribed by her prior physician. These five patients needed help, and they realized that prescription drugs were risky and not the answer. They all returned to my office between six and eight weeks after their first visit, and our findings are listed on the next page.

They wiped out their cardiovascular high-risk status, and many of their other problems cleared up as well. Peggy's anemia went away. Eugene was no longer fatigued. Keith's heartburn disappeared, so he was able to stop taking antacids and acid-blocking medication, and his allergies started to improve. In just six weeks, Peter, who had suffered from angina, was now walking more than 2.5 miles a day without any pain. He couldn't believe how his heart symptoms melted away so quickly after only a few weeks of following my nutritional advice. Perhaps most importantly, all five of these patients were enthusiastic about life again.

PEGGY	BEFORE	AFTER
Total cholesterol	249	150
Triglycerides	169	105
LDL	157	80
HDL	58	49

MARIA	BEFORE	AFTER
Total cholesterol	283	168
Triglycerides	90	79
LDL	183	98
HDL	91	52

EUGENE	BEFORE	AFTER
Total cholesterol	247	156
Triglycerides	72	42
LDL	191	104
HDL	51	44

KEITH	BEFORE	AFTER
Total cholesterol	238	158
Triglycerides	165	79
LDL	152	99
HDL	52	43.5

PETER	BEFORE	AFTER
Total cholesterol	164	126
	(on a	(off a
	statin)	statin)
Triglycerides	210	179
LDL	119	54
HDL	32	36

When you adopt a program of nutritional excellence to reverse or prevent heart disease, you need to be prepared for some astonishing effects and benefits: namely, that you will prevent and reverse almost all other diseases simultaneously. For example, your digestion will improve, and you'll get rid of your heartburn, hemorrhoids, and constipation. You will eliminate your headaches, gain more energy, and age more slowly. But the most important benefit is that you will also lower your risk of other serious diseases, especially dementia, strokes, diabetes, and cancer.

My mission is to encourage all people to adopt a Nutritarian diet-style, with the addition of appropriate exercise. I recommend this regardless of a person's risk factors or cholesterol level, because most Americans die of either cardiovascular disease or cancer. The

Nutritarian diet, with moderate exercise, protects against all leading causes of death and promotes a long life.

My Advice Versus Conventional Authorities

The new guidelines for the use of statins from the American College of Cardiology (ACC) and the American Heart Association (AHA), developed in conjunction with the National Heart, Lung, and Blood Institute, are very different from my recommendations because they do not stress lifestyle interventions. If these ACC/AHA guidelines were applied as directed, the number of people using cholesterol-lowering drugs would increase significantly.

Gone are the recommended LDL cholesterol targets—specifically, those that suggest physicians treat patients with high LDL cholesterol to less than 100 mg/dl or for patients with known CAD to less than 70 mg/dl. According to the expert panel, there is simply no evidence from randomized, controlled clinical trials to support treatment to a specific target (one that is that low). As a result, the new guidelines make no recommendations for specific LDL cholesterol targets for the prevention of heart disease. This means that doctors should prescribe these drugs to all people at risk for heart disease, regardless of the results of blood tests.

The new treatment guidelines emphasize four major patient groups that should be treated with these drugs because of their higher risk:

1. Individuals who already have documented heart disease

2. Anyone with an LDL cholesterol level higher than 190 mg/dl, such as those with familial hypercholesterolemia

3. All people with diabetes aged 40 to 75 years old

4. Individuals without evidence of heart disease but who have a high ten-year risk of heart attack according to a risk calculator that considers age, race, blood pressure, cholesterol, blood sugar, weight, and family history

These new, complicated recommendations have lots of problems. In particular, there are problems with treating everyone, without taking into account their level of fitness, their percentage of visceral fat, and whether they have adopted a therapeutically effective diet. But the main issue is that these treatment guidelines emphasize drugs, not food and exercise, as the solution. But diet is the cause of heart disease, and taking drugs will do little to stop needless suffering and needless death as long as the diet stays the same.

Many medical authorities and researchers disagree with these guidelines and believe that the risk calculator overestimates risk and places people on statins who are unlikely to benefit from them. A recent study put the ACC/AHA calculator to the test with real people and found that over a ten-year follow-up, the calculator overestimated risk by 78 percent.[35] This 2015 study, along with many earlier studies that reached similar conclusions, points to a serious problem: *Millions of people on statins will not gain any benefits from the drugs, but they can incur substantial risks over the ensuing decades of their lives.* Some commentators have glossed over the issue of overestimated risk, implying that some overtreatment with statins isn't important. However, the rationale for risk prediction is precisely to distinguish between those patients who are reasonably likely to benefit from drug therapy and those whose probability of benefit is marginal or absent and would incur needless risk through the use of medication.

The Benefits of Statins Are in Serious Doubt

Doctors need to make it crystal clear to their patients that food is the cause of, and should be the primary treatment for, heart disease. Everything else is window dressing. Most people who take cholesterol-lowering medications still experience cardiac events, advancement of their disease, and even death from their heart problems.

A critical 2010 meta-analysis investigated all studies performed on patients with high cholesterol but no history yet of heart disease. Researchers analyzed eleven randomized controlled trials involving 65,229 participants and found no reduction in all-cause mortality with the use of statins in these high-risk patients.[36] This speaks loudly to the relative ineffectiveness of statins when you consider that almost all high-risk patients have significant atherosclerosis many years before heart disease rears its ugly head.

Researchers are now questioning the early studies on statins and are even questioning the benefits shown with meta-analysis that includes studies before 2005, when almost all of the studies were conducted by pharmaceutical companies.[37] They exposed the fact that recent studies, done by researchers without such conflicts of interest, have not replicated those benefits. These scientists explain:

New penal regulations on clinical trials came into effect [in the European Union, or EU] in 2004. After 2004–2005, all clinical trials, performed by scientists relatively free of conflict of interest with pharmaceutical industries, reported that statins were effective in lowering LDL-C [LDL cholesterol], but no significant beneficial effects were observed for the prevention of CHD [coronary heart disease]. Currently, the majority of scientists continue to claim that statins are effective in preventing CHD, but these claims are based on meta-analyses of reports, including those published before the EU regulation (mostly in 1990s). However, our group did not adopt the results of industry-supported publications as reliable in our cholesterol guidelines.

It is not controversial that people with the greatest risk, the most advanced heart disease, and the highest cholesterol levels benefit the most from statins. But obviously, the amount of protection offered by aggressive statin therapy is limited, and the conventional dietary advice offered by most dietitians, physicians, and other health professionals falls short in offering significant long-term protection.[38] Even when patients with more substantial risk are stratified according to risk and the most at-risk patients are treated, the benefits are limited. The real benefits of superior nutrition are almost always ignored in favor of the limited benefits of drugs.

Even exercise alone produces positive results that are at least as good as those with medication. In a meta-analysis, which included 305 randomized controlled trials with 339,274 participants, and which compared conventional statin use and drug guidelines to exercise alone, there was no significant difference in mortality.[39] There were no definitive differences between drug and exercise interventions in coronary heart disease, heart failure, and prediabetes. The researchers concluded, "Our findings reflect the bias against testing exercise interventions and highlight the changing landscape of medical research, which seems to increasingly favor drug interventions over strategies to modify lifestyle."

Drugs have become the mainstay of cardiology, and the new ACC/AHA clinical practice guidelines further foster their aggressive and excessive use. Among the absurdities of the new guidelines is that all middle-age black males—regardless of whether they eat healthfully or not—are now "racially profiled" as meeting the criteria for treatment with statin drugs.

The troubling reality is that a huge population is already taking these drugs. According to the National Center for Health Statistics, more than 50 percent of men in the United States between the ages of 65 and 75 are on these statin drugs already.[40]

Facts About Statin Drugs

1. When statins are used for primary prevention (that is, treating cholesterol levels with no heart disease apparent), no mortality benefit has been shown. Your chances of dying prematurely are the same.

2. As of 2015, no statin drug has been compared with lifestyle interventions for the prevention of cardiovascular disease.

3. Both weight gain and diabetes increase in statin users, and physical activity is lower, likely secondary to impairment of exercise tolerance.[41]

4. The risks of statin drugs are more serious than we have previously thought.

A 2010 study that analyzed the medical records of two million statin users reported increases in the risk of liver dysfunction, muscle-related side effects, acute kidney injury, and cataracts associated with statin use.[42] Muscle breakdown, called *rhabdomyolysis,* and associated pain can be very serious, leading to kidney and liver damage. But even in those people with no such noted or detectable side effects, muscle injury occurs, blunting the fitness benefits of exercise.[43]

Larger doses of statin drugs are associated with a greater likelihood of side effects, and additional risk factors such as the use of other drugs, older age, and the presence of diabetes and high triglyceride levels also increase the likelihood of adverse effects.[44] In addition to known adverse effects, debate continues over whether statins may have detrimental effects on brain function.[45] Approximately 17 percent of people who take a statin experience an adverse effect, including sexual dysfunction, exertional fatigue, decreased energy, memory problems, depression, and insomnia.[46]

Although statins may have a place in medical therapy for some high-risk patients with very high cholesterol levels, people who adopt a Nutritarian diet-style rarely need them. But the main problem with statins is that they promote weight gain and diabetes, the very conditions an expert panel considers to put people at high risk and the major risk factors for premature cardiac death.[47] Not all statins are associated with diabetes, but the ones that generally lower cholesterol the most are the most diabetes-promoting.

For women, statin drug use packs a double whammy, with an increased risk of certain breast cancers along with the increased risk of diabetes. Research funded by the U.S. National Cancer Institute found that women aged 55 to 74 who had been on statins for ten years or more had an 80 percent increased risk of developing invasive ductal carcinoma, which accounts for 80 percent of breast cancers. It also found an almost doubled occurrence of invasive lobular carcinoma, which accounts for 10 percent of breast cancers.[48]

Overall, this is a doubling of breast cancer occurrence in these statin-treated women. Since statins increase insulin levels and IGF-1 (and often body weight), it is reasonable to expect to see a rise in these hormonally sensitive cancers. However, the degree of rise was still shocking, even to the research scientists.

The link between statins and diabetes is even more established by observational data from the Women's Health Initiative trial that show a 48 percent increase in the risk of new-onset diabetes associated with statins in postmenopausal women—and this was found with all statin drugs.[49] A 2013 study of almost five hundred thousand Canadians found that the overall odds of developing diabetes were higher with higher-potency statins: Lipitor resulted in a 22 percent higher risk, Crestor users had an 18 percent increased risk, and Zocor showed a 10 percent increased risk.[50] This was followed by a study in Europe confirming that all statins increased risk proportional to adherence and dose.[51] However, it is still most likely that some statins are more diabetes-promoting than others, especially the stronger ones.

HIGHER RISK OF DIABETES	LOWER RISK OF DIABETES
Zocor (simvastatin)	Pravachol (pravastatin)
Lipitor (atorvastatin)	Lescol (fluvastatin)
Crestor (rosuvastatin)	Mevacor (lovastatin)

Many physicians and scientists share the sentiment that statins need to be used less, not more. As John Abramson of Harvard Medical School and cardiologist Rita F. Redberg pointed out in an opinion piece in the *New York Times* called "Don't Give More Patients Statins":

This announcement [that more people should take statins] is not a result of a sudden epidemic of heart disease, nor is it based on new data showing the benefits of lower cholesterol. Instead, it is a consequence of simply expanding the definition of who should take the drugs—a decision that will benefit the pharmaceutical industry more than anyone else. . . . According to our calculations [the new guidelines] will increase the number of healthy people for whom statins are recommended by nearly 70 percent. . . . Instead of converting millions of people into statin customers, we should be focusing on the real factors that undeniably reduce the risk of heart disease: healthy diets, exercise and avoiding smoking. Patients should be skeptical about the guidelines.[52]

Over the past thirty years, the number of people taking drugs has continuously risen; some physicians even argue that *all* people should take statins in the United States. This is not altogether illogical, since cardiovascular disease is our number one killer. But statins don't offer nearly as much protection against overall mortality as people think.

Statins are only somewhat effective for people who have advanced heart disease. But for people who have less than a 20 percent risk of getting heart disease in the next ten years, statins not only fail to reduce the risk of death, but also fail to reduce the risk of serious illness. The studies that medical authorities and physicians use to justify the benefits of statins in lower-risk populations are highly biased because they use the avoidance of angioplasty and bypass surgery as benefit endpoints instead of overall serious events and death from all causes.

As we saw in Chapter 2, angioplasty is an overused procedure that does not extend life span in stable cardiac patients. Using drugs to avoid this procedure, when it may never have been indicated to begin with, is not justified. This is explained in an article by Dr. Abramson and his Harvard research associates published in the *British Medical Journal*:[53]

The best indication of the net effect of a treatment on overall health is the total number of serious adverse events—which include deaths from all causes, hospital admissions, prolongations of admission, cancer, or permanent disability. Only three of the five largest trials (JUPITER, ASCOT, and LIPID) reported data on serious adverse events, none of which found a reduction associated with statins in this population. After all-cause mortality, "hard" cardiovascular endpoints—cardiovascular death, myocardial infarction, and stroke—are the most reliable because they minimize subjective input and are least vulnerable to bias in adjudication.

With no reduction in all-cause mortality and no evidence of reduction in total serious adverse events for patients with five-year cardiovascular risk of <10%, the net benefit-harm equation has zero overall benefit and ignores the clear evidence of harm that has been demonstrated in clinical trials and observational studies. A retrospective cohort study found that 18% of statin-treated patients had

*discontinued therapy (at least temporarily) because of statin-related
adverse events. Forty percent of the adverse events were related to
musculoskeletal symptoms.*[54] *At the same time, 18% or more of this
group experienced side effects, including muscle pain or weakness,
decreased cognitive function, increased risk of diabetes, cataracts or
sexual dysfunction.*

And wait—it gets worse. Research scientists are finding eventual
damage to the heart from statin use, possibly even increasing the risk
of heart failure with long-term use. Supporting these findings is that
these drugs interfere with muscle function, even in people without
muscle complaints or lab findings of muscle breakdown.

Remember, the heart is a muscle, and over years, it may be subtly
damaged, just like skeletal muscles. This may be an important reason
why statins fail in primary prevention. As patients take the statins for
many years, starting earlier in the disease process, more dangers accrue
as the years go by. Researchers argue that this is a probable reason why
statins have been associated with greater mortality in recent trials.[55]
Their findings include the following:

- Statins inhibit synthesis of vitamin K2, which is important in
  preventing coronary calcifications.

- Statins are mitochondrial toxic, depleting coenzyme Q10, heme
  A, and adenosine triphosphate production, leading to muscle degeneration. This can have long-term negative effects on the heart
  muscle, even without muscular complaints.

- Statins inhibit selenium-containing protein synthesis, creating
  cardiac muscle stress, which leads to cardiomyopathy and heart
  muscle disease.

Risks of Statin Drugs Summarized

The risks of taking statin drugs include the following:
- Breast cancer
- Cataracts

- Cognitive problems
- Diabetes
- Heart failure
- Kidney injury
- Liver dysfunction
- Myopathies (muscle damage)
- Reduced physical fitness
- Weight gain

Even more dangerous is the false sense of reassurance that is created when physicians prescribe medications and do not aggressively insist on lifestyle modifications. The overuse of cholesterol-lowering and blood pressure medications discourages patients from taking the steps that actually reduce cardiovascular disease and can save lives.

Statins give the illusion of protection to many people who would be much better served if their doctors insisted that they exercise more, eat more carefully, and lose weight. This advice falls on deaf ears when patients think drugs can do the same thing. Too many people think that because drugs lower their cholesterol levels, they don't have to change their diet.

A member of the ACC/AHA guidelines committee essentially gave a similar opinion when that person discussed the lack of evidence for LDL level targets and admitted that this is one main reason why the targets have been dropped from the current guidelines. They noted that cholesterol lowered by drugs does not have the same effect as cholesterol lowered by nondrug methods, such as diet and exercise.

The problems with statins do not, in any way, lessen the importance of lowering "bad" cholesterol. However, it makes it clearer that we have to lower it with the *right food,* not the *right drugs.*

I call the prescription pad the "permission" pad—because when medications offer a solution to a problem, patients invariably dismiss the necessity of changing their diets and think they have permission to eat whatever they want.

You should always review any guidelines and recommendations with your doctor, because he or she will know your health history and details. But I have a different set of criteria than such guidelines and most doctors, because I generally advise people who have agreed to follow my aggressive nutritional plan that reverses heart disease and radically lowers ox-LDL and its associated risks.

Under my standard of care, it would be exceedingly rare that a person would meet the criteria for statin use—probably fewer than one in a hundred patients. Those with LDL cholesterol levels between 120 and 160 mg/dl, despite dietary excellence, could use a natural cholesterol-lowering agent such as plant sterols and pomegranate punicalagins added to their protective diet (see Chapter 10). Alternatively, they could opt for a more expensive or less utilized test for measuring ox-LDL. This would better ascertain risk and aid in medical decision-making to determine whether a statin would be indicated.

What About Aspirin?

You might be wondering at this point whether you should take just aspirin. Not so fast! As with other drugs, you never get something for nothing. All drugs have risks, and if you live in a manner in which you avoid the need for medication, you protect yourself from those risks. It is true that most heart attacks are caused by clots enlarging within the blood vessel, and aspirin can interfere with blood clotting, thereby reducing the risk of developing clots. However, people who are eating right already have a much lower risk of developing a clot because of their favorable diet. Aspirin has risks that can be severe and even deadly, so you need to be careful.

In recent years, scores of studies have questioned the conventional notion that taking aspirin is a good thing to do because it prevents heart attacks and reduces the risk of developing pancreatic and colon cancers. But aspirin does bad things, too. Since a healthy diet is protective against these cancers, why take a risk with aspirin?

A large 2009 study on diabetics without known heart disease who were taking aspirin showed a dramatic increase in deaths: a 17 percent increased death at age 50, and a 29 percent increase by age 85 for those on aspirin.[56] Diabetics with advanced heart disease did demonstrate a survival advantage with the use of aspirin. This was immediately followed by a 2010 study confirming that in lower-risk people who did not have advanced cardiovascular disease, aspirin did not reduce the number of vascular events such as heart attacks and strokes and did not enhance life span. In fact, the group treated with aspirin had more hemorrhagic strokes, and no benefits to compensate for that.[57]

A Japanese clinical trial involving more than fourteen thousand patients aged 60 to 85 with heart disease risk factors such as hypertension, high cholesterol, and diabetes found that taking a daily aspirin provided no protection against heart disease deaths or nonfatal heart attacks or strokes compared with taking a placebo for five years.[58] The trial was stopped early after researchers determined that aspirin provided no benefits. Of note in this study was a significant increase in the risk of bleeding requiring transfusion or hospitalization in the aspirin-treated group.

"Aspirin is indicated for patients at high, short-term risk," such as those who had a heart attack, stroke, or procedure to open a clogged heart artery, wrote Dr. J. Michael Gaziano, of Brigham and Women's Hospital, and Dr. Philip Greenland, of Northwestern University Feinberg School of Medicine, in an editorial that accompanied the study. "On the other hand, patients at very low risk of vascular events should not take aspirin for prevention of vascular events, even at low dose."[59]

However, a person eating the dangerous SAD, or DAD as I call it, may be better off with aspirin despite the increased risk for bleeding because of its mild heart benefits and some protection it offers against colon cancer in this cancer-prone population. The bottom line is that unless you have advanced heart disease, have had a recent cardiac event or a stent placed, or have another reason that makes you at heightened risks of clot formation, you are better off eating healthfully and not taking aspirin.

If all the physicians in the United States gave their patients the information contained in this book about reversing heart disease through superior nutrition and about the drawbacks of medical care, we would be faced with an interesting set of outcomes. Most patients would get well; their heart disease would resolve and not require medical services. So doctors and hospitals would lose most of their business, and pharmaceutical companies would lose billions of dollars. People would have to be retrained for new careers, as a multibillion-dollar industry involving hospitals, health-care workers, drugs, and medical supply and equipment manufacturers would lose most of their customers. It's not a likely scenario, but I'm sure you can imagine the economic and social uproar that would occur. Obviously, there is, and will continue to be, strong resistance to this approach.

That said, the science doesn't lie, and the choice is yours to make.

CHAPTER FOUR

The Nutritional Path to Reversing Disease

To assure superior nutrition that maximizes health and longevity, the goal is to achieve an adequate nutrient density in your diet and also to make sure that all the raw materials your body needs to maintain excellent health are supplied in the most favorable amounts.

After reviewing the preponderance of evidence on these issues, the vast majority of nutritional scientists, and physicians who have no predetermined agendas or biases, would be forced to agree on these three dietary principles:

1. Vegetables, beans, seeds, nuts, and fruits are health-promoting foods.

2. Excessive amounts of animal products increase chronic disease risk.

3. Refined carbohydrates promote chronic disease and lead to people becoming overweight and obese.

Of course, we have all heard that green vegetables are good for us. But they are better for us than you might have thought and are intimately related to the prevention and reversal of heart disease.

We tend to minimize scientifically proven effects that these food choices have on our health. Eating a Nutritarian diet is not a fad; eating healthfully is the single most effective preventative and therapeutic intervention available to us. It is the best "prescription" any doctor can make. And if we take it seriously and follow the advice, the results can alter our lives.

In this chapter we look specifically at the foods that can literally help save your life—and how.

Vegetables, Especially Cruciferous Vegetables

Greens, especially the cruciferous kind (such as kale, cabbage, and bok choy), are as close to a miracle food as we can get. These vegetables are known for their anticancer effects but are also powerfully associated with a lower risk of death from cardiovascular disease and all other causes. Other types of produce also play important roles in safeguarding our health and maintaining an ideal weight.

Green leafy vegetables are the foods with the highest nutrient density, and it is no surprise that greater intake of such greens is associated with a reduced risk of cardiovascular disease compared with other vegetables.[1] They are also very low in calories, yet high in protein, calcium, and fiber compared with the calories they contain. Greens are the healthiest high-protein foods on the planet because they are so rich in a wide spectrum of other nutrients, too. These vegetables are key to increasing our intake of plant protein and reducing our intake of animal protein in order to enhance life span.

For example, a cup of chopped frozen broccoli contains about 50 calories and has about 6 grams of protein and 6 grams of fiber. This means that about half of the calories come from protein. A cup of raw broccoli has about 30 calories and about 3 grams of protein. Likewise, a cup of frozen cooked kale has about 40 calories and 4 grams of protein, and a cup of raw kale has only about 30 calories. The point is, these vegetables are so low in calories that you cannot eat too much of them, and they are so rich in nutrients, the more you eat, the better.

The more you eat green, the more you get lean.

Specifically, a greater consumption of cruciferous vegetables—a family of vegetables also known for their anticancer effects—is most powerfully associated with a lower risk of death from both cardiovascular disease and all causes.[2] In fact, when 134,796 adults were followed for years (women were followed for a mean of 10.2 years and men for 4.6 years), a linear inverse association was revealed between eating these green vegetables and cardiovascular mortality. This means that the more greens eaten, the fewer heart attacks and stroke deaths, with no leveling off of the trend. All vegetables were linked to increased protection from premature death, but green cruciferous vegetables offered the most protection. One hundred grams of vegetables is about a cup, so eat up!

CRUCIFEROUS VEGETABLES AND LONGEVITY GRAPH

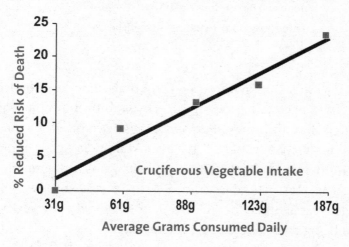

Oxidative stress is known to be a significant contributor to the development of cardiovascular disease. *Oxidation* means more unstable compounds that can inflame our cells and lead to premature aging and chronic disease. Our antioxidant defenses are activated by a combination of plant-derived compounds and the body's own antioxidant enzymes. Green cruciferous vegetables contain *glucosinolates*, which, when chewed, form phytochemicals called *isothiocyanates* (ITCs) in the mouth. These ITCs signal the body to produce its own protective antioxidant enzymes by activating a protein called Nrf2.

CASE HISTORY: PROOF FROM A PATIENT

A 44-year-old man (6 feet tall, 216 pounds, BMI 29 kg/m²) with a history of high cholesterol and hypertension had blood pressure measurements averaging 140/90 mmHg, in spite of blood pressure medication used. He suffered from angina manifesting as chest tightness and pressure on exertion, as well as night sweats for about a year. He also became short of breath almost immediately when he tried to exercise.

He committed fully to a Nutritarian diet-style in August 2011. Over the next two months, he lost 35 pounds (181 pounds, BMI 24 kg/m²), and his blood pressure normalized to around 110/60 mmHg. His total cholesterol decreased from 216 to 161 mg/dl. His night sweats, chest tightness, and shortness of breath resolved during these two months. Three years later, his weight had dropped even more and he continued to be free of symptoms, to have normal blood pressure and cholesterol, requiring no medications.

Nrf2 is a transcription factor, a protein that can increase or decrease the expression of certain genes. It works by binding a specific sequence present in genes called the *antioxidant response element*. In the presence of certain phytochemicals, Nrf2 is activated to induce cells to produce natural antioxidant enzymes and to protect against inflammation.[3] In other words, green vegetables control the "on" and "off" switches for the protective machinery in our cells. This machinery defends our vessels from being damaged or aging prematurely.

The more you eat green, the more life span you glean.

For example, one study on sulforaphane (an ITC found in broccoli) showed that, once activated, Nrf2 suppresses the activity of adhesion molecules on the endothelial cell surface to prevent binding of inflammatory cells and therefore retard the development of atherosclerotic plaque.[4] Another study showed that sulforaphane and other ITCs, by activating Nrf2 in endothelial cells, maintained vascular elasticity and inhibited oxidative aging of the blood vessels.[5] ITCs also help to main-

CRUCIFEROUS PLANT CELL

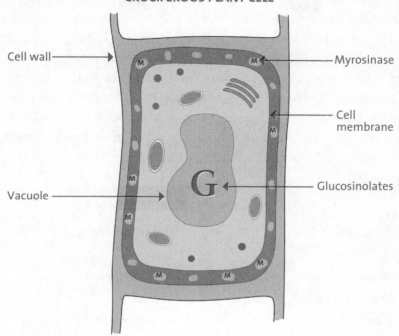

Cell wall — Myrosinase

Cell membrane

Vacuole — Glucosinolates

tain the integrity of the blood-brain barrier, a vascular system that is crucial for proper brain tissue function.[6] Nutritional science indicates that these green foods are essential for excellent heart health and promotion of maximum life span.

If you have high blood pressure or heart disease and are looking to reverse it, eating lots of green cruciferous vegetables—both raw and cooked—will aid your recovery. Remember, because the reaction that produces the necessary ITCs occurs in the mouth, the better you chew the vegetables, the more ITCs are formed. The enzyme that drives this biochemical reaction (named *myrosinase*) is housed in the cell membrane, and when you chew, it gets released and mixes with glucosinolate. Because myrosinase can be deactivated by heat or cooking, it is important to eat some raw cruciferous vegetables every day and chew them exceptionally well. Shred some red cabbage or Chinese cabbage on your salad, add a little arugula or watercress, or use a bit of ground mustard seed for flavor.

If you eat cooked broccoli, kale, bok choy, or other cruciferous vegetables later in a meal, the myrosinase you ate from the raw vegetables will make the cooked veggies produce more ITCs. When you cook soups with added greens, make sure to process the greens in a blender first, while they are still raw, and then add them to the soup liquid. Blending the greens before they are heated will allow the ITCs to be formed. Note that if you had added them to the soup first, cooked them until soft, and then blended them, the myrosinase would have been deactivated and fewer ITCs would be formed.

COMMON CRUCIFEROUS VEGETABLES

Arugula	Collard greens
Bok choy	Kale
Broccoli	Mustard greens
Brussels sprouts	Radish
Cabbage	Turnip greens
Cauliflower	Watercress

Other phytochemicals that can activate Nrf2 include anthocyanins (found in berries), epigallocatechin gallate (EGCG) (found in green tea), and resveratrol (found in grapes and peanuts).[7] Exercise may also activate Nrf2.[8] In contrast, smoking suppresses the protective actions of Nrf2. Human endothelial cells exposed to the blood of smokers compared with that of nonsmokers showed decreased Nrf2 expression, which reduces antioxidant defenses.[9] It is not surprising that smoking and green vegetables have opposite health effects! Maybe smokers should think about lighting up some broccoli—on the stove—instead.

The Allium Family: Onions and Garlic

The allium family of vegetables includes onions, garlic, leeks, chives, shallots, and scallions. Epidemiological studies have found that increased consumption of allium vegetables is associated with decreased risk of oral, esophageal, colorectal, laryngeal, breast, ovarian, and prostate cancers. For example, one large European study found between a 50 to 88 percent risk reduction for multiple cancers for participants who consumed the greatest quantities of onions or garlic.[10] That is amazing!

Allium vegetables are rich in cancer-fighting *organosulfur compounds*. As with the cruciferous vegetables and ITCs, the beneficial organosulfur compounds are produced when the cell walls of the vegetables are broken down by chopping, crushing, or chewing. These compounds are thought to be mostly responsible for the cancer-protective effects of allium vegetables, and their action and presence are enhanced when the vegetable is raw—either chewed well or blended.

In scientific studies, organosulfur compounds were shown to prevent the development of cancers by detoxifying carcinogens and halting cancer cell growth.[11] In studies of breast cancer cells, garlic and onion phytochemicals caused cell death or halted cell division, preventing cancer cells from multiplying.[12] These rich phytonutrients also fight heart disease effectively.

Epidemiological studies show an inverse correlation between garlic consumption and the progression of cardiovascular disease. Numerous studies and clinical trials have confirmed the ability of garlic to reduce the risk factors associated with cardiovascular disease by

• Inhibiting enzymes involved in cholesterol synthesis

• Decreasing platelet aggregation

• Preventing oxidization of LDL cholesterol

• Increasing the antioxidant status of the vascular tissues[13]

Onions have similar effects. Onions are natural anticlotting agents because they possess substances with fibrinolytic activity and can suppress platelet-clumping. The anticlotting effect of onions closely correlates with their sulfur content. Onions and garlic, and their allium family members, are rich in polyphenols, which include flavonoids and quercetin. Yellow and red onions are richer in these antioxidant compounds than white onions, and shallots are especially high in polyphenols. Red onions are also particularly rich in anthocyanins (which are also abundant in berries) and quercetin.[14]

Onions and the other vegetables of the allium family can be added to any vegetable dish for both great flavor and excellent health benefits. As with the green cruciferous vegetables, those in the allium family must be eaten raw and chewed well or chopped finely before cooking to initiate the chemical reaction that forms the protective sulfur compounds.

When you cut onions and your eyes begin to tear, it's because the onions are creating these anticancer sulfur compounds. Don't discard too much of the outer layer of the onion or the part close to the root, because that is where the flavonoids are most highly concentrated. A good strategy is to remove the outermost paper shell, but not the part right under that—and use as much of the area around the root as possible. To maximize protective compounds and minimize eye irritation when chopping onions, do the following:

- Make sure that the onion is cold before you cut it. (Tip: Put it in the freezer for five minutes.)
- Cut the end of the root off with the root facing away from you.
- Preserve as much of the onion adjacent to the root as possible.
- Cut or chop the onion finely, or put it in a blender or food processor before cooking.
- Eat some raw onion every day.

Berries, Cherries, and Pomegranates

Berries, cherries, and pomegranates are not just tempting and delicious—they also have a host of unique and beneficial properties that are essential for protecting your health.

- Berries and cherries are high in nutrients, phytochemicals, and fiber.
- Berries have the highest nutrient-to-calorie ratio of all fruits.
- Berries are some of the highest antioxidant-rich foods in existence.
- Cherries, which are a stone fruit, are also rich in flavonoid antioxidant compounds.[15]

Flavonoids occur as pigments in fruits and flowers. Berries, cherries, and pomegranates are abundant in flavonoids, which are concentrated in their skins and give rise to their deep hues of red, blue, and purple.[16] Flavonoids are thought to have a number of additional beneficial effects in the body beyond their antioxidant capacity. In fact, flavonoids are believed to contribute to health primarily by their ability to modify cell-signaling pathways, rather than through their antioxidant capacity. Flavonoids affect pathways leading to changes in gene expression, detoxification, inhibition of cancer cell growth, and proliferation and inhibition of inflammation and other processes related to heart disease.[17]

Several studies have shown that high flavonoid intake lowers the risk of heart disease by up to 45 percent because of the cell-signaling actions of flavonoids.[18] Flavonoids in berries, cherries, and pomegranates—and other pomegranate polyphenols—appear to act in several different ways to maintain heart health. These include reducing inflammation; improving blood lipid, blood pressure, and blood sugar levels; and preventing plaque formation.[19] For example, not only do blueberries lower blood pressure in a way similar to medications, but a recent study showed a 68 percent increase in blood nitric oxide levels among women who consumed blueberry powder.[20] Nitric oxide relaxes and protects blood vessels.

Blueberries, strawberries, and blackberries all have been shown to slow or reverse age-related cognitive decline in animal studies, and blueberries have now been tested for their effect on human memory.[21] Older adults with mildly impaired memory were given wild blueberry juice as a supplement. After as few as twelve weeks, measures of learning and memory had improved.[22]

The antioxidants in cherries have been shown to protect brain cells against oxidative stress, implying that eating cherries may help to prevent neurodegenerative diseases like dementia.[23] In people with mild memory complaints, those who drank pomegranate juice daily performed better on memory tasks compared with placebo and displayed an increase in brain activation, as measured by functional magnetic resonance imaging (fMRI).[24]

It might surprise you to know that berries and cherries may help you sleep. Berries and tart cherries are one of the few food sources of the hormone and antioxidant melatonin, which regulates the sleep-wake cycle in the human brain.[25] Tart cherry juice supplementation has been associated with improvements in sleep quality.[26] These anti-inflammatory effects could also benefit people suffering from gout.[27]

In summary, berries, cherries, and pomegranates are important components of a natural, high-nutrient diet. I recommend eating them regularly to provide the body with protection against free radicals, inflammation, heart disease, and cancers. Include them as part of your variety of fruits, in addition to a bounty of vegetables, beans, nuts, and seeds. Together, these plant foods can provide you with an abundant and varied mix of antioxidants, further protecting your health. Because berries, cherries, and pomegranates are not available year round—or can be expensive when purchased out of season—using frozen fruit is a reasonable alternative.

Tomatoes, Tomato Paste, and Tomato Sauce

Carotenoids are a family of more than six hundred phytochemicals, including alpha-carotene, beta-carotene, lycopene, lutein, and zeaxanthin. Carotenoids are abundant in green and yellow-orange vegetables and fruits and help to defend the body's tissues against oxidative damage.[28] The levels of carotenoids in your skin are a good indicator of your overall health because they parallel the levels of plant-derived phytochemicals that have been absorbed into your tissues. I use a carotenoid skin testing method to noninvasively track my patients' progress as they adopt a Nutritarian diet. You can even see this yourself; within about six months of following a nutrient-rich diet, you will see your skin and hands looking healthier and younger, with a bit of a protective orange, tannish glow.

In a study of more than thirteen thousand American adults, low blood levels of carotenoids were found to be a predictor of earlier death.

Lower total carotenoids, alpha-carotene, and lycopene in the blood were all linked to increased risk of death from all causes. It is important to note that of all the carotenoids, very low blood lycopene was the strongest predictor of mortality.[29]

Lycopene is the signature carotenoid of the tomato. The lycopene in the U.S. diet is 85 percent derived from tomatoes.[30] In the human body lycopene is found circulating in the blood and also concentrates in the male reproductive system, hence its protective effects against prostate cancer.[31] In the skin, lycopene helps to prevent ultraviolet damage from the sun, protecting against skin cancer.[32] Lycopene is known for its anticancer properties, but it has also been intensively studied for its beneficial cardiovascular effects.

Many observational studies have found a connection between higher blood lycopene levels and lower risk of heart attack. For example, a study in men found that low serum lycopene was associated with increased plaque in the carotid artery and tripled the risk of cardiovascular events compared with higher levels.[33] In a separate study, women were split into four groups according to their blood lycopene levels; those in the top three groups with the highest levels were 50 percent less likely to have cardiovascular disease compared with those in the group with the lowest levels.[34]

A 2004 analysis from the Physicians' Health Study data found a 39 percent decrease in stroke risk in men with the highest blood levels of lycopene.[35] New data from an ongoing study in Finland have strengthened these findings with similar results. A thousand men had their blood carotenoid levels tested and were followed for twelve years. Those with the highest lycopene levels had the lowest risk of stroke; they were 55 percent less likely to have a stroke than those with the lowest lycopene levels.[36] Previous data from this same group of men found that higher lycopene levels were associated with a lower risk of heart attack as well.[37]

How Does Lycopene Work?

Lycopene is an extremely potent antioxidant; its antioxidant capability is said to be double that of beta-carotene and ten times that of vitamin E.[38] Several studies that gave supplemental tomato products to volunteers found that the subjects' LDL particles were more resistant to oxidation. LDL oxidation is an early event in atherosclerotic plaque formation, and lycopene helps to prevent this.[39]

Another study found improved endothelial function after just two weeks of a tomato-rich diet. *Endothelial function* refers to the ability of the endothelium (the inner lining of blood vessels) to properly regulate blood pressure. Oxidative damage can impair endothelial function.[40] Similarly, a randomized controlled trial using lycopene supplements in patients with cardiovascular disease also reported enhanced endothelial function. The patients assigned to lycopene supplementation showed improved endothelial function (measured by forearm blood flow) of 63 percent after eight weeks, whereas the placebo group saw no improvement.[41]

Lycopene also has non-antioxidant actions that studies show may protect against cardiovascular disease. First, there is evidence that lycopene may inhibit HMG-CoA reductase, the enzyme responsible for making cholesterol (this is also the enzyme that cholesterol-lowering statin drugs inhibit).[42] As you might expect, trials that added extra tomato products to subjects' diets reduced their blood cholesterol levels. Second, a meta-analysis of twelve trials found that daily supplemental tomato products (approximately 1 cup of tomato juice or 3 to 4 tablespoons of tomato paste) reduced LDL cholesterol by 10 percent. This effect is comparable to that obtained with low doses of statin drugs (with no risk of side effects).[43] Lycopene also has several anti-inflammatory actions and can prevent excessive proliferation of vascular smooth muscle cells.[44] These are the cells that comprise the majority of blood vessel walls, so excessive growth of these cells can lead to vessel stiffening and enhance plaque development.

Of course, lycopene is not the only nutrient found in tomatoes; they are also rich in vitamins C and E, beta-carotene, and flavonol antioxidants, just to name a few.[45] Single antioxidants usually don't exert their protective effects alone; we learned this lesson from clinical trials of beta-carotene, vitamin C, and vitamin E supplements, which did not reduce cardiovascular disease risk.[46] It is the interaction between phytochemicals, in the complex synergistic network contained in plant foods, that is responsible for their health effects. We cannot replicate this in a pill.

Of all the common dietary carotenoids, lycopene has the most potent antioxidant power. But combinations of carotenoids are even more effective than any single carotenoid, because they work synergistically.[47] Blood lycopene, as used in many of these studies, is simply a marker of high tomato product intake. Similarly, high alpha-carotene and beta-carotene levels are markers of high green and yellow-orange fruit and vegetable intake. It is clear that colorful fruits and vegetables provide significant protection from cardiovascular disease.

In a given year, a typical American will eat about 92 pounds of tomatoes.[48] Enjoy those 92 pounds, and even add some more! Add fresh, juicy raw tomatoes to your salads; include diced or unsulfured sun-dried tomatoes in soups; and enjoy homemade tomato sauces and soups. Be mindful of the sodium content of ketchup and other tomato products; choose the low-sodium or no-salt-added versions. No-salt-added, unsulfured dried tomatoes are also great. Diced and crushed tomatoes in glass jars are preferable to those in cans to avoid ingesting the endocrine disruptor bisphenol-A (BPA) or other can lining material.

Also keep in mind that carotenoids are absorbed best when accompanied by healthy fats—for example, in a salad with a seed- or nut-based dressing.[49] Lycopene is also more absorbable when tomatoes are cooked. One cup of tomato sauce contains about ten times the lycopene of a cup of raw, chopped tomatoes, so enjoy a variety of both raw and cooked tomatoes in your daily diet.[50]

The Importance of How and When You Eat

The exposure to these disease-fighting phytochemicals in colorful plant foods aids not just in the recovery from heart disease, but also in the reduction of body fat. When the reversal of heart disease is being discussed, the other critical nutritional issue is weight loss. It is vital that anyone who strives to lose weight—and achieve a reversal of heart disease—never regains that excess weight. The rapid regain of weight can be associated with the deposition of visceral fat and vulnerable plaque.

For people who are overweight, losing fat is not enough to cause heart disease to reverse. Achieving reversal requires both superior nutrition, with a favorable micronutrient exposure, and the removal of excess body fat. It is both the removal of fat and the nutritional integrity of the body's tissues that enable the atherosclerosis to resorb and resolve. The critical issue here is that eating the right type of food helps reduce and control appetite.

People overeat because of many different social, emotional, recreational, and addictive reasons. A major cause of excessive caloric intake is a hunger drive that directs people to consume more calories than they require. One of the common barriers to weight loss is the uncomfortable sensation of hunger that drives overeating and makes dieting fail, even in people who are obese from overconsumption of calories.

My twenty-five years of experience in this field of study, supported by research papers I have published, have documented that enhancing the micronutrient quality of the diet, even in the context of a substantially lower caloric intake, significantly mitigates the experience of hunger.[51]

In a 2010 study of 768 participants, we found that the better they adhered to the NDPR dietary approach, the more likely their hunger sensations were transformed. Ninety percent of those adhering 90 percent to the NDPR (Nutritarian) dietary style reported a change in their perception of hunger. The uncomfortable physical and emotional symptoms of hunger gradually resolved after people embraced this diet. We observed this reduction in the drive to overeat to be strongly correlated with the degree of adherence to the diet—meaning that the healthier the diet, the less strong the drive to overeat.

A diet high in micronutrients decreases food cravings and overeating behaviors. Sensations I call *toxic hunger*—such as fatigue, weakness, mental fog, loss of attentiveness, stomach cramps, fluttering, tremors, irritability, and mild headaches—are commonly interpreted as hunger. These sensations resolve gradually for the majority of people who adopt an NDPR diet. A new, nondistressing sensation, which I have labeled "true" or "throat" hunger, replaces these toxic hunger symptoms.

It is well documented that a diet low in antioxidant and phytochemical micronutrients leads to heightened oxidative stress and a buildup of toxic metabolites.[52] When a diet is low in dietary antioxidants, phytochemicals, and other micronutrients, intracellular waste products such as free radicals, advanced glycation end products, aldehydes, lipofuscin, and lipid A2E accumulate.[53] Other studies have demonstrated an adverse effect of low-micronutrient foods containing higher amounts of simple carbohydrates, fats, and animal products on the levels of inflammatory markers, metabolic by-products, and oxidative stress in the body.[54] Put more simply, your risk factors for heart disease increase when you are eating a diet that does not include an abundance of nutrient-dense foods.

It has also been shown that a higher intake of nutrient-rich plant foods decreases measurable inflammatory by-products.[55] When a diet is low in micronutrients and plant phytochemicals, inflammatory by-products build up in the body. It is well established in the scientific literature that these toxic metabolites contribute to disease[56] and can be associated with typical withdrawal symptoms, including headaches.[57] Heightened elimination of these waste products may create symptoms that can feel similar to withdrawal from drug addiction.

I call the eating and digesting phase of the digestive cycle the *anabolic phase*. When digestion ceases, the *catabolic phase* begins. This is when the body is using the stored energy reserves and can most efficiently heal, repair, and self-clean. During this phase cellular waste products and toxins are more effectively mobilized and eliminated, leading to the uncomfortable symptoms perceived as hunger. There is no need for additional calories at the initial part of the catabolic phase. In fact, the body has just finished storing all the calories from the most recent meal. Nevertheless, because these uncomfortable symptoms are relieved by eating, they drive overeating behavior and are a major factor leading to obesity.

Healthful eating is more effective for long-term weight control because it modifies and diminishes the sensations of withdrawal-related hunger, enabling overweight individuals to be more comfortable, even while consuming substantially fewer calories.

Anabolic Phase ⟶ Catabolic Phase

Digestive and Absorptive Period ⟶ Utilization of Stored Energy

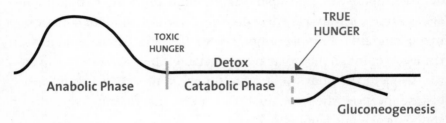

The glucose curve rises during and immediately after a meal, as digestion is in its anabolic phase. The glucose in the blood not immediately burned for energy is stored as glycogen, primarily in the liver and muscle tissues. Then, as the blood glucose falls to baseline, these glycogen stores are gradually broken down to release glucose into the blood, keeping the glucose curve steady to fuel the body's and brain's needs. This is the catabolic phase of digestion but is also called *glycolysis,* since glycogen is being used for energy, and liver detoxification is enhanced.

As soon as food has been eaten, digested, and assimilated and the postprandial (after-meal) glucose returns to baseline, the catabolic utilization of glycogen reserves and fatty acid stores begins. True hunger normally increases in intensity as glycogen stores are diminishing toward the end of the catabolic phase. True hunger does not occur at the start of the catabolic phase, when glycolysis begins and the body's energy reserves are high; those symptoms (toxic hunger) are withdrawal symptoms caused by the elimination of cellular waste products that accumulate from an unhealthy diet.

In contrast, true hunger, which occurs hours later when glycogen stores are nearly depleted, prevents gluconeogenesis. *Gluconeogenesis* is the utilization of muscle tissue for needed glucose after glycogen stores have been depleted. True hunger protects lean body mass but does not fuel fat deposition. It exists to protect lean body mass from being used as an energy source.

Evidence suggests that overweight individuals build up more inflammatory markers and oxidative stress when fed a low-nutrient meal, compared with normal-weight individuals.[58] The heightened inflammatory potential in people who have a tendency toward obesity is marked by increasing levels of lipid peroxidase and malondialdehyde and reduced activation of liver detoxification enzymes.[59]

This supports my clinical experience that people who are prone to obesity experience more withdrawal/hunger symptoms. The resulting heightened discomfort drives them to eat frequently and overconsume calories. It is a vicious cycle promoting continuous (anabolic) digestion, frequent feedings, and increased intake of calories.

GLUCOSE CURVE OF CONTINUOUS ANABOLIC ACTIVITY

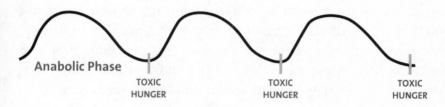

Anabolic Phase

TOXIC HUNGER   TOXIC HUNGER   TOXIC HUNGER

Chronically overweight people in the typical American food environment feel "normal" only by eating too frequently or by eating a heavy meal. They can feel okay only if they continue digesting food right up to the beginning of the next meal. They need excess calories in order to feel normal. This frequent eating prevents the utilization of glycogen and body fat that would normally occur during the catabolic phase, making weight gain inevitable.

An NDPR diet, after an initial phase of adjustment during which a person experiences toxic hunger because of withdrawal from proinflammatory foods, can result in a sustainable eating pattern that eliminates this major impediment to weight loss.

When our bodies have acclimated to a noxious or toxic agent, it is called addiction. When we stop consuming the toxic agent, such as caffeine or nicotine, we feel ill, as the body tries to mobilize cellular wastes and repair the damage caused by exposure to the toxic agent. This is called withdrawal.

Suppose you drink three cups of coffee or caffeinated soda per day. If your caffeine level dips too low, you will get a withdrawal headache. Having another cup of coffee or soda makes you feel better because it retards detoxification, or withdrawal. In other words, the caffeine withdrawal symptoms spur you into drinking more caffeine products to manage those symptoms.

Likewise, toxic hunger is heightened by consuming caffeinated beverages, soft drinks, and processed foods. It occurs after a meal is digested and the digestive tract is empty. It makes people feel extremely uncomfortable, so uncomfortable that they feel they need to eat or drink a caloric load for relief. We have a population of food-addicted people who have complicated emotional eating patterns.

The first step to unwinding this complex problem of excess eating and excess weight is to eat healthfully—with the expectation that it will be tough to do for the first few days. With time, it will get easier both physically and emotionally. However, without committing to a healthful, high-nutrient eating style, you will find that this vicious cycle of diet and weight-loss failure is almost impossible to remedy.

The Facts About Fish, Fish Oil, and Omega-3 Fatty Acids

A 2012 review and meta-analysis looked at all the best "randomized clinical trials evaluating the effects of omega-3s from fish or fish oil on life span, cardiac death, sudden death, heart attack, and stroke."[60] Overall, the researchers found no protective benefit for all-cause mortality, heart disease mortality, sudden cardiac death, heart attack, or stroke.

In the past, some studies have shown cardiac benefits from fish and fish oil and others have not. Today, with larger numbers of people studied for longer periods of time, the benefits have been tempered.

The disease-causing SAD cannot be made less risky—in any significant sense—by taking fish oil supplements, aspirin, or statin drugs. We have to face the reality that the quality of our diets is too powerful an anti-health modulator to overcome with a few pills.

However, it is helpful to analyze in depth the contradictory studies on the long-chain omega-3 fatty acids DHA and EPA, which account for the supposed benefits of fish and fish oil. Examining the details of hundreds of these studies indicates that both a deficiency and excess of these long-chain omega-3 fats can be harmful. A review of these data demonstrates this effect—and indicates, specifically, that too much fish oil can be problematic.

The idea that all this fish oil may not be a great idea first came to light in 2003 after the second Diet and Reinfarction Trial (DART-2) was published.[61] The earlier DART trial had shown a clear benefit from fish oil over the short term, right after a heart attack. However, this second trial was one of the first studies on fish oil that followed people with heart disease for many years. It randomized into four groups 3,114 men who were younger than 70 and had angina. The four groups were:

1. Those who were advised to eat two portions of oily fish weekly, or to take three fish oil capsules daily (3 grams)

2. Those who were advised to eat more fruit, vegetables, and oats

3. Those who were given both the above types of advice

4. Those who were given no specific dietary advice

Mortality was ascertained after three to nine years. The researchers determined that the group who were supposed to eat more fruits and vegetables did not comply well with their diet, but the group advised to eat more fish and take fish oil did. Researchers found that this group had a 25 percent increased risk of death and more than a 50 percent increased risk of sudden cardiac death. The excess risk was largely found among the subgroup given fish oil capsules.

There is clearly a problem with taking 3 grams of fish oil a day—that is a lot of fish oil! One problem with fish oil is that it is vulnerable to oxidative damage, or rancidity. The second problem is the high amount recommended to this group. I have reviewed all the studies on this issue, and the tremendous number of differences found among them demonstrates that the exposure to some fish or a small amount of fish oil seems to offer benefits. However, the minute you start taking high doses (more than 1 gram) of fish oil, problems seem to occur and negate many of the benefits.

It seems that a dietary deficiency in EPA and DHA is not life span–favorable, but on the other hand, too much may be not favorable, either.

Consider this 2013 study, which I think is one of the best to evaluate the risks and benefits of DHA-EPA adequacy. It evaluated the risk of death in 2,692 individuals between 70 and 80 years of age, following their blood levels of these beneficial fats.[62] These individuals did not have a history of heart disease. Total mortality, as well as fatal and non-fatal heart attacks and strokes, was tracked for sixteen years. This study was particularly informative because it relied on blood tests to determine the levels of these two fatty acids, rather than just a self-reported dietary history. Study researchers concluded that higher blood levels of omega-3 EPA and DHA were associated with lower total mortality, especially heart disease deaths.

This study found that adequate blood levels of EPA and DHA had important longevity-promoting benefits, especially in reducing the risk of arrhythmic cardiac death by almost 50 percent. The result was more than two years of longer life in the highest quintile of study subjects.

Another recent study corroborated this finding: that an adequate, but not excessive, amount of EPA and DHA was life span–favorable. In a multiethnic cohort of 2,837 U.S. adults, blood levels of polyunsaturated fatty acids and dietary intake were examined. For the following ten years, cardiovascular events, deaths, and strokes were monitored. Analysis of the data found that both dietary and circulating EPA and DHA were associated with about half as many cardiovascular events such as heart attacks.[63]

The main point is that we need EPA and DHA in our diets. But it is important to recognize that levels that are too low or too high can place us at increased risk of cardiovascular events. Of course, the need to determine safe and beneficial levels holds true, in most cases, for other nutrients that the body requires. My guidelines are supported by the preponderance of evidence on this issue and my review of not merely a few, but hundreds of trials.

Consider atrial fibrillation, a common cardiac arrhythmia, and whether omega-3 fatty acid plays a role. A review of all the data about this issue shows a similar pattern. DHA deficiency may increase the risk of developing atrial fibrillation in later life, but taking more, once adequacy is reached, does not increase protection. And it's important to note that too much fish oil may actually increase the risk of developing atrial fibrillation.

For example, two studies confirmed that blood levels demonstrating DHA adequacy were related to a reduced incidence of atrial fibrillation.[64] One study in 2009 followed people who did not have atrial fibrillation for an average of 17.7 years to discover who would develop this most common arrhythmia. Researchers found a 38 percent decreased incidence of atrial fibrillation in participants whose blood work showed adequate levels of DHA. The other study in 2012 confirmed these findings, demonstrating a graded and linear association with higher DHA levels in the blood and lower incidence of atrial fibrillation.

However, these findings were directly contradicted by three other studies which showed that ingesting too much fish or fish oil can moderately increase the risk of atrial fibrillation. Nevertheless, a detailed analysis of the data in these studies reveals a U-shaped association, demonstrating that both too little and too much can moderately increase risk. So all these data really are not contradictory or confusing, as they consistently demonstrate that research participants who are deficient in omega-3 fatty acids (as documented by blood work) had more atrial fibrillation, and those ingesting too much fish or fish oil also had moderately increased risk.[65]

There is also some evidence that ingesting too much fish oil may increase the risk of prostate cancer. A report from researchers at the Fred Hutchinson Cancer Research Center in Seattle compared blood samples from 834 men diagnosed with prostate cancer with samples from 1,393 men who didn't have the disease. Men whose blood samples were in the top 25 percent of omega-3 fatty acid content were 43 percent more likely to have been diagnosed with prostate cancer than men whose blood samples were in the lowest 25 percent of omega-3 content.[66]

The findings were published online in the *Journal of the National Cancer Institute* but were highly criticized as not being definitive due to too many unknown variables about the effect of prostate cancer on these blood levels. Nevertheless, caution here is indicated, especially since a meta-analysis of this issue showed a 15 percent greater risk of prostate cancer with the highest levels of EPA-DHA.[67] We must consider these other potential risks that are being suggested from overusing fish oil supplements or eating too much fish.

Omega-3 Fatty Acids: What You Need to Know for Maximum Heart Health and to Prevent Dementia and Depression

Being conservative and cautious here, I suggest taking supplemental DHA and EPA if you are not eating fish regularly, but do not overdo supplementation. I prefer an algae-based DHA and EPA in a relatively low dose to prevent deficiency, so you can be assured it is free from environmental contaminants that can be found in fish and fish oil. Supplementing is an important concern when following a vegan diet for therapeutic benefits. Even though the risk of heart disease for a vegan would be exceedingly low, there is the potential risk of developing depression and dementia from fatty acid deficiency, especially from chronically low EPA and DHA.

More than a dozen epidemiological studies have reported that reduced levels of long-chain omega-3 fatty acids are associated with increased risk of age-related cognitive decline or dementia such as Alzheimer's disease.[68] DHA promotes the growth and maintenance of nervous tissue and improved cognition. In animal models, DHA adequacy prevents the amyloid accumulation commonly seen in Alzheimer's patients. Most critically, human clinical trials also show increased brain shrinkage with aging in people who have lower blood levels of DHA, evaluated eight years after initial DHA measurements.[69] The hippocampus area in the brain plays an important role in memory and usually begins to atrophy before symptoms of Alzheimer's appear. This area of the brain was found to be particularly vulnerable to shrinkage associated with a low omega-3 index (3.4 percent compared with 7.5 percent). (The omega-3 index is a measure of the levels of EPA plus DHA in red blood cells.)

This is of particular concern considering the large number of un-supplemented vegans who demonstrate deficiency as measured by the omega-3 index.[70] In this study, 166 healthy vegans showed a wide range in DHA-EPA levels, which did not correlate with the amount of short-chain omega-3 intake. That means that more alpha-linolenic acid from flaxseeds and walnuts did not translate into higher levels of EPA and DHA, suggesting that the major variation was primarily due to genetic differences in conversion enzymes.

A significant percentage of the vegans had levels less than 3 percent (as shown in the graph), suggesting serious risk of later-life brain com-promise. This study also demonstrated that a low-dose, algae-derived supplement of only 265 milligrams of EPA (88 milligrams) plus DHA (177 milligrams) was sufficient to normalize the omega-3 index results on subsequent blood tests.

OMEGA-3 INDEX IN VEGANS

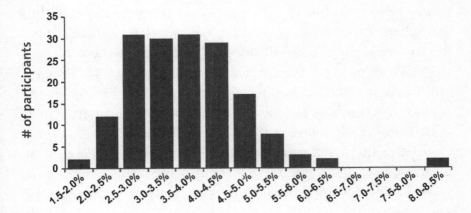

My two and a half decades of clinical experience treating vegans who have some failure to thrive on a vegan diet have repeatedly demon-strated a percentage whose lack of DHA and EPA resulted in an episode of depression or anxiety depressive disorder. These findings are consistent with a meta-analysis demonstrating that people with depression com-monly have lower EPA and DHA levels.[71] DHA deficiency in depressed patients, relative to healthy controls, is linked to anxiety and depression. The low omega-3 fatty acid status commonly observed in patients with major depressive disorder may reduce the effectiveness of the most commonly used medications for this disorder, called selective serotonin reuptake inhibitors (SSRIs).[72] Supplementation with DHA-EPA, especially EPA, has been shown to be helpful for people with depression.[73]

Not merely DHA but other common deficiencies could additively increase depression risk. Low vitamin D (best measured with a 25-hydroxy vitamin D blood test) can also exacerbate the risks of dementia and depression and has been associated with diminished global cognitive function and greater decline over four years. In this study, people with 25-hydroxy vitamin D higher than 30 ng/ml showed insignificant decline; those with levels of 20 to 29 showed moderate decline; and those with levels less than 20 showed severe decline.[74] These findings were matched almost perfectly in another study.[75] It is important to pay attention to all these factors (because of the varied needs of individuals) to assure that people who are counting on longevity-promoting dietary advice are not left with some irreversible loss of memory and brain function. I see many patients who eat healthfully and follow the advice of nutritional leaders, yet they still have low levels of these important nutrients, placing them at needless risk.

When following a vegan or near-vegan diet, it may also be important to assure that zinc requirements are optimized. Zinc levels and needs can vary among individuals, with some people requiring more than is biologically accessible through a vegan diet.

A meta-analysis of seventeen studies measuring zinc levels demonstrated that zinc concentration averaged 1.85 umol/l lower in depressed subjects versus controls, and greater depression severity was associated with greater relative zinc deficiency.[76] The research also corroborates my clinical experience that women are more susceptible to depression from low and borderline zinc intake compared with men.[77] I have found that supplemental zinc, added to the antidepression protocol, has been extremely effective, especially in speeding up the response to therapy and ameliorating anxiety associated with depression or anxious depression. Some studies corroborate this experience.[78]

Understanding Failure to Thrive in a Small Percentage of Vegans

A number of important trials have confirmed the benefits of dietary supplementation with omega-3 fatty acids, not only in several psychiatric conditions, but also in inflammatory, autoimmune, and neurodegenerative diseases. It is unfortunate, but understandable, that many vegans, when they develop emotional disorders or symptoms, have been turned away from the vegan diet and returned to eating meat and fish. However, the most unfortunate part is that they often swing back to the other extreme, consuming a diet too high in animal products (which has a new constellation of risks) instead of understanding their deficiencies and repairing them conservatively.

A diet-style that most effectively reverses heart disease is vegan or near-vegan. But in our valiant efforts to win the war against this defeatable foe, we must make sure that we don't ignore other potential nutritional risks. Though this discussion of the issue only touches on some main concerns, it has become apparent from my clinical experience that an unsupplemented, low-fat vegan diet should ignite a spark of caution. This diet-style is not natural to our genetic heritage and has not been pursued for generations. Its promotion as the "perfect" diet for all can result in a failure to thrive in some children and can be unsafe for pregnant and nursing women. In addition, an unsupplemented vegan diet can increase the risk of developing depression and later-life dementia and increase the risk needlessly for some people with advanced heart disease.

We must always err on the side of caution when scientific results are not definitive or are controversial. Very little in the world of nutritional science is known with 100 percent certainty. We always need to consider the preponderance of the evidence within a conservative framework that is informed by broad clinical experience.

My very busy clinical practice, which caters to this population of vegans and health seekers, may shine a different light on some of these issues. I have communicated with other medical professionals who have similar practices and have reported similar or identical findings.

Certainly, vitamin B12 is the most important supplement to use for someone eating a vegan or near-vegan diet, or for an aging population. It is also important to assure a source of iodine in the diet, since many of us do not use iodinated salt or eat seaweed regularly.

Plant proteins are preferable to animal proteins, and less animal protein is invariably more favorable to health, so it is unusual to have to be concerned with people's protein needs. Vegetables, beans, seeds, and nuts supply plenty of protein, even for athletes. The rare individual may require more plant protein or some animal products to account for digestive idiosyncrasies, especially as concerns the amino acids taurine and carnitine. Being alert to patients' unique needs is important, especially as protein assimilation diminishes with advanced aging. When these requirements are evident, a small amount of animal products suffices. (See Chapter 7 for more about protein.)

Without a predetermined philosophy or agenda, we must use a clear, unbiased evaluation of today's science, in conjunction with assessment of the broad spectrum of individual needs, to assure outcomes that are invariably favorable.

In Chapter 8, I walk you through everything you need to know to put nutritional science into action in your kitchen to transform your health. The science is clear that the nutritional protocol described here is the single most effective way to prevent and reverse heart disease. But first we turn to one of the most important topics related to heart disease: fat.

CHAPTER FIVE

Fat-Food Nation:
The Science of Fat

Have you heard that saturated fat is good, not bad? Cholesterol and eggs are good, not bad? Lots of people in the media and on the Internet have jumped on this bandwagon. "Eat Butter" claimed *Time* magazine's cover on June 23, 2014. Mark Bittman's March 2014 column in the *New York Times* rhapsodized, "Butter Is Back."

A 2014 meta-analysis in the *Annals of Internal Medicine* concluded, "Current evidence does not clearly support cardiovascular guidelines that encourage high consumption of polyunsaturated fatty acids and low consumption of total saturated fats."[1] The media ran with it.

And why wouldn't they? There is a strong desire of not merely the producers of meat, butter, and eggs to claim their products are safe, but also the meat-and-butter-eating public and media to distort and misinterpret information to justify their eating preferences. Low-carbohydrate, Paleo, and other high-meat-diet advocates proudly tell their followers that this research has exonerated saturated fat and proved that the connection between saturated fat and heart disease was just a myth. The overall message is that everyone now has free rein to eat all the meat, butter, and cheese they want with no consequences.

These statements and headlines are sensationalized misinterpretations of the science. They do a serious disservice to an already nutritionally confused and unhealthy public for whom heart disease and cancer are the leading causes of death. Promoting the view that foods rich in saturated fat, such as meat, butter, and cheese, are harmless requires ignoring an overwhelming amount of evidence linking increased meat consumption to a higher risk of death. It also requires ignoring much additional evidence showing that saturated fat–rich meals impair endothelial function, raise cholesterol, and lead to populations with higher rates of both heart disease and cancer.[2]

CASE HISTORY: PROOF FROM A PATIENT

It would be easy to blame my health problems on heredity because I've been heavy since childhood. I have a history of obesity, heart disease, and diabetes on both sides of my family. Over the years, I tried many diets, but they didn't work well or for long. I reached a top weight of 263 pounds on my 5-foot-4-inch frame and resigned myself to forever being a plus-size woman. I avoided seeing doctors because, although they lectured me about my weight, the only solution they offered was a calorie-restricted version of the standard American diet, which made me feel always hungry and miserable.

At age 56, I had a stroke. After almost a month in the hospital and a rehab center, I returned home diagnosed with type 2 diabetes, high blood pressure, high cholesterol, arteries that were about 65 percent blocked, and a low thyroid level. To control all these ills I was given a bunch of prescription medications, which I was expected to take for the rest of my life. About a year after the stroke, I was diagnosed with a serious form of tachycardia and ended up having two stents for a 95 percent blockage, and even more prescriptions.

My husband searched the Internet for ways to help me become healthier and found Dr. Fuhrman's website. He read *Eat to Live,* which claimed dramatic results through dietary changes. I was skeptical about trying yet another diet, but since I could no longer be in denial about my weight and health, I agreed. Because I was still in a wheelchair, my husband had to prepare meals for both of us. Although he only had a little weight to lose, he joined me on the diet, assured by Dr. Fuhrman's website that a high-nutrient, vegetable-based diet would also be healthy for him. I quickly shed pounds, and my lab tests improved. Although my diabetes was controlled to the satisfaction of my doctors, Dr. Fuhrman said the first priority was to get rid of it completely with nutritional excellence. No physician I had seen ever mentioned this as a possibility.

About a year and a half later, I was no longer diabetic and had no further heart problems. My current weight is around 130, slightly less than half my maximum. I have gone from a plus-size 24W/26W to a misses' size 8/10, which is a smaller size than I have ever worn in my adult life. As hard as it is to imagine, the last time I was this weight, I was younger than 12. I also no longer snore and my energy and stamina have increased. Although I didn't fully recover from the stroke, maybe about 90 percent, there are things I can do more easily now than before when I was just fat. My husband and I both have more immune resistance. We used to catch every bug that came around, but now we're rarely sick.

It's been many years since I started the Nutritarian diet, and I have maintained my weight loss and have had no diet-related medical problems. Even though I don't take any medication for diabetes or statins for cholesterol, my most recent lab results show my fasting blood sugar at 75 mg/dl, total cholesterol at 144 mg/dl, and triglycerides at 61 mg/dl. I owe all these positive changes to Dr. Fuhrman's program. I still have a hearty appetite, but I'm no longer addicted to food.

Charlene Vanderveen

Those who support these false claims have not scrutinized all the evidence on this topic or have allowed their judgment to be impaired by cognitive biases, such as food preference, status quo bias, and the "bandwagon" effect. Plus, multiple interventional studies now show that heart disease not only can be prevented, but also can be reversed by avoiding animal products. In contrast, not one study shows that the reversal of plaque or elimination of cardiac deaths is possible with a diet high in animal products. Don't believe in fairy tales.

Glossary

Saturated fats—some naturally occurring fats are called saturated because all the carbon atoms are single bonds. It is well established that eating more saturated fats raises cholesterol. These fats are solid at room temperature and generally are recognized as a significant cause of both heart disease and cancer. Saturated fats are found mainly in meat, fowl, eggs, and dairy. The foods with the most saturated fat are butter, cream, meat, and cheese. Palm oil and coconut oil have higher amounts of saturated fat compared with other plant fats. Almost half the saturated fat in coconut oil is lauric acid, a medium-chain triglyceride that is safer than other saturated fats. But just because coconut oil is not as bad as butter doesn't mean it's a health food.

Unsaturated fats are a mix of monounsaturated and polyunsaturated fat. Eating unsaturated fats lowers cholesterol when substituted for saturated fats, but excessive amounts may promote cancer and obesity. Examples of unsaturated fats are the fats in nuts and seeds such as flaxseeds, sunflower seeds, macadamia and pistachio nuts, almonds, walnuts, and cashews as well as avocados and olives.

Monounsaturated fats are fats with only one double bond in the carbon chain. They are liquid at room temperature and are thought to have health benefits. The supposed health benefits of these fats appear when these fats are used in place of dangerous saturated fats. Monounsaturated fat is found in avocados, almonds, peanuts, and most other nuts and seeds. Keep in mind: No fats that are extracted from whole foods (oils), such as olive oil and almond oil, even if they are monounsaturated, should be considered health food because they are low in nutrients and contain 120 calories per tablespoon, promoting weight gain. When you consume the entire food containing monounsaturated fat, you get a significant amount of important fat-binding fibers and nutrients that are lost when the oil is extracted. It is always best that our fat intake come from whole food, not oil.

Hydrogenated fat—hydrogenation is a process of adding hydrogen molecules to unsaturated fats, which makes plant oils, which are liquid at room temperature, solidify. An example is margarine. These fats are also called *trans* fats. The hardening of the fat extends its shelf life so that the oil can be used over and over again, such as to fry potatoes in a fast-food restaurant, or added to processed foods such as crackers and cookies. While hydrogenation does not make the fat completely satu-rated, it creates *trans* fatty acids, which act like saturated fats. These fats raise cholesterol, and evidence is accumulating that demonstrates the harmful nature of these manufactured fats and their relation to both cancer and heart disease. Avoid all foods whose ingredients con-tain partially hydrogenated or hydrogenated oils.

Cholesterol is a waxy fatlike substance found in all cells of our bod-ies. Our bodies produce the amount we need. It is also found in animal foods such as meat, fowl, dairy, and eggs. It is known that too much of certain types of cholesterol in our blood promotes heart disease. Eating cholesterol does raise unfavorable blood cholesterol somewhat, but not as much as eating saturated fats and *trans* fats. The amount of cholesterol in plants is so negligible that you should consider them cholesterol free.

Low-Density Lipoprotein (LDL) Cholesterol—cholesterol cannot dis-solve in the blood, so it needs proteins (called *lipoproteins*) to transport it to where it needs to go. LDL cholesterol is one of five lipoproteins, but this one has the most affinity for the inside of blood vessels, especially when oxidized. LDL cholesterol is the bad guy that promotes the plaque that leads to blockages and heart attacks. Thus, the more LDL choles-terol you have in your blood, the greater your risk of heart disease.

High-Density Lipoprotein (HDL) Cholesterol—HDL cholesterol is the "good" cholesterol and carries cholesterol back to the liver for removal from the body. So higher HDL helps keep cholesterol from building up in the walls of the arteries. Individuals with a ratio of total to HDL cho-lesterol higher than 4 are considered to have an exceptionally high risk of developing heart disease. So, the higher your HDL cholesterol, the better. However, people with exceptionally low LDL cholesterol do not have to worry about their HDL level. You don't need the garbage collec-tors when there is no garbage.

Docosahexaenoic Acid (DHA) Fat—DHA is a long-chain omega-3 fatty acid that is made by the body, but it can also be found in algae and fish, such as salmon and sardines. DHA is used in the production of anti-inflammatory mediators that inhibit abnormal immune function and prevent excessive blood clotting. DHA is not considered an essential fat because the body can manufacture sufficient amounts if adequate short-chain omega-3 fatty acids are consumed (flaxseeds, walnuts, soybeans, leafy green vegetables). However, because of genetic differences in enzyme activity and because of excess omega-6 fats, many people who do not consume fish regularly are deficient in this important fat.

Arachidonic acid is a long-chain omega-6 fatty acid produced by the body, but it is also found in meat, fowl, dairy, and eggs. Products formed from excessive amounts of this fatty acid have the potential to increase inflammation and cause disease. They may increase blood pressure, thrombosis, vasospasm, and allergic reaction. They are linked to arthritis, depression, and other common illnesses.

Triglycerides comprise the largest proportion of fats (lipids) in the diet, in the adipose tissue, and in the blood. Immediately after a fatty meal, triglyceride levels rise in the bloodstream. We store triglycerides in our fatty tissues and muscle as a source of energy and gradually release and metabolize them between meals according to the energy needs of the body. Only a small portion of triglycerides is found in the bloodstream. High blood triglyceride levels reflect increased body fat stores. High triglycerides further promote and contribute to atherosclerosis in people with high cholesterol.

Body fat—*visceral fat* is the fat stored within the abdominal cavity around important internal organs, including the heart. It is associated with a number of serious health concerns, including high blood pressure, diabetes, and heart disease. *Subcutaneous fat* is the fat stored directly under the skin layers and is easily discernable by pinching the skin. It is widely distributed over the body but can accumulate preferentially in the buttocks and abdominal area.

Saturated Fat, Carbohydrates, and Heart Disease

Saturated fats are called *saturated* because they are saturated with hydrogen atoms. Saturation with hydrogen atoms makes the molecules in the fat fairly straight, so that they can be packed closely together, making these fats solid at room temperature. Monounsaturated and polyunsaturated fats can't pack as closely together, making them liquid at room temperature. The solid *trans* fats and saturated fat are the fats most closely associated with fat in your heart.

All fat-containing foods contain a combination of all three types of fat. Meat, eggs, and dairy products are generally the richest in saturated fat. Fish is somewhat higher in polyunsaturated fat because of the omega-3 content. Plant sources of fat, such as nuts, seeds, avocado, and vegetable oils, are higher in monounsaturated and polyunsaturated fats and lower in saturated fats. The exceptions are coconut and palm oil, which are high in saturated fat. The major sources of saturated fat in the SAD are cheese, conventional desserts, chicken, processed meats, and red meat.[3]

Saturated fat is thought to affect heart disease risk primarily through its effects on blood cholesterol levels. Research dating back to the 1950s and 1960s showed that adding saturated fats to the diet increased cholesterol when compared with adding polyunsaturated fats.[4] More recent human studies have consistently confirmed that saturated fat elevates blood cholesterol to a greater degree than monounsaturated or polyunsaturated fat.[5]

The 2014 meta-analysis that sparked the headlines extolling the virtues of saturated fat included thirty-two observational studies of dietary fat intake, seventeen studies of circulating fatty acids, and twenty-seven randomized controlled trials supplementing with omega-3 fatty acids. The authors found a decrease in CAD risk associated with long-chain omega-3 intake and an increase in risk for *trans* fat intake. No significant differences in risk were found for monounsaturated fat, omega-6 fat, or saturated fat.[6]

Does this mean that saturated fat poses no risk? Of course not. Both the interpretation of the data and the distortion of the findings by meat-promoting websites and the media demonstrate a troubling bias that permeates our society and hopes to maintain the present status quo of dietary-induced disease.

Replacing saturated fat with polyunsaturated fat decreases heart disease risk a bit, but replacing saturated fat with refined carbohydrate does not.

When saturated fat intake is studied, "replacement nutrients" are a crucial piece of the puzzle.[7] If you reduce the amount of foods rich in saturated fat in your diet, you must replace those foods with some other source of calories. In the 1970s, 1980s, and 1990s, when Americans were encouraged to reduce saturated fat–rich foods such as meat, dairy, and processed baked goods, most people didn't replace them with vegetables and other whole plant foods; instead, they replaced them with bread, pasta, white rice, and low-fat (and high-sugar) processed baked goods—*foods that cause disease just as much.*

The critics who claim that saturated fat poses no health risks have it wrong; it's not that saturated fat isn't harmful, it's that refined carbohydrates are just as bad. It is no surprise that no reductions in heart disease risk were found with lower saturated fat intake when people who ate smaller amounts of red meat and butter ate *more* white flour, processed cereals, and sugar instead! Plus, animal products have other detrimental properties besides fat, such as excess protein, iron, and carnitine (discussed below in more detail), all of which also promote atherosclerosis. Even the lower-fat animal products need to be reduced for serious heart disease protection, regardless of their fat content.

It is evident that this recent, highly publicized meta-analysis doesn't tell the whole story.

Analyses that paid the proper attention to replacement nutrients reported that while replacing saturated fat with (processed) carbohydrates did not reduce heart disease risk, replacing saturated fat with polyunsaturated fat from foods such as nuts, seeds, and avocados did reduce risk. Of course, those results weren't as highly publicized, since they couldn't spark any headlines trumpeting "meat, butter, and cheese are good for you!"

A pooled analysis published in 2009 found that replacing 5 percent of calories from saturated fat with polyunsaturated fat was associated with a 13 percent decreased risk of coronary events and a 26 percent decreased risk of coronary deaths. However, replacing 5 percent of calories from saturated fat with refined carbohydrates slightly increased risk of coronary events and had no effect on coronary deaths.[8]

Another meta-analysis, published in 2010, analyzed randomized controlled trials (which contained intervention studies that were excluded from the new meta-analysis) that replaced saturated fat calories with polyunsaturated fat calories in subjects' diets for at least one year. This analysis found an average decrease in total cholesterol of 29 mg/dl and reported that each 5 percent increase in polyunsaturated fat calories reduced CAD risk by 10 percent. A notable finding in this analysis was that the longer the duration of the intervention diet, the greater the benefit; for each additional year, the intervention groups lowered their risks another 9.2 percent.[9]

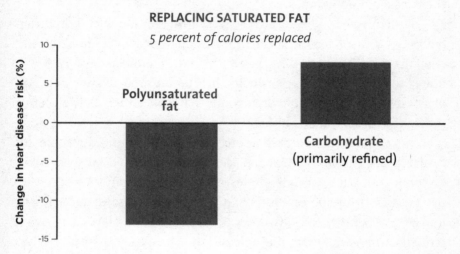

REPLACING SATURATED FAT

5 percent of calories replaced

The conclusion reported in the 2014 meta-analysis that got all the play in the press doesn't accurately reflect the preponderance of evidence from prevailing science. To repeat its conclusion: "Current evidence does not clearly support cardiovascular guidelines that encourage high consumption of polyunsaturated fatty acids and low consumption of total saturated fats." A more appropriate conclusion would have been:

Current evidence does not clearly support the benefits
of low consumption of saturated fats if those calories are
replaced with high-glycemic carbohydrates.

High-Glycemic Versus Low-Glycemic Carbohydrate Foods

The main reason that the meta-analysis of these observational studies suggested that replacing saturated fat with carbohydrates does not reduce heart disease risk was that these studies did not evaluate the quality of the carbohydrate eaten. We need to be more specific about the type of carbohydrate.

White bread and beans are two very different foods and on different ends of the glycemic spectrum. Although very little research has been done on replacing saturated fat with different classes of carbohydrate foods, one study has evaluated heart attack risk relative to intake of saturated fat and carbohydrate foods that have either a low glycemic index or a high glycemic index.[10]

The researchers followed more than fifty thousand people for twelve years and found that replacement of saturated fat with high-glycemic-index (GI) carbohydrates increased heart attack risk by 33 percent (see the graph opposite), but replacement of saturated fat with low-glycemic-index carbohydrates decreased risk. It makes sense that refined carbohydrates would increase risk, since they increase triglycerides and small LDL particles and promote insulin resistance.[11] Several studies have associated higher dietary glycemic index or glycemic load with a greater risk of cardiovascular disease.[12]

> Polyunsaturated and monounsaturated fats are a bit better for you than saturated fats, but this does not make them *good* for you.

Studies show that unsaturated fats are not as bad as saturated fats, but we have to be careful here because the oil derived from these unsaturated fats is not a health food. I discuss this more later, but for now the key is this: It is the reduction of foods high in saturated fat and the replacement of them with vegetables, beans, nuts, and seeds that demonstrates marked benefits. In other words, whole nuts and seeds have powerful cholesterol-lowering and cardiovascular benefits compared

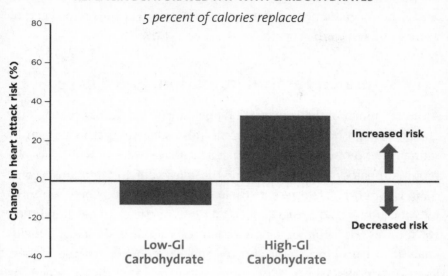

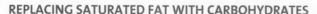

REPLACING SATURATED FAT WITH CARBOHYDRATES

5 percent of calories replaced

with the fats extracted from those foods (the oils). These study subjects consumed processed oils to increase unsaturated fat intake, so the full benefit of replacing saturated fat–rich animal foods with whole plant foods was not measured or realized. Plus, nuts and seeds have been shown to offer additional cardiovascular and life span benefits not related to their effects on lowering cholesterol.

These studies, and the way they were reported by the press, not only confused people, but they also obscured the dangers of high-glycemic carbohydrates. The interesting learning point here is that some of these studies suggest that refined carbohydrates are actually *worse* than saturated fats for the heart.[13]

Which is *the* worst doesn't really matter, except in reinforcing the dietary admonition to stay away from white bread, white rice, sugar, and sweeteners—all of which can increase the risk of heart disease. It's too bad that it is not headline-grabbing to say that to protect against heart disease, nuts and seeds should be a major source of dietary fat. Several clinical studies have observed beneficial effects of diets high in raw nuts to lower LDL cholesterol levels.[14] For example, in one study using a diet rich in nuts and seeds and vegetables, LDL cholesterol was lowered 33 percent in just six weeks.[15] But more importantly, nuts and seeds have been demonstrated to offer a dramatic degree of protection against sudden cardiac death.[16]

Saturated Fat, Inflammation, and Cancer

Although much of the conversation about saturated fat has centered on cholesterol and heart disease, evidence also suggests that foods rich in saturated fat promote cancer. Saturated fats have been shown to provoke proinflammatory gene expression, the release of inflammatory compounds, or both.[17] Two recent studies found associations between saturated fat intake and breast cancer, and one of these studies implicated red meat as the saturated fat–rich food responsible.[18] Similarly, a meta-analysis of thirty-five studies on the subject reported that the highest levels of saturated fat intake in women were associated with a 19 percent increase in breast cancer risk. This analysis also implicated meat.[19]

Eating saturated fat increases the storage of visceral fat in your body. One study fed participants muffins to make them gain weight; those who ate muffins made with palm oil (saturated) gained more visceral fat than those who ate muffins made with sunflower oil (polyunsaturated).[20] Researchers have also found more visceral fat in subjects who ate butter (saturated).[21]

To develop an optimal diet, one has to simultaneously consider thousands of studies on human nutrition, including the awareness that saturated fat–rich diets also promote insulin resistance, which is a contributing factor to developing diabetes, heart disease, and cancer.[22] Red and processed meats also contain a significant amount of arachidonic acid, an omega-6 fatty acid shown to increase risk of breast tumors in animals by promoting inflammation.[23] Another consideration is that animal protein itself also increases the risk of cancer by increasing circulating levels of IGF-1, which promotes tumor growth.[24]

Inflammation is also increased by carnitine (in red meat) and choline (in eggs, dairy, and meat) because they are metabolized by gut bacteria into a proinflammatory compound called trimethylamine-N-oxide (TMAO), and chronic inflammation is known to contribute to cardiovascular disease and cancer.[25] Well-done red meat and processed meat also expose us to dietary carcinogens such as heterocyclic amines and N-nitroso compounds.[26] In addition, red meat contains large amounts of heme iron, which promotes oxidative stress—another contributor to cardiovascular disease and cancer.[27] This is one of the reasons why more meat in the diet enhances LDL oxidation, and higher iron levels in the blood correlate with higher heart disease death.[28]

Oxidation of LDL cholesterol is an early and important step in the development of cardiovascular disease and one of the reasons that antioxidant-rich foods are protective.[29]

Meat and Butter Are Not Health Foods

Proponents of meat-heavy diets are incorrect when they say that there is no clear link between red meat intake and cardiovascular disease. The Nurses' Health Study was one of many studies that implicated both full-fat dairy and red meat in increasing heart disease risk. Also in the Nurses' Health Study, replacing one daily serving of red meat with one daily serving of nuts was associated with a 30 percent reduction in risk of CAD.[30]

In addition, there is a significant link between red meat intake and stroke. An analysis reporting on five studies of red and processed meat in a diet and stroke risk found substantial increases in ischemic stroke risk (the most common type of stroke): For each 100-gram increment of red meat eaten daily, risk rose 13 percent. Similarly, there was a 13 percent increase in risk for every 50-gram increment of processed meat eaten daily.[31] Moreover, red meat intake has an indisputable link to colon cancer.[32]

Full-fat dairy products are additional major sources of saturated fat in the SAD. Seventy percent of the fat in milk is saturated, and dairy fat also contains some naturally occurring *trans* fat.[33] Substantial evidence from human trials shows that whole milk and butter intake increase total and LDL cholesterol.[34] Evidence also links higher intake of dairy products to prostate and ovarian cancers.[35] The key to preventing and reversing cardiovascular disease is to eat foods that have positive benefits, avoiding all negative influences. It is important to remember that all dietary insults are cumulative and can prevent recovery.

The Importance of Nuts and Seeds
to Heart Health

Nuts and seeds are heart warming!
They are rich in nutrients, protect against
heart disease, and reverse disease.

Epidemiological studies have consistently shown that nut consumption is beneficial for heart health. Eating five or more servings of nuts per week is estimated to reduce the risk of CAD by 35 percent.[36] Long-term studies have shown that eating nuts and seeds protects against sudden cardiac death, reduces total and LDL cholesterol and inflammation, and is also associated with longevity.[37] A 2010 review pooled the data from twenty-five clinical studies that compared a nut-eating group with a control group: It was shown that eating 1, 1.5, and 2.4 ounces of nuts per day was associated with a reduction in LDL cholesterol of 4.2 percent, 4.9 percent, and 7.4 percent, respectively.[38] Similarly, substantial evidence from human trials shows that avocado consumption improves blood lipid levels.[39]

It is true that many people have inappropriately maligned fat. Some have even suggested that nuts are an unhealthy or unfavorable food because of their high fat content. However, recent cumulative evidence unequivocally points to the fact that frequent consumption of nuts protects against heart disease and promotes longevity.

The best and largest cohort studies in nutritional epidemiology, such as the Adventist Health Study, the Iowa Women's Health Study, the Nurses' Health Study, the Physicians' Health Study, and the CARE Study all confirm that eating nuts and seeds is associated with a 30–50 percent decreased risk of CAD death, primarily sudden cardiac death, and dramatic decreases in all-cause mortality.

Not only did the Nurses' Health Study demonstrate that nuts substituted for carbohydrate foods reduced cardiac death by 30 percent, but even more compelling was the fact that the substitution of nut fat for saturated fat was associated with a 45 percent reduction in heart disease death. Researchers concluded that "given the strong scientific evidence for the beneficial effects of nuts, it seems justifiable to move nuts to a more prominent place in the United States Department of Agriculture Food Guide Pyramid." Nuts and seeds have been linked to protection from cardiovascular disease in hundreds of studies. Even in those that include various dietary patterns and different ethnicities, there is no controversy regarding the protective effects of nuts and seeds.[40]

Nuts and seeds grow on deep-rooted trees and are naturally packaged in protective shells. They retain their nutrients well after being picked, and their rich mineral, fiber, flavonoid, and sterol contents result in about half the heart attack rate in regular consumers of nuts compared with nonconsumers.[41] The majority of today's evidence simply does not support the idea that there is a health or therapeutic advantage of extreme fat restriction by excluding seeds and nuts from a diet in an effort to lower weight, improve diabetic parameters, or reverse heart disease.

For example, in the Physicians' Health Study, which followed 21,454 male physicians for seventeen years, the most dramatic relationship between any food and survival was the reduced mortality associated with nut consumption two or more times per week compared with no consumption of nuts or seeds. In this study, nuts and seeds had antiarrhythmic and antiseizure effects and were associated with a 60 percent reduction in sudden cardiac death.[42] These benefits are not limited to meat-eating populations; significant life span benefits are seen in nut-eating vegans as well. In the oldest Seventh-Day Adventists (older than 84) a 39 percent decrease in heart disease death was demonstrated when researchers compared those people with higher nut/seed intake (five times weekly) with those with lower nut/seed intake.[43]

When you include more calories from nuts and seeds in your diet, you reduce high-glycemic calories, further increasing their therapeutic potential and leading to further reductions in hemoglobin A1c and lipids.[44] Observational studies on this topic demonstrate that people who eat nuts regularly tend to have a lower BMI than those who don't eat nuts and more weight loss compared with equal calories of carbohydrates in the diet.[45]

Interventional studies corroborate these findings. For example, a study demonstrated a 62 percent greater reduction in BMI and 50 percent greater reduction in waist circumference in a group given nuts instead of more carbohydrates.[46] The main reasons that nuts contribute to weight maintenance are because they make you feel full and they increase the oxidation of fat. Also, all of their calories are not accessible for absorption (15–20 percent are lost), which increases stool fat.[47]

This is a very interesting issue because eating nuts, even though they are high in fat, decreases fat absorption to such a degree that it can substantially lower the fat digested and absorbed from one's total diet. One recent study determined that when the stool fat loss from eating nuts is considered, the usable calories from an ounce of almonds amount to only 129, not the 170 calories they actually contain.[48] These researchers demonstrated that previous studies underestimated the amount of nonabsorbable fat from nuts, leading to overestimates in the caloric content of nuts by about 32 percent. They also demonstrated that some fats from other foods are not absorbed as well after nuts are eaten, further diminishing available calories.

It has been shown repeatedly that nuts and seeds do a lot to enhance your health, as you can see from all the research that supports this list showing that nuts and seeds do the following:

Lower cholesterol[49]

Lower triglycerides[50]

Prevent gallstones[51]

Prevent or improve diabetes[52]

Lower blood pressure[53]

Lower body weight and body fat[54]

Prevent stroke[55]

Prevent dementia[56]

Prevent cancer[57]

Reduce all-cause mortality and extend life span[58]

The Adventist Health Study confirmed that nut consumption was one of the most dramatic features accounting for extended life span benefits, a variable producing a greater benefit than being a vegan.[59] In other words, vegans generally lived the longest, but only if they ate seeds and nuts regularly. Those vegans who did not eat nuts and seeds did not live as long as the intermittent meat eater (flexitarian) who ate them. Nuts alone account for a 5.6-year difference in life span in the Adventist Health Study data, meaning that people who did not regularly eat nuts and seeds lived shorter lives.

Multiple potential mechanisms exist for the life span benefits of nuts and seeds, including the effects of polyphenols, sterols, vitamin E fragments, nitric oxide promoters, and cancer inhibitors as well as enhanced micronutrient absorption of phytonutrients from other foods due to eating nuts and seeds in the same meal.

Over the past twenty-five years while treating thousands of patients who suffered from high blood pressure, diabetes, and advanced heart disease, I have observed marked benefits from including these foods in their diets. Excluding nuts and seeds in favor of more low- or mid-quality carbohydrates is undoubtedly unfavorable for those medically or metabolically challenged with chronic disease and would presumably increase mortality risk. For maximum benefits, you should incorporate nuts and seeds into meals, rather than having them merely as a snack. (In the rare case of the individual who consumes them excessively, rather than for replacement calories, their use would need to be curtailed, as discussed in Chapter 8.)

Oil Is Not a Whole, Natural Food and Does Not Grow on Trees

Although vegetable oils (such as olive, sesame, soybean, and canola oils) are relatively low in saturated fat and higher in unsaturated fats, you should use these processed foods minimally or not at all. Oils lack the beneficial factors that whole nuts and seeds contain. Nuts and seeds contain fiber, minerals, antioxidants, and other phytochemicals in addition to healthy fats that contribute to cardiovascular health.[60] Most of these nutrients are missing in refined oils. It has been noted that the effect of nuts on LDL cholesterol is greater than that which would be predicted on the basis of their fatty acid profile (which is what is in the oil). Also, regularly using oils promotes weight gain and could lead to an excess of omega-6 fatty acids, which can be a problem.

All oils, including olive oil, contain 120 calories per tablespoon, and those tablespoons of fat calories can add up fast. Ounce for ounce, oil is one of the most fattening, calorically dense foods on the planet. It packs more calories per pound (4,020) than butter (3,200). Oil will add fat to already plump waistlines, heightening the risk of disease, including diabetes, heart disease, and cancer.

Certainly, it is better to use olive oil rather than butter or margarine, but it can still sabotage your successful weight-loss results. Using oil in the preparation of meals makes losing weight more difficult, and many people will not lose weight at all. A small amount of olive oil would be acceptable in an otherwise high-nutrient diet, if someone is also thin and physically active. However, for many overweight individuals, oil adds another 300 to 700 calories to the daily menu. These low-nutrient calories impede the goal of achieving superior health and weight loss, especially when seeds and nuts are the preferable source of fat calories. To continue to eat foods prepared in oil and maintain a healthful, slender figure, dieters must carefully count calories and eat tiny portions—not something I recommend because it cycles dieters back to the typical formula for failure of trying to eat thimble-size portions of food.

Along the same lines, eating beet sugar does not have the same biological effects as eating a beet. One is dangerous because the nutrients and fibers have been removed, and the other supports health. Like the beet sugar, oil is a processed food; the nutrients and fiber have been removed. Consuming walnut oil has a different biological effect than eating whole walnuts. Sesame seed oil has a different biological effect compared with eating sesame seeds. Olive oil contains few nutrients (except a little vitamin E) and a negligible amount of phytochemical compounds compared with the calories supplied. All oils are rapidly absorbed and enter the bloodstream so quickly and with such concentration that they cannot be burned for energy and are therefore stored as fat. The average American consumes about 400 calories from fattening oil a day—a large contributor to high body fat in oil-consuming populations.

Nuts and seeds contain fewer calories per tablespoon than oil, and their fat calories are not all absorbed. Some of the fats in nuts and seeds stay bound to the fibers and pass into the stool. The rest of the fats are slowly absorbed, satiating hunger and encouraging fatty acid oxidation, meaning they are burned for energy. They are rich in sterols, stanols, fibers, minerals, lignans, and other health-promoting nutrients. Numerous scientific studies link them to a slimmer waistline and longer life span, especially for prevention of heart disease and cancer.[61] Eating even a small amount of nuts or seeds helps you feel satiated, stay with your eating program, and have more success at long-term weight loss. Seeds give you all the advantages of nuts, plus more. They are generally higher in protein than nuts and have many additional important nutrients, such as omega-3 fats and anticancer lignans.

Oils, like other processed foods, have their fibers and most nutrients removed, are weight-promoting, and do not have the health benefits of seeds and nuts.[62] In fact, a recent study compared a traditional Mediterranean diet with one that substituted nuts for the oil and found that atherosclerotic plaque regressed only in the diet containing the nuts; it did not regress in the control diet or oil-heavy Mediterranean diet.[63]

The Mediterranean diet was further evaluated in Spain, where 7,216 men and women were randomized to include either nuts or olive oil in their diets. The nut group, which consumed more than three servings of nuts a week, had a 39 percent reduced all-cause mortality (compared with the oil users) over the average 4.8 years of follow-up.[64] You will find that in the Nutritarian program the delicious texture and flavor of whole nuts and seeds are used to make dressings and sauces that taste even better than oil-based dressings and sauces. Best of all, the result is superior health.

Walnuts, Hemp Seeds, Chia Seeds, and Flaxseeds Are Strongly Recommended

Walnuts, hemp seeds, chia seeds, and flaxseeds have the most favorable omega-3 content of all nuts and seeds. I believe that everyone should eat these superfoods every day. Walnuts in particular have been associated with a host of positive biological effects, such as improved cardiovascular parameters, enhanced brain viability with aging, reduced cardiovascular deaths, and longer life span. They have even been shown to prevent aging of the brain by reducing the oxidant load on brain cells and improving nerve cell–to–nerve cell signaling and neurogenesis.[65] There is no question that including walnuts in a cardio-reversal protocol is valuable.

Studies have also shown that walnuts remove cholesterol from the body, lower LDL cholesterol and triglycerides, and increase HDL cholesterol.[66] They also lower LDL particle number and serum glucose, both very favorable features for cardiac protection. Furthermore, they have been shown to increase endothelial function and enhance vascular elasticity.[67] No other food or medicine can do even a few of these things, yet walnuts do all of them simultaneously.

The omega-3 alpha-linolenic acid content of flaxseeds, hemp seeds, chia seeds, and walnuts is also beneficial. Omega-3 fatty acids have clear benefits for cardiovascular health.[68] Omega-3 and omega-6 fatty acids regulate the inflammatory response, and although some omega-6 fat is necessary, evidence suggests that excessive intake of omega-6 and low intake of omega-3 (characteristic of Western diets with added cooking oils) may promote a chronic inflammatory state that contributes to cardiovascular disease and cancer. Higher omega-6 intake has been linked to increased cancer risk, whereas higher omega-3 intake is often linked to decreased risk.[69] Keep in mind: though the excess omega-6 from oils is stored in the body, the omega-6 in nuts and seeds should be burned off for energy, therefore, unless one is overeating, they would not contribute to omega-6 excess in the body's tissues. I recommend that about half of your nut and seed intake come from these higher–omega-3 nuts and seeds, specifically flaxseeds, hemp seeds, chia seeds, and walnuts.

FLAXSEEDS DRAMATICALLY LOWER HIGH BLOOD PRESSURE

Eating more fruits and vegetables lowers blood pressure and reduces the risk of stroke.[70] People can avoid the risky side effects of prescription drugs to lower blood pressure by eating natural foods that are effective at lowering blood pressure, such as tomato paste, pomegranates, and berries.[71] But the food with the most powerful ability in this arena are flaxseeds, because their blood pressure–lowering effectiveness has been shown to exceed that of most medications.

A prospective double-blind placebo-controlled randomized trial gave people 30 grams of flaxseeds in their regular food. Six months later, these people were found to have systolic blood pressure lowered by 10 mmHg and diastolic blood pressure by 7 mmHg; for those with elevated systolic blood pressure (above 140 mmHg), those in the flaxseed-eating group saw a drop of 15 mmHg compared with those not eating flax.[72]

Most drugs do not lower blood pressure this much, and it is important to note that studies on natural foods that lower blood pressure also show a reduction in stroke risk that drugs cannot replicate. For example, another study that followed more than one thousand middle-aged men for more than twelve years found a greater than 55 percent reduction in overall stroke and a 59 percent reduction in ischemic stroke (the most common type) with a higher intake of tomato products.[73] Plus, the synergistic combination of flaxseeds, other seeds and nuts, tomatoes, and berries in the diet is even more powerful than each one alone.

High Cholesterol Is Not Harmless

It cannot be denied that exposure to higher amounts of saturated fat raises cholesterol levels; too many studies document this relationship. However, some saturated fat and cholesterol skeptics believe and promote the idea that high cholesterol does not matter. The people with this alternative agenda who try to exonerate meat and saturated fat seek out observational studies, with only minor differences in dietary quality, that weaken the association between diet and death. Although it is impossible to deny the connection between the consumption of animal products and high cholesterol, such cholesterol skeptics make an effort to deny that animal products and high cholesterol play a significant role in increasing a person's risk of developing heart disease and dying from heart disease.

One of the strategies they use to persuade people that it is okay to eat more butter, cheese, and meat is to argue that LDL cholesterol is not a good marker for disease risk because the oxidized version of LDL (ox-LDL) is the true "bad" cholesterol. They also claim that those people who have low cholesterol have a higher risk of death from certain causes such as cancer. Neither of these claims holds up to scientific scrutiny.

It has become abundantly clear over the past decade that ox-LDL is more important than native LDL in atherogenesis (the process of plaque formation in the inner lining of arteries). The oxidant state and the formation of ox-LDL not only promote plaque but also are strong factors in plaque instability and acute coronary syndromes.[74] However, it is the consumption of vegetables and nuts that lowers ox-LDL and oxidation in general, not the consumption of fat and meat products. In fact, diets low in oils and saturated fats have been shown to reduce LDL oxidation.[75] Similarly, diets that include nuts and seeds also lower LDL oxidation because of the phenolic antioxidants and other beneficial compounds they contain.[76]

Cholesterol skeptics can make these claims because ox-LDL could get a bit worse with less saturated fat and more refined carbohydrates and polyunsaturated oils in the diet. Saturated fats may be more resistant to oxidation than polyunsaturated oils, but you don't get ox-LDL to optimal levels unless you almost eliminate both oils and saturated fats from the diet. It is important to note that the high-fat, high–meat-and-butter advocates and the cholesterol skeptics never can show that their preferred diet is safe or protective against heart disease; they merely point to the fact that the standard, and outdated, dietary guidelines to cut back on saturated fat do not offer significant protection against heart disease.

So the minor differences in oxidation that occur from switching one type of fat for another do not lead to a viable solution for the prevention of heart disease. Instead, we have to eat primarily plant produce, eliminate oil and most animal products from our diets, and use nuts and seeds as our primary source of fat. Just because a study can show that ox-LDL can worsen as saturated fats are decreased and more refined carbohydrates are consumed does not mean that the disease-causing ox-LDL can be reduced to safe levels by eating more saturated fat. The only way to reduce ox-LDL to safe levels and to prevent and even reverse heart disease and open up clogged arteries is to eat a diet of high-antioxidant-containing produce.

We likely will always find some vocal people who want to believe anything, no matter how unsubstantiated, so they can rationalize why they don't need to change their diets and can continue to eat their pre-ferred foods with abandon. Unfortunately, the gravity of this irrespon-sible messaging is significant, and such people perpetuate the epidemic of heart disease and cancer in this country, creating needless deaths in those whom they influence.

The fact is, even slightly higher cholesterol levels maintained for many years can damage a person's heart and increase risk of prema-ture death. Because a high cholesterol level reflects an unhealthy di-etary pattern, it does not necessarily mean that drugs designed to lower cholesterol will lessen mortality in such people, because they still are eating the unhealthy diet. In addition, we don't really know all of the negative effects that will accumulate from medications taken through-out most of a person's adult life.

Consider this important study that tracked about fifteen hundred people at age 55 who had lived with eleven to twenty years of high cholesterol.[77] Researchers followed these adults for up to twenty years past age 55 to see how their high cholesterol affected their risk of heart disease. The results showed that for every ten years a person had high cholesterol early in life, the risk of heart disease death for that person doubled. Those whose cholesterol was elevated for eleven to twenty years had quadruple the risk of heart disease death compared with those who had low cholesterol levels. The researchers defined high cholesterol conservatively as an LDL higher than 130 mg/dl. The cho-lesterol skeptics have no leg to stand on. The researchers concluded: "The duration of time a person has high cholesterol increases a per-son's risk of heart disease above and beyond the risk posed by their current cholesterol level. Adults with the highest duration of exposure to high cholesterol had a four-fold increased risk of heart disease, compared with adults who did not have high cholesterol."

The data from this study showed that for every ten years a person has borderline elevated cholesterol (LDL between 120 and 130 mg/dl), the risk of heart disease increases by nearly 40 percent. Many other studies confirm these findings and document increased heart-related deaths, and also increased overall mortality, for people who have high cholesterol levels for many years.[78] In fact, researchers who conducted a 2011 study that followed participants for forty-six years concluded the following:

> A strong and graded relation was found between the cholesterol level and total mortality, with the men with a cholesterol level ≤4 mmol/L (154 mg/dl) having the lowest mortality. In all, the men with the lowest cholesterol gained the most life years. However, no association was found with the cholesterol level in the year 2000 (when 16% were using statins) and subsequent mortality. The lowest (≤4 mmol/L) cholesterol value in midlife also predicted a higher score in the physical functioning scale of RAND-36 in old age. In conclusion, a low total cholesterol value in midlife predicts both better survival and better physical functioning in old age.[79]

This tells us that achieving lower cholesterol levels near the end of life with the use of statin drugs did not correlate with increased life span. However, *earning* a low cholesterol level through healthy eating earlier in life did not merely extend life span, but also offered a better quality of life. Cholesterol levels typically drop toward the end of life as our health deteriorates, making it appear erroneously as if there is a relationship between lower cholesterol and death; this confuses the clear relationship between high cholesterol throughout life and increased risk of premature death.

The risks of high cholesterol cannot be denied. However, taking a cholesterol-lowering drug starting at age 70 is not going to offer significant protection for someone who has eaten poorly for seventy years and continues to eat poorly. Cholesterol-lowering drugs started late in life have only a limited effect on protecting against future cardiac events. Cholesterol skeptics use cholesterol levels near death to show that even people with treated lower cholesterol levels still have high rates of cardiac deaths. However, every study that considered cholesterol level over many years shows an excellent correlation between higher cholesterol levels maintained for a large segment of life and an early cardiac death.

The only conclusion is that for optimal protection and maximum life span, we need to eat healthfully and *start* eating healthfully as early in life as possible.

Egg Consumption, Cholesterol, and Diabetes

Eggs are a confusing and difficult food to analyze, because they are very high in cholesterol. Thus they bring forth strong opinions on both sides of the issue. We know that eating cholesterol does not raise blood cholesterol as much as eating saturated fat, but as we've seen, that does not make it harmless. I am always amazed by the definitive statements people make about complicated nutritional issues without carefully reviewing all of the scientific literature and evidence. The efforts to promote eggs as healthful and without risk certainly demonstrate the effectiveness of the food industry and the aligned interest of others who want to exonerate the risk associated with their preferred foods. But an unbiased look at the evidence demonstrates otherwise.

When we review recent studies conducted on eggs and scrutinize the data, we see that the most carefully done studies—with adequate control of confounding variables and with the largest number of participants—show that egg consumption increases the risk of cardiovascular diseases in a dose-response manner, especially in patients with diabetes. This means that the more eggs eaten, the higher the risk. For overweight individuals, the risk of developing diabetes goes up considerably with egg consumption. This was the conclusion of a recent meta-analysis that pooled the results of fourteen studies involving 320,778 individuals; it demonstrated a 30–40 percent increased risk of cardiovascular death for diabetics with higher egg intake.[80]

The results of this meta-analysis were further supported by another 2013 meta-analysis which indicated that for people with diabetes, the risk of CAD was 54 percent higher in those in the highest category of egg intake.[81] The most significant and largest long-term studies examining this issue were ominous and certainly did not exonerate eggs. The Physicians' Health Study and Women's Health Study followed more than twenty thousand men (mean follow-up, 20 years) and thirty-six thousand women (mean follow-up, 11.7 years), respectively. A study combining data from these prospective investigations found that men eating seven or more eggs per week were 58 percent more likely to be diagnosed with type 2 diabetes, and women 77 percent.[82]

Another 2013 meta-analysis pooled findings from the Cardiovascular Health Study, the Physicians' Health Study, the Women's Health Study, and the Adventist Health Studies. It found that the highest category of egg consumption was associated with a 42 percent increase in diabetes risk. Specifically among diabetic subjects, a 69 percent increase in cardiovascular disease risk was associated with eating one or more eggs a day.[83]

But a small 2015 study showed the opposite. It reported a *decrease* in type 2 diabetes risk associated with increasing egg intake, up to four eggs per week, at which point the protective effect plateaued. Those consuming four eggs a week showed a 38 percent decrease in risk (measured at ten years of follow-up). This study was performed on a population of men in Finland, ages 42–60 at baseline. Scientists have questioned the impact of this study because the group with the higher egg intake was more likely to be younger, with less likelihood of smoking and less heart disease and hypertension; they also had a notably higher fiber and lower carbohydrate intake. With such a healthier cohort, it may not be the four eggs eaten every week that made them healthier. Even the authors acknowledged that replacement of "low-quality carbohydrates" with eggs in this population could be the factor in the findings of reduced risk.[84]

Clearly this small study should be viewed as an outlier, because it is not consistent with all the others demonstrating a real risk from regular egg consumption. Even though fasting cholesterol does not increase substantially due to cholesterol intake, the heightened level of cholesterol in the bloodstream after a meal containing eggs is significant. The authors of a 2010 review on eggs and cardiovascular risk astutely pointed out that we are in a nonfasting state for much of the day and that a meal containing eggs increases blood cholesterol and other lipids and oxidative stress after that meal for many hours, contributing to heart attack risk. They recommend that people with heart disease or who are at risk of heart disease avoid eggs.[85]

It is not just the high cholesterol in egg yolks but also the fact that eggs are high in choline that may ignite a spark of caution. Choline promotes microbial production of TMAO in the gut. This proinflammatory compound is linked to risk of cardiovascular disease in humans and has been shown to drive atherosclerosis in animals.[86] The bottom line is that similar to other animal products, eggs are not without risk and not the food to recommend to people who are overweight, are diabetic, or have heart disease.

Can Cholesterol Be Too Low?

When it comes to CAD, there may be no such thing as total blood cholesterol levels being too low, especially when those low levels are earned by eating healthfully and are not the result of disease. There was some controversy years ago about whether to strive for lower cardioprotective cholesterol levels after several studies in the 1980s noted that depression, suicide, hemorrhagic stroke, cancer, and death from other causes were higher in some groups with very low cholesterol levels. Recent investigations studying larger populations, however, have not confirmed these questionable findings.

When investigators looked more carefully at the individual characteristics of the studied populations, they were able to explain the earlier findings. This issue is complicated because these studies evaluated individuals who were eating the SAD, which is rich in saturated fat and other components of animal products that raise cholesterol and low in plant-derived antioxidants, phytochemicals, and essential fatty acids that improve cholesterol ratios. They found that many people who demonstrated very low cholesterol levels, while following the modern, cholesterol-promoting diet, actually had a compromised health status or undetected chronic disease that caused the low cholesterol level.

For instance, we know that cancer causes the liver to produce less cholesterol. Low cholesterol may be associated with cancer but does not cause it. Researchers showed that cholesterol starts to fall up to eight years before a person dies from cancer. They also demonstrated that people with the greatest drop in cholesterol in a four-year period (who did not improve their diets to lower their cholesterol) were those most likely to develop cancer.[87] The low cholesterol did not cause the cancer; the cancer caused the low cholesterol. Cancer can exist in the body many years before it can be detected or diagnosed. People who work to lower their cholesterol levels by avoiding saturated fats and eating a high-nutrient diet with lots of raw vegetables, cooked green vegetables, and beans do not have a pathological condition causing their low cholesterol. They *earned* it.

This is why in rural China, where people eat nearly a vegetarian diet, average cholesterol levels are very low, as are cancer rates. People with the lowest cholesterol in the China Study actually had the lowest cancer rates as well. Obviously, there is a difference between people who have low cholesterol because their diet-style earns it and those whose cholesterol seems unjustifiably low on a modern heart-disease-promoting diet that almost everyone in the West eats. This demonstrates that low cholesterol is not associated with cancer in those eating a diet that keeps their cholesterol low. Very low cholesterol in a person eating a cholesterol-promoting diet may be a sign of disease, such as cancer, especially if the cholesterol level dropped very low later in life after being high.

As another example, excessive consumption of alcohol and the resultant liver damage lowers cholesterol, too. Men who are heavy drinkers have low blood cholesterol levels. Lung disease, certain types of cancers, and many other illnesses also suppress appetite; and when people eat less, their blood cholesterol levels drop even farther. The earlier studies that showed some increased risks with low cholesterol did not account for the fact that bad health habits and poor health can cause low cholesterol in an unhealthy segment of the population.

There is no evidence to suggest that earning a low blood cholesterol with excellent health habits will increase your risk of disease. Low cholesterol is a sign of good health. But if a person has a very low blood cholesterol level while consuming a diet rich in meat, cheese, and saturated fat, his or her doctor should be alerted to look for a hidden cancer, addiction to alcohol, cigarette or drug use, emotional disorder, or other disease. These illnesses may cause an unearned, very low cholesterol level.

In the past, it was thought to be good enough if a person had a cholesterol level that was better than average. About twenty years ago, doctors advised their patients to strive for a total cholesterol lower than 200 mg/dl. Eventually, this advice was found to be inadequate, and now we know that it is not very good to be average in a population that is so prone to developing atherosclerotic heart disease. On autopsy, almost all American adults demonstrate significant CAD;[88] even 78 percent of young trauma victims who died before the age of 35 demonstrated significant atherosclerosis on autopsy.[89]

If you eat standard American food, you will inevitably develop standard American diseases.

If we want to rival the low cholesterol of populations that eat mostly natural plant foods and do not have heart disease, we must try to attain total cholesterol numbers lower than 150 mg/dl. The average total cholesterol level in rural China, as documented in the Cornell China Study, was 127 mg/dl.[90] Heart attacks were rare, and both cancer and heart disease rates plummeted as cholesterol levels fell, which reflected a very low consumption of animal products. The lowest occurrence of heart disease and cancer occurred in the group that consumed plant-based diets with less than two servings of animal products per week.

It is important to note that some people do have genetically low cholesterol that is not earned by a superior diet; this does not necessarily mean that anything is wrong with their health. It may just be genetics. On the other hand, if your cholesterol is high, you should start to worry because you could be at increased risk for heart attack and cancer. It is imperative that you change your diet immediately. Most people with high cholesterol created those high levels by eating the unhealthy SAD that too many of us still eat.

How Does Saturated Fat Impact Cholesterol?

Some authors and online sources claim that the increase in LDL due to a diet high in saturated fats is unimportant because saturated fat also increases HDL, or the "good" cholesterol. This is not true. Higher HDL may be mildly beneficial, but the lower HDL levels observed with lower amounts of saturated fats in the diet were noted only in those diets that replaced saturated fat with high-glycemic carbohydrates, not monounsaturated and polyunsaturated fats.[91] Multiple studies on using whole nuts and seeds as a major fat source in place of saturated fats have demonstrated dramatic improvements in HDL levels and other cardiovascular parameters.[92]

There are some claims that if a food is high in stearic acid, a particular type of saturated fat, it will not affect cholesterol levels. Different subsets of saturated fat have different effects on cholesterol. Lauric, myristic, and palmitic acids increase total and LDL cholesterol levels, but stearic acid does not.[93] However, since foods containing saturated fat contain a mix of these fatty acids, it isn't possible to consume only one of them. For example, palm shortening, unsweetened chocolate, lamb, veal, and beef tallow are some of the richest sources of stearic acid, but they are also high in palmitic acid.[94] Overall, foods high in saturated fat elevate LDL cholesterol levels.

Another popular claim made by those who aim to justify eating meat and butter is that saturated fat does not increase the small, dense LDL particles that are considered more dangerous than larger LDL particles.[95] A study of men following either a low- or high-saturated-fat diet for six weeks found that higher saturated fat was associated with larger LDL particles and higher total LDL cholesterol levels.[96]

A similar study started with two weeks of a high-saturated-fat diet and then switched to the use of olive oil, canola oil, or sunflower oil for four weeks. A small reduction in LDL particle size was seen with all three oils compared with the high-saturated-fat diet. However, even the authors of this study reported that these small changes did not lessen disease risk and that the slight tendency toward larger LDL particles did not offset any of the risk associated with the overall increase in LDL due to increased saturated fat intake.[97] It is important to recognize that diets high in refined carbohydrates increase small, dense LDL via elevating plasma triglycerides.[98] Minimizing the intake of refined carbohydrates to keep triglycerides in the favorable range is most likely the best way to reduce small, dense LDL particles. In other words, these arguments do *not* show that eating more fat is healthful but merely demonstrate the dangers of high-glycemic, refined carbohydrates— and with that there is no debate.

What About Plant Saturated Fats, Like Coconut?

Another common question is whether plant sources of saturated fat, such as coconut, are as harmful as animal sources, such as red meat. Coconut and palm fats do raise total and LDL cholesterol levels. In one study, participants ate a diet containing equal amounts of total fat from coconut (rich in saturated fat), walnuts (rich in polyunsaturated fat), or almonds (rich in monounsaturated fat) for three weeks each; blood cholesterol was measured after each diet phase. Total cholesterol was 7 percent and 5 percent lower with the almond and walnut diets, respectively, compared with the coconut diet; LDL was 10 percent and 9 percent lower. HDL cholesterol was unchanged.[99] This means that eating coconut oil and even coconut does not offer the metabolic and cardiovascular benefits that walnuts and almonds do.

With the widespread awareness of the dangers of *trans* fat, some packaged foods have relied on palm oil, a highly saturated fat, to replicate the functional characteristics of hydrogenated oils. Palm oil has been shown to have similar effects on total and LDL cholesterol levels as *trans* fat (partially hydrogenated soybean oil).[100] Although coconut and palm oils may not be as bad as fat from butter and meat, you should not consider them to be health foods.

However, saturated fat and LDL cholesterol should not be viewed in a vacuum. Other heart disease–promoting qualities accompany the saturated fat exposure in meat, including harmful exposure to excess carnitine, iron, and animal protein without fiber and protective phytochemicals and phytates. So clearly, the exposure to some saturated fat in coconut does not have the same overall cardiovascular risk as that of saturated fat–rich meats.

At the same time, these questions are almost irrelevant, because as we've seen, all oils are calorically dense and fattening compared with the whole foods from which they are extracted. Oils efficiently spike caloric intake upward when used liberally in cooking. Remember, coconut—and especially coconut oil—has never been shown to lower blood pressure, lower cholesterol, encourage reversal of heart disease, or reduce cardiac death, as we have seen with nuts and seeds, particularly walnuts.

Don't sabotage your weight-loss goal with oily dressings and sauces.

Vegetables and salads are very low in calories. However, if you cover these healthy low-calorie foods with a few tablespoons of a high-fat, high-calorie, oil-based dressing, you turn vegetables and salads into weight-promoting foods. I know you have been told that olive oil is healthy food, but in reality, it is not. Keep in mind, oil is processed food; it is not a natural whole food. Oils, even if they are monounsaturated, should not be considered health food because they are low in nutrients and contain 120 calories per tablespoon, promoting weight gain.

Sure, olive oil and almond oil are improvements over animal fats and margarine, but they still contribute to our overweight modern world. Overweight Americans consume an average of 3 tablespoons of oil in their daily diets, commonly adding an extra 250–500 calories to their food intake each day. You need to reach a thinner, ideal weight to achieve maximum protection against and to reverse heart disease. Use oil, even olive oil, sparingly or not at all; certainly, do not have more than 1 teaspoon per day.

As an alternative to oil, you can make great-tasting salad dressings from raw nuts and seeds, such as walnuts, pecans, cashews, sunflower seeds, sesame seeds, pistachios, and avocados. I recommend these nut- and seed-based salad dressings instead of those based on refined oils because they help ensure that we get these "good" fats delivered along with their antioxidants and phytochemicals and other health-supporting benefits. Remember, the key is to use nuts and seeds to *replace* the oil used in salad dressings, sauces, and dips, not *in addition to* it. Plus, these nuts and seeds function as low-glycemic replacement calories that are beneficial for diabetics and people who are overweight and can replace all the meat, cheese, butter, and refined carbohydrates that people were eating before.

I often mix fresh fruit with a little vinegar and a small amount of nuts or seeds to make delicious, heart-healthy, nutrient-rich dressings. I include many of my favorite dressing recipes in Chapter 9.

The Take-Home Message About Fat

The bottom line is this: Americans still need to eat more wholesome plant foods and fewer animal products and oils. Saturated fats have not been shown to be safe and healthy, so we should minimize in our diets those foods that are rich in saturated fat. The major source of fat intake in our diets should be seeds and nuts, not meat, dairy, butter, and cheese. We should eat less saturated fat–rich food in favor of more beans, intact whole grains, vegetables, nuts, and seeds. We also should pay attention to increasing our omega-3 fat intake by including chia seeds, flaxseeds, hemp seeds, and walnuts in our diets. Finally, we should avoid excess omega-6 fatty acid by limiting our intake of animal fats and cooking oils.

CHAPTER SIX

Salt Is a
Four-Letter Word

There's table salt, sea salt, Celtic salt, Peruvian Pink, Hawaiian Black Lava, Himalayan, and *fleur de sel*. But whatever marketers call it, whatever it costs, and whatever its pedigree, salt is simply sodium chloride (NaCl)—and despite trendy claims to the contrary, it's bad for you.

The excessive level of sodium in the modern American diet has caused an epidemic of high blood pressure. This high blood pressure is dangerous, because it puts a strain on the heart muscle and can lead to ischemic or hemorrhagic stroke, kidney damage, heart attack, or cancer. The human body was designed to get its optimal level of sodium from a natural diet, but most Americans consume about *six times* what they need.

Avoiding processed foods and excess salt doesn't have to mean that you're condemned to a life of bland food. When you dial back the salt, your palate readjusts, and you start to taste and appreciate the wonder of natural flavors. Your heart (and the rest of your internal organs) will reward you with improved health and longevity—and your taste buds will thank you, too.

If you live in the United States, your lifetime probability of developing high blood pressure is around 90 percent.[1] This is a sobering statistic, since high blood pressure increases a person's risk of developing heart disease, as well as kidney failure and stroke. Lowering high blood pressure decreases the risk of stroke and heart failure.

After many years of high salt exposure, blood pressure starts to rise. By the time this occurs, cutting down on salt does not so easily resolve the problem. When high levels of salt are consumed, more fluid is retained in the body and must be carried by the blood vessels, which increases both blood pressure and the load on the heart. With a higher circulatory volume, more pressure is exerted on the blood vessel walls. After decades, the walls react to this stress by thickening, stiffening, and narrowing. Like pushing water through a smaller opening at the end of a hose, this raises resistance and requires higher pressure to move blood to the organs. The heart now has to pump against this high-pressure system.

Lifting heavy weights in the gym causes muscles to become larger. This same phenomenon happens to the heart, with one notable exception: There is no break, no time for the heart muscle to recover from the stress. This 24/7 activity causes the heart to enlarge (called *hypertrophy*) and become more prone to irregular beating (arrhythmia) and heart failure.

High salt intake also promotes scarring of the heart muscle, called *cardiac fibrosis,* which further increases the risk of arrhythmia. More and more mechanisms of damage from salt have become increasingly defined in recent years.[2] Similarly, the kidneys, which each contain around one million tiny, delicate filters comprised of tiny blood vessels, lose their function from the excessive blood pressure. This leads to *hypertensive nephrosclerosis,* a major cause of kidney disease.

Numerous observational studies and randomized controlled trials document the fact that high sodium intake increases blood pressure.[3] The evidence has been called "overwhelming."[4] A recently published large long-term lifestyle intervention study showed that a 25–35 percent reduction in dietary sodium over ten to fifteen years resulted in a 25–30 percent lower risk of cardiovascular problems.[5]

It is estimated that a 50 percent decrease in sodium consumption in the United States could prevent at least 150,000 deaths annually.[6] According to a meta-analysis of sixty-one studies, the lower an individual's blood pressure (at least down to 115/75 mmHg), the lower the risk of stroke or heart attack.[7] There was no threshold below which the risk

CASE HISTORY: PROOF FROM A PATIENT

Even in just two months, I saw incredible results. At the start of Dr. Fuhrman's program, I was overweight with a blood pressure around 160/110, which was difficult to bring down. I took up to five blood pressure medications at the same time and it was still barely normal. I was barely fitting into my 52-inch-waist pants. My cardiologist told me I had developed atrial fibrillation, probably due to severe obstructive sleep apnea.

I read *Eat to Live* and started on the program. Two months later, I had lost 40 pounds and 4 inches off my waist. My blood pressure came under control, and my sleep apnea and atrial fibrillation were gone. The good news is that, except for some lagging energy levels during the first two weeks, it has been nearly effortless. Now, two years later, my blood pressure is excellent with no medications, I don't snore anymore, I have lost a ton of weight, and my heart problems are gone. It is not exaggerating to say that Dr. Fuhrman saved my life.

Jeff Rowan

did not decrease. This steadily decreasing risk of stroke or heart attack is based on the assumption that the lower blood pressure numbers are earned through healthy eating, exercise, and salt avoidance and are not simply medicated downward.

But it is not all about blood pressure. Many different studies show the interesting finding that high salt intake is linked to increases in all-cause mortality and that salt's death-hastening effects occur in people who are not "salt sensitive" to its blood pressure effects.[8] High sodium intake predicts overall mortality and risk of CAD independent of other cardiovascular risk factors, including blood pressure.[9]

How Much Salt Should We Eat?

If we just ate natural foods without added salt, we would most likely consume about 500–750 milligrams of sodium a day. Real food, by which I mean whole food, supplies the perfect amount of minerals people need to maximize their health.

The human body was designed to function on natural food, and early humans did not consume salt. Our Stone Age ancestors ate a diet consisting mainly of fruit, vegetables, nuts, seeds, fish, insects, and wild game. All of the sodium that humans require, as well as the other minerals we need, is present in those natural foods. This eat-what-you-can-find diet continued for approximately one hundred thousand generations, during which time salt was not added to food.

Today, most areas of the world consume ten times as much sodium as would be found in a natural, unsalted diet. Our species developed agriculture around three hundred generations ago. Approximately ten generations ago (starting in the mid-eighteenth century), the Industrial Age changed our diet by revolutionizing the agricultural sector. Farmers learned how to maximize crop output and make meat and dairy more affordable—and available year-round.

What I call the Processed Food Era started just two to three generations ago, after World War I. This was when people started buying convenience foods because commercially baked goods, as well as processed foods made tasty with salt, sugar, and preservatives, became cheap and widely available. But the skyrocketing rates of illness that have been caused by this modern diet demonstrate that our bodies still live with the "thrifty genes" that were selected over a long period, during which our ancestors lived with low salt intake, periods of starvation, and caloric inadequacy.[10] These genes were selected to conserve sodium, not get rid of it.

Almost all Americans, as well as most people in modern industrialized societies, consume excessive amounts of salt. This means that we have to look at isolated or primitive populations to accurately see the long-term outcome of low salt intake.

It is still possible to find pockets of people living on mostly natural-food diets that do not contain added salt. Tribes in New Guinea, the Amazon Basin, the highlands of Malaysia, and rural Uganda all eat very little salt. Hypertension is unheard of in these regions, and blood pressure does not rise steadily with age, as it does in the United States and other countries with high salt intakes. The most elderly members of these populations have blood pressure readings like those we see in children. When salt is introduced into these salt-free cultures, however, blood pressure climbs.[11]

Medical anthropologists know that all people from cultures that do not use salt as a condiment experience almost no increase in blood pressure, even into old age. By contrast, blood pressure rises significantly over many years in all human populations in which salt is added to food in significant quantities. One can easily see that most people who live in societies that add salt to their diet end up with high blood pressure sooner or later.

Some people claim that they are not salt sensitive, because they have low blood pressure even on a high-salt diet. But over years of use, the high salt intake takes its toll, and almost everyone eventually develops high blood pressure. About 70 percent of Americans have hypertension by the time they are in their 60s, and of those who are lucky enough to escape it up to age 65, 90 percent will still develop high blood pressure if they live past 80.[12]

At that point, it is not so easy to cut out the salt and fix all the damage. For maximal disease prevention, sodium levels should probably be less than 1,000 mg/day—which is about the normal level for our biological needs. Ultimately, high-sodium diets lead to high blood pressure, which causes an estimated two-thirds of strokes and almost half of all heart attacks.

According to the National Institutes of Health, consuming less sodium is one of the most important ways to prevent cardiovascular disease.[13] Certainly, maintaining a healthy, slim body weight, eating a nutrient-dense diet rich in vegetables and fruits, and not smoking are also critical factors in preventing disease. But lowering sodium intake is equally important, because a high level of sodium in the diet ranks as a primary killer in our modern, toxic food environment. Most people overlook this fact until it is too late.

Most of the world's population today consumes 2,300–4,600 milligrams of sodium daily (1–2 teaspoons of salt). Average adult sodium intake in the United States is around 4,000 milligrams for every 2,000 calories consumed. The average American consumes more than 2,500 calories a day. Natural foods contain less than half a milligram of sodium per calorie. If you are trying to keep the sodium in your diet to a safe level, avoid foods that have more sodium than calories per serving. It would be impossible to consume too much sodium if you ate a healthy diet of real food in its natural state. Except for some sodium-wasting medical conditions or rare individuals, it would be unusual for anyone to require more sodium than is present in real food in its natural state.

Cutting out salt is so important because it can usually lead to high blood pressure being reversed without drugs. Even the Centers for Disease Control and Prevention reports that salt and high blood pressure kill far more Americans than tobacco (or anything else).[14] Almost 70 percent of all Americans, including everyone older than 40, should cut their salt intake by nearly two-thirds, to 1,500 milligrams.

Medications cannot do nearly what diet improvement and salt reduction can do. More and more physicians and scientists have begun to recognize this. Just cutting out salt can return the blood pressure to normal in most cases, which can reduce the risk of heart disease by at least 70 percent.

Is More Salt Good for You?—The Latest "News"

You may have read recent articles in some newspapers or Internet sites about studies questioning the need for people to watch their salt intake. These articles claim that it is more longevity-promoting to eat *more* salt, not less. An editorial in the *New England Journal of Medicine* questioned the accuracy of the data and admitted that this new information, released in 2014, undermines current recommendations to reduce salt intake.[15]

It is clear that salt interests and processed food manufacturers contribute to, and support, those who deny that salt is dangerous. It is also clear that they fund scientific studies in an attempt to demonstrate that salt intake is not a disease risk. Clearest of all is the fact that they will continue to do so.

In other words, even though hundreds of studies confirm and demonstrate increased blood pressure with increased salt intake, mysteriously, in this new study, these higher blood pressures did not translate into a higher risk of heart disease and strokes. The study suggests that using less salt can even make things worse.[16] It seems that just as we are gaining a bit of traction in encouraging healthier behaviors, a "study" comes along to tell people that they might as well give up and go back to eating whatever they want. They are told that nothing matters. Just as with the saturated fat fiasco (discussed in Chapter 5), something fishy is going on here.

Whenever you see study results claiming that consuming butter, salt, sugar, and animal fat is good for you, rather than bad, you must look carefully at how the researchers arrived at this conclusion and what the overwhelming preponderance of evidence shows. Remember, there are always deniers who can be very popular and who can write books claiming that what you eat doesn't matter.

Of the recent studies that led to the misleading findings on salt, two of them used data from the ongoing Prospective Urban Rural Epidemiology (PURE) study.[17] These two 2014 studies, let's call them Study A (salt) and Study B (potassium), estimated sodium and potassium intake on the basis of a single morning urine collection. Then the subjects were followed for an average of only 3.7 years, which essentially makes the results worthless. The accepted standard for assessing sodium intake is twenty-four-hour urine collection on multiple occasions through the study and then following participants for at least ten years.

The results from Study A showed that the group with salt intake (estimated as a result of that one measurement) of less than 3 grams a day actually had more deaths than the group consuming 3–6 grams a day. That is great news for all you salt lovers out there, but this study, though adding a confusing ingredient to the pot, does not indicate that more salt is actually better than less salt.

Not only was one urine test the determinant of salt use (whereas multiple direct measurements are needed to ascertain intake more accurately), but also consider that it is not uncommon for people who are ill or have medical issues to eat less food and therefore consume less salt. Plus, the number of people in the lowest salt cohort was only

4 percent of participants, indicating that this group included the sicker people to begin with. They were not a population that was eating a low-salt diet; they were people who had eaten a high-salt diet much of their lives and then lowered their salt intake for a reason. Researchers did not identify this factor in their study results.

Other factors indicate that Study A's information was distorted:

- More than 40 percent of the participants were from China and other countries where high salt use is almost universal.

- The participants came from countries with a lower standard of medical care.

- The participants came from countries where life span is significantly lower than in the United States.

- In these countries, many of the "walking ill" are not officially diagnosed with a medical condition.

For Study A to have any validity, the period of study would have to be significantly lengthened. In addition, the deaths occurring for the first five years after salt intake measurements were made would have had to be excluded from analysis to make sure that people who were already sickly were excluded from the results. But in this case, these were the only deaths used for analysis.

For example, people with congestive heart failure or other undiagnosed medical conditions that affect appetite and salt intake have a limited life span, despite the reduction in their appetites and salt intake. In the high-salt-consuming populations studied, those with the lowest sodium in their urine were likely those with a reduced appetite due to diseases not yet diagnosed, such as cancer.

This study's results imply that people who are losing weight or eating less food have a higher risk of mortality. But these results are skewed because they don't exclude the participants with medical issues that cause them to lose weight, have less appetite, and be less active.

These results are similar to the contradictory results of other studies indicating that being slim is unhealthy while ignoring the fact that people with serious illnesses lose weight during the last five years of their lives. We know that being slim is the secret to longevity, if slimness is maintained throughout life. In other words, you have to follow younger, healthier individuals for many years rather than for just three to four years to ascertain the benefits and risks of being on a long-term low-salt diet.

Study B was also based on just one urine collection and observed that people who consumed less potassium and more sodium had higher blood pressure on average. This was particularly true in those who were older and had elevated blood pressure to begin with.

The study did demonstrate the obvious: Blood pressure is lower with lower sodium intake and higher potassium intake. However, it did not show these blood pressure benefits translated into fewer deaths because it used the same cohort of participants as Study A. We know that high blood pressure is one of the most powerful predictors of earlier mortality, as demonstrated by hundreds of other studies. The fact that this studied cohort did not show that lower blood pressure resulted in lower death rates demonstrates the obvious flaws inherent in the study design that confusingly skewed the results of both these published papers.

The questionable claims being made by the authors of these two PURE articles, suggesting that a low salt intake may somehow be dangerous, undermines public health efforts to reduce salt intake to prevent high blood pressure. This is particularly troubling because the preponderance of credible scientific data continues to show that elevated blood pressure is the single greatest heart disease risk factor in most populations and is caused predominantly by long-term sodium intake worldwide higher than 2,000 mg/day.

Contrast this research with a huge study on salt published in the *New England Journal of Medicine*, also in 2014.[18] This was a comprehensive meta-analysis that evaluated data from sixty-six countries and 107 randomized intervention trials that analyzed the potential effect of limiting dietary sodium intake to that recommended by the World Health Organization (WHO)—2,000 mg/day.

This meta-analysis was more robust than the ones based on the PURE data, in that it used twenty-four-hour urine samples and dietary records, and corroborated both. Unlike Study A and Study B, it also took the duration of the intervention into account. The study determined that if the WHO's sodium target were implemented, approximately 1.65 million cardiovascular deaths every year would be prevented. Even more dramatic was the study's calculation showing that cardiovascular deaths would be reduced by another 40 percent if the reference intake were lowered from 2 grams to 1 gram of sodium a day. Researchers used the data collected to determine that that reduction would prevent 2.3 million deaths, 40 percent of which would occur before the age of 70. This study confirmed that when populations are studied in the long term, the lower the sodium intake, the better.

The average sodium intake worldwide in 2010 was 3,950 mg/day, which is nearly double the WHO recommendation and nearly triple what is now recommended by the American Heart Association (1,500 mg/day). In their global meta-analysis of controlled intervention studies, these researchers also noted that reducing dietary sodium lowered blood pressure in all adults, with the largest effects seen in older individuals, those of African descent, and those with preexisting high blood pressure. The researchers acknowledged that this data may underestimate the full health effect of excessive sodium intake, which is also linked to a much higher risk of nonfatal heart disease, kidney disease, and stomach cancer—the second most deadly cancer worldwide.

Keep in mind that all scientific studies are done on the people eating the same disease-promoting diet that everyone else is eating in the modern world. Therefore, the results are considered "normal," but since the studies are really observing ubiquitous poor health, the results can be confusing. We can't really determine what is ideal until we do studies on people who are eating optimally. I hope that in the future more research will be performed on people who choose to eat and live more naturally and safely.

Salt Takes a Huge Toll on Society

The association between high blood pressure and salt intake is clear. The following list and supporting research show the extent of salt's toll on society:

- The high blood pressure that results from a lifetime of salt exposure is a major cause of the 1.5 million heart attacks each year.[19]

- Salt reduction by 1,200 milligrams a day is estimated to prevent fifty-four thousand to ninety thousand heart attacks each year in the United States.[20]

- High blood pressure is the leading risk factor for stroke, which is the main reason people end up in nursing homes.[21]

- Hypertension is a leading cause of kidney failure.[22]

- High blood pressure is a major risk factor for senility.[23]

- High blood pressure is a leading cause of heart failure.[24]

- Heart failure is a leading reason for hospital admissions in the United States.[25]

- High blood pressure increases the risk of developing atrial fibrillation—the most common heart rhythm disorder.[26]

- Excess salt and meat are two of the major causes of kidney stones.[27]

- Cancers of the stomach, esophagus, and kidneys are all promoted by excessive salt intake.[28]

- Excess salt intake promotes more headaches and heartburn.[29]

Unfortunately, most of the medical community gives only a tiny bit of lip service to preventing or treating high blood pressure through improved diet, weight loss, and exercise. Your doctor may say to you, "You need to lose weight and eat less salt." However, without offering an effective program, definitive guidelines, and supportive educational materials, such advice is sure to fail. Most doctors use the "prescription pad approach" to treating hypertension, and the minute the pad comes out of the drawer, it is assumed that a patient will not make adequate lifestyle changes. Offering medication gives people the mistaken impression that their blood pressure is adequately addressed and that they are free to continue the same disease-promoting lifestyle that caused their high blood pressure in the first place. Inevitably, people find that their conditions worsen over time; they have to increase their medication dosage, and their rate of aging and the potential for developing disease is accelerated.

If drugs were not available, most of us would be forced to curtail our dietary indiscretions, reduce our salt intake dramatically, lose weight, and exercise. If drugs were not dispensed as the primary solution for high blood pressure, maybe the entire population could be educated about the importance of superior nutrition and salt avoidance at a young age. Who knows? But as it is, people still deserve to be given a chance to truly protect themselves with a low-sodium, cardioprotective diet and appropriate exercise. I'm sure that many people would choose this route with the appropriate information, education, and support.

What About Natural Salts and Sea Salts?

Salt, or sodium chloride, can be mined from the ground or harvested from the sea. But all salts, whether from the sea, a salt mine, or salt marshes, trace their origins to the ocean, which has covered various parts of the earth throughout history. *Table salt,* the most commonly used salt, is refined to remove impurities and contains some additives, such as talc and silica aluminate, to prevent it from caking. Table salt is usually iodized. *Coarse salt* is the same as table salt but has larger crystals.

But these days we've moved beyond the simple table salt. *Sea salt* is mostly distilled from seawater and can be finely or coarsely ground. *Celtic salt* is an expensive version of sea salt that is harvested by solar evaporation of water taken from the Celtic sea. If that doesn't sound impressive enough, you can go for the even more expensive and rare *fleur de sel,* which is said to form only when the wind blows from the east over the salt marshes in Guérande, France.

And it doesn't stop there. Peruvian Pink and Hawaiian Black Lava salt can be yours for about twenty dollars for a 4-ounce bottle. On the

Internet, you can also find "The Original Himalayan Crystal Salt," said to be "white gold" because it contains eons of stored sunlight. The website refers to the hidden stored information of 250 million years of bioenergy locked within the crystals, waiting to be released.[30]

All of these products, however, are just sodium chloride—NaCl— in different sizes, shapes, textures, and prices. The different flavors that people perceive are mostly related to texture. Sea salts, for instance, are composed of larger, flakier crystals, and when you bite into a larger crystal of salt, the flavor is different. However, when you cook with sea salt, any differences disappear because the salt dissolves into the liquid ingredients. Some salts marketed as sea salts are mined from regular salt deposits and are not ground as finely, to maintain larger chunks.

Devotees of sea salts and specialty salts claim that they taste better and are nutritionally superior because of the trace amounts of minerals they contain. But the truth is that salt is salt, and the presence of a tiny amount of minerals (such as a hundredth of a milligram) within a salt does not make excess sodium less damaging.

Even if the salt did contain a larger amount of minerals, would those minerals make excess consumption of sodium beneficial? It is the tremendous magnitude of sodium exposure that makes it a risky food. The risk of sodium exposure is not made harmless by a tiny bit of minerals that might be contained in the salt.

No type of salt provides any significant nutritional benefit. Even the so-called mineral-rich salts contain more than 98 percent NaCl. The amounts of trace minerals that specialty salts may supply are negligible and have no significant effect on human health. For example, Celtic salt contains 2,400 milligrams of sodium per teaspoon, the same as almost all other salts. If you consumed a half-teaspoon with your food—taking in a whopping 1,200 milligrams of extra salt—would you have consumed a significant amount of trace minerals? Of course not. The mineral contribution would be completely insignificant compared with the food you eat.

Your best source of minerals is food. Vegetables contain all the trace minerals humans need, in the amounts that are meaningful to human health, as the chart makes clear.

CELTIC SALT AND SPINACH COMPARED

NUTRIENT	CELTIC SALT (½ T.)	SPINACH (1 C.)
Calcium, mg	5.3	245
Potassium, mg	3.8	839
Magnesium, mg	13.5	157
Phosphorus, mg	0.002	102
Iron, mg	0.08	6.4
Zinc, mg	0.0001	1.4
Copper, mg	0.0001	0.3
Fluoride, mcg	0.01	68
Manganese, mg	0.02	1.7
Selenium, mcg	0.0001	2.7

There are two groups of minerals: *major minerals* and *trace minerals*. We need more than 100 mg/day of the major minerals—calcium, phosphorus, magnesium, sulfur, potassium, sodium, and chloride. We need trace minerals in smaller amounts (less than 100 mg/day). Trace minerals include iron, iodine, zinc, selenium, copper, chromium, manganese, and molybdenum. Sea salt does not contain iodine; it is added to table salt. Sea salts provide dangerously high amounts of sodium, and they do not supply the trace minerals humans need in anything even resembling adequate amounts.

A peculiar phenomenon has led some alternative health authorities and health groups to sell and promote salt to their clientele. Their message is that some of these special salts are good for you, and as for the amount you consume: the more, the better. They often deny that the special salt they recommend raises blood pressure. Often, the health claims made are astounding—especially when you consider the known dangers associated with salt consumption.

Rather than supplying the body with trace minerals, these natural salts actually remove minerals from the body, because the body has to excrete the excess sodium consumed. For example, it is well known that as excess salt is eliminated in the urine, calcium is leeched from the body. An extra 1,000 milligrams of sodium excreted in the urine would carry with it about 20 milligrams of calcium. This amount that is lost is much more than any salt product could possibly supply.[31]

Sodium in Processed Foods Versus Natural Foods

If a serving of a food contains 100 calories, in its natural state it would not have more than 50 milligrams of sodium. So if you see that 100 calories of food contains 200 milligrams of sodium per serving, you know that 150 milligrams of sodium were added to what was naturally found in the food. I suggest that people not add more than 300–500 milligrams of extra sodium to their day's dietary intake over and above what is provided naturally. This allows you to have one serving of something each day that has some sodium added to it, such as a whole grain pita bread or tomato sauce. But remember: All other foods you consume should contain only the sodium that Mother Nature put there.

As much as possible, avoid foods that have labels—that is, foods that are packaged and processed. But if you do eat a food that has a label, read the Nutrition Facts before you buy it. Keep in mind that a product that claims to have "reduced sodium" or be "light in sodium" may still contain very high levels. These are the guidelines that food manufacturers must follow when making such sodium claims:

Sodium Free—less than 5 mg per serving

Very Low Sodium—35 mg or less per serving

Low Sodium—140 mg or less per serving

Reduced Sodium—at least 25 percent less than the regular product

Light in Sodium—at least 50 percent less than the regular product

SODIUM CONTENT OF SAMPLE FOODS

FOOD	SODIUM (mg)	FOOD	SODIUM (mg)
Apple (1 item)	1	Pasta sauce, marinara (1 C)	1,100
Banana (1 item)	1	Pasta sauce, low sodium (1 C)	40
Orange (1 item)	0	Salad dressing, Italian (2 T)	486
Strawberry (1 item)	2	Salad dressing, Italian, light (2 T)	250
Broccoli, uncooked (1½ C)	44	Soy sauce (1 T)	1,029
Celery, raw (1½ C)	122	Soy sauce, low sodium (1 T)	600
Carrots, raw (1½ C)	126	Tomato juice (8 oz)	656
Kale, boiled (1½ C)	45	Tomato juice, low sodium (8 oz)	24
Lettuce, romaine (5 C)	22	Bread, whole grain (2 slices)	253
Spinach, boiled (1½ C)	189	Cereal, Cheerios (1 C)	214
Kidney beans, boiled (1 C)	2	Oats, cooked in water (1 C)	2
Kidney beans, canned (1 C)	770	Chicken breast (4 oz)	84
Kidney beans, canned, no salt (1 C)	30	Ham (2 slices)	739
Cashew butter, unsalted (2 T)	5	McDonald's Quarter Pounder with cheese	1,176
Cashews, raw, unsalted (¼ C)	4	Chicken filet sandwich with cheese	1,238
Cashews, roasted, salted (¼ C)	219	Biscuit with egg, cheese, and bacon	1,260
Sunflower seeds, unsalted (¼ C)	1	Cheese pizza (2 slices)	672
Sunflower seeds, salted (¼ C)	131	Potato puffs (1½ C)	1,432
Vegetable broth, canned (1 C)	940	Pretzel, soft (1 item)	1,615
Vegetable broth, canned, low sodium (1 C)	140		

Since natural foods do not contain much sodium, where does all this salt in the American diet (and diets around the world) come from? It turns out that the salt you add at the table or during cooking is just the tip of the salt block. Only about 11 percent of the salt in the SAD comes from salt added at home. Processed and restaurant foods account for 77 percent, and the remaining 12 percent occurs naturally in foods. Processed foods can contain 1,000 milligrams (or more) of sodium per serving, and many typical restaurant meals contain 2,300–4,600 milligrams![32]

It's not just the usual fast-food villains that are piling on the sodium; seemingly innocent, healthy foods can be part of the problem, too. One cup of canned vegetable broth can provide 940 milligrams of sodium, and 1 cup of canned beans can rack up 770 milligrams. Two tablespoons of Italian dressing on your salad adds 486 milligrams, and 1 cup of regular pasta sauce could include 1,100 milligrams. (See table on the previous page for other foods and low-sodium options.)

Sodium levels vary widely across brands for the same product. Some brands have 50–200 percent more sodium than their competitors. The "same" product, marketed in different countries, will also have different sodium levels. For instance, a publication of the Center for Science in the Public Interest called "Salt: The Forgotten Killer" pointed out that Nabisco saltines sold in the United States have 40 percent more sodium per serving than those sold in Canada.[33]

Why are processed foods so loaded with sodium? Because salt heightens flavor, reduces bitterness, and enhances sweetness. Salt is perfect for processed foods. It is cheap, it keeps foods from becoming discolored, and it extends shelf life. It also binds water and makes foods weigh more, so you sometimes pay more for a heavier package.[34]

When food companies conduct consumer research, they find that unless their food products are salty enough, people do not like the way they taste. As consumers, we have gotten used to higher and higher levels of salt. After years of exposure to high-salt foods, our taste buds have lost their sensitivity to sodium, and we have lost some of our ability to taste other subtle flavors in real food. Therefore, we find that all food tastes too bland unless it is oversalted. Everything tastes flat to a population that heavily salts their food, demands packaged foods, and consumes restaurant meals that contain lots of salt.

Salt, Strokes, and Other Health Problems

A heart-healthy diet and low cholesterol
can increase risk of hemorrhagic stroke.

There are two types of stroke: *ischemic* or *embolic strokes* caused by clots, and *hemorrhagic strokes,* typically more devastating, caused by a broken vessel that bleeds into brain tissue. Ischemic strokes are like heart attacks of the brain and are related to our atherosclerosis-promoting dietary habits, but the hemorrhagic stroke can occur with little or no atherosclerosis present.

In fact, hemorrhagic strokes occur more frequently in people who have low cholesterol. They are much more common in Asia because of that population's high salt consumption. The combination of high salt and low saturated fat is highly related to hemorrhagic strokes. For example, in Japan hemorrhagic strokes were found to be three times more common in people with total serum cholesterol levels less than 160 mg/dl compared with those who had higher levels, even though the higher levels were associated with an increased risk of ischemic stroke.[35]

High salt consumption may also be potentially more dangerous for vegans, vegetarians, and those who have "earned" a low cholesterol because of their careful diets. We know that high cholesterol levels are associated with an increased risk of coronary heart disease. But at very low cholesterol levels, the risk of hemorrhagic stroke increases as the risk of heart attack decreases.

Studies have suggested that low serum cholesterol could enhance the vulnerability of small intraparenchymal cerebral arteries and lead to the development of stroke in the presence of hypertension.[36] The plaque-building process that results in atherosclerosis and premature death may in some way protect the fragile blood vessels in the brain from rupture caused by years of high blood pressure.

That said, there is a very simple solution to this issue, and that is to keep salt intake relatively low so a hemorrhagic stroke becomes almost impossible to happen. However, a person who is vegan, or near-vegan, and is consuming a very high-salt diet could be at a significantly increased risk of hemorrhagic stroke, especially since that person will often live longer and not have a life-ending heart attack first. To protect against heart attacks, ischemic strokes, and hemorrhagic (bleeding) strokes, we must radically curtail salt consumption as we eat a cardioprotective diet.

And there's even more bad news about salt.

In addition to hypertension, excess salt intake may be related to other health problems. As we've already seen, salt increases the body's excretion of calcium, which could lead to loss of bone mass and osteoporosis.[37] Diets high in salt appear to cause higher rates of infection with *Helicobacter pylori*, the bacterium that causes stomach ulcers. Salt has also been shown to be associated with higher rates of stomach cancer.[38] In addition, numerous studies have shown salt to be associated with asthma; a reduction in salt intake can improve breathing.[39] Some of these studies seem to indicate that salt has a stronger negative effect on the lungs of boys.[40]

There is good reason to call salt "the forgotten killer." Although it is easy to get distracted with other diet-related topics that dominate the headlines, it is vital to be aware that high sodium levels can be deadly. Eating a healthy, plant-based diet composed of unprocessed whole foods—without salt—is the best protection we have.

Add Flavor—By Reducing Salt

The natural flavor of food without added salt is an acquired taste. It may not happen immediately, but your taste preferences *will* change and you will learn to prefer food without salt.

Be creative and use other flavoring agents. Try herbs, spices, onion, roasted and raw garlic, lemon or lime juice, vinegar, or (salt-free) lemon pepper to add flavor. Experiment with fresh herbs and not merely the dried versions. Fresh mint, cilantro, and dill add interesting flavors. I use many types of salt-free herbal seasoning blends, which are widely available in both supermarkets and specialty stores. Condiments such as ketchup, mustard, soy sauce, teriyaki sauce, and relish are high in sodium, so read the labels, choose low-sodium versions, and use them sparingly to keep salt intake down.

You can enhance the flavor of vegetable dishes without adding salt. Here are some good combinations of veggies and herbs/spices suggested by the Palo Alto Medical Foundation:[41]

Asparagus: Garlic, lemon juice, and vinegar

Corn: Pepper, green pepper, pimiento, and fresh cilantro

Cucumbers: Dill weed, chives, and vinegar

Green beans: Lemon juice, marjoram, dill weed, nutmeg, pepper, and oregano

Greens: Onion, garlic, pepper, and vinegar

Peas: Mint, pepper, parsley, and onion

Potatoes: Dill, parsley, onion, green pepper, chives, and pimiento

Squash: Onion, nutmeg, ginger, mace, and cinnamon

Tomatoes: Basil, garlic, oregano, marjoram, and onion

Try making your own seasoning blend. Here's an example: Mix together 1 teaspoon ground celery seed, 1 teaspoon crushed garlic, and the following crushed dried herbs: 2½ teaspoons marjoram, 2½ teaspoons summer savory, 1½ teaspoons thyme, and 1½ teaspoons dried basil. You can also add dehydrated onion, oregano, chili powder, cumin, or any other favorite flavor.

The bottom line: A healthy diet, which includes much less salt than what most of us eat, protects us, not just against heart disease, but against most other chronic diseases. Hypertension, diabetes, angina, and strokes are not natural for the human species; rather, they are the inevitable outcome of all the nutritional stresses we put on our bodies.

CHAPTER SEVEN

Comparing Cardioprotective Diets

B esides my guidelines offered here and in my other books describing the Nutritarian diet, several other dietary guidelines promise to prevent heart disease through better nutrition such as the U.S. Department of Agriculture (USDA)–approved DASH diet and the Mediterranean diet. Other nutritional experts have also offered plans with documented reversal of heart disease such as Nathan Pritikin, Dr. Dean Ornish, and Dr. Caldwell Esselstyn. All of these diets have some basic—and beneficial—similarities, such as an emphasis on plant-based nutrition and the restriction of animal products and oil. But some of these diets are too permissive to adequately protect your health, allowing too much animal products, oil, and sugar. Some of the diets needlessly forbid healthful foods, such as nuts and seeds, and permit nutritional deficiencies. In this chapter I examine some popular reasonable diets and compare their strengths and drawbacks.

Preventing and reversing heart disease with nutritional excellence is not a theory; it is a proven modality with benefits that cannot be achieved with medications or surgery. Only a diet consisting predominantly of whole plant foods has been scientifically demonstrated to reverse heart disease and potentially remove the risk of future cardiac events, as documented in numerous peer-reviewed journals (discussed and referenced in this chapter).

I argue that nutritional excellence is *powerfully effective,* whereas drugs, invasive procedures, and surgical interventions are marginally effective at best—and in many instances, they are harmful. Let's put this in perspective by comparing the effects of dietary interventions with the aggressive use of cholesterol-lowering drugs (in combination with the more moderate or standard dietary recommendations from the American Heart Association).

The Reversal of Atherosclerosis with Aggressive Lipid Lowering (REVERSAL) study was a double-blind randomized trial comparing the effects that two different statins, administered for eighteen months, had on atherosclerotic burden, measured by intravascular ultrasound.[1] At thirty-four centers in the United States, 654 patients were randomized to moderate lipid-lowering treatment using 40 mg pravastatin or intensive treatment with 80 mg atorvastatin.

Changes in the burden of fatty plaque present inside the coronary arteries (atheromas) showed a significantly lower progression rate in the intensive treatment group. However, this study did not demonstrate regression of atherosclerosis in either group, but merely the slowing of progression or the lack of progression in the most aggressively treated patients.

Let's compare the results of the REVERSAL study with those seen in patients undergoing intensive dietary therapy. We'll see that dietary therapy is more effective and definitively shows the reversal, not merely the reduction, of progression. Dietary therapy also shows a heightened degree of protection from future cardiac events compared with aggressive, conventional cardiology care or drug therapy.

Let's look at the studies on nutrition and lifestyle for the reversal of heart disease, the effectiveness reported from such interventions, and the similarities and differences of the various approaches. My clinical experience over the past twenty-five years is also important because the nutritional reversal of heart disease and diabetes has been my full-time specialty.

I have experience with thousands of patients who have reversed their cardiovascular disease. I have treated thousands of people with high blood pressure, diabetes, and advanced heart disease. These people have demonstrated that when a treatment plan that combines nutritional excellence and appropriate exercise is applied in a private practice setting, the results are profound. We can effectively cure these medical problems and significantly extend life. Only a few physicians in the United States have had this long-standing, cumulative clinical experience in successfully applying these methods.

> This emphasis on curing medical problems through
> nutritional excellence is not "alternative medicine,"
> nor is it integrative medicine. Emphasizing nutritional
> excellence is *progressive* medicine; it is *correct* medicine.

CASE HISTORY: PROOF FROM A PATIENT

I had two heart attacks, one in October 1999 and the other in September 2000; stented both times.

I was on lots of different medications over the years, typically two for high blood pressure, a statin for high cholesterol, a proton-pump inhibitor for heartburn, and aspirin. My weight fluctuated between 200 and 215 pounds during thirteen years when I also suffered from kidney stones, hernia, enlarged prostate, indigestion, joint pains, and blurred vision as a result of medication side effects. In 2009, my lipid profile off statins showed cholesterol of 307, triglycerides of 499, and HDL of 30.

In the fall of 2012 at the age of 69 I read all of Dr. Fuhrman's books and watched lots of his DVDs and started the Nutritarian diet. It worked so effectively I was able to stop all the medications six weeks after I started the program. Now all my pains and medical problems are gone, and I don't need medications for my heart, cholesterol, or high blood pressure. I lost more than 50 pounds and now weigh 148. My wife also lost 35 pounds and transformed her health too. My total cholesterol in September 2014 was 168, LDL 111, triglycerides 86, and HDL 48. My blood pressure runs about 120/65. I use no medications.

Jim Alfieri

Dietary intervention is lifestyle medicine. Unfortunately, patient care should have been at this place long ago. I hope that in the near future, dietary intervention becomes the norm. This is where medicine *would* go if it were not driven by financial incentives, if it were not influenced by social and political forces that focus on fueling profits and favor the status quo. Of course, everybody is enthralled with high-tech medical science and places it on an undeserved pedestal, even when it is not very effective.

In this chapter I aim to establish the gold standard of dietary intervention for heart patients. The right diet is paramount in maximizing the years of life you can enjoy. I review the dietary features required for effective prevention and treatment of heart disease and address again some unfavorable dietary trends and claims. I then look at various diets with reported benefits to the cardiovascular system to analyze their effectiveness, strengths, and weaknesses. This is an important preliminary step before I explain the ideal way to eat to reverse disease.

It is important to remember that only plant foods contain antioxidants and phytochemicals and have anti-inflammatory effects. And we have to recognize that certain plant foods, such as raw vegetables, are more anti-inflammatory than others. These protective effects are essential for reversing heart disease; therefore, these foods need to be emphasized.

High Protein Means High Death Rates

All cardioprotective diets must be rich in nutritional factors from plants that enable cellular repair and reduce inflammation. Furthermore, they all must be considerably lower in animal products or be vegan because many studies show that animal products promote heart disease.[2]

We have already discussed the 2012 study (referenced above) that followed forty-three thousand women for an average of 15.7 years and found a 60 percent increased risk of cardiovascular events in those adhering to a low-carb, high-protein dietary pattern.

The researchers also documented a gradual and persistent increase in the subjects' risk of developing cardiovascular disease or suffering cardiac death as the consumption of animal products increased and the consumption of carbohydrates decreased.

I mention this again here because, so frequently, false claims are made that high-protein diets offer cardiovascular and metabolic benefits. A promoter of this type of high-protein diet may reference a study showing weight reduction and the resultant lowering of cholesterol (mostly from the exclusion of refined carbohydrates). But what they *can't* show is a reversal of atherosclerosis or a lowering rate of death from cardiovascular disease after subjects follow a diet in which animal products are consumed excessively, even if the diet doesn't include any refined carbohydrates. The point of bringing this up again is to make sure you understand that heart attack incidence increases gradually as the consumption of animal products increases gradually. So even moderate amounts of animal products increase cardiovascular death and can prevent the reversal of present atherosclerosis.

No study has ever shown that a diet with a significant amount of animal product–based foods can reverse atherosclerosis—and no study ever will show that. Too much evidence demonstrates the opposite.

Not even a case series of a small number of individuals on a Paleo, or animal protein–based, diet has ever shown a reversal of advanced heart disease. Even though hundreds of books are written, lots of big words are thrown around, and lots of claims are made to the contrary, it is all just hot air. These meat-based diets are the problem, not the solution. Just as our discussion in the last chapter of all the boutique salts that have appeared on the market concluded that salt is salt, the same is true of meats—lean, grass-fed, free-range, or wild—meat is meat. And this holds true when we consider the supposed "benefits" of meat for cancer prevention, too.

When presented with overwhelming evidence that diets high in meat and animal fat are dangerous, the Paleo crowd sometimes responds by denying the evidence. Paleo proponents argue that the dangers are associated only with consumption of commercial meat, not wild or pasture-fed animals. This is not true.

Much of the research showing the risks of having too much animal products in the diet is based on studies of hundreds of different countries and populations, especially low- and middle-income populations that tend to eat naturally raised animal products.[3] Countries with populations that consume mostly grass-fed animals still have among the highest rates of heart disease and cancer in the world.

Uruguay, home of the gaucho, is a country where people are renowned for their skills in raising cattle. It is one of the world's top consumers of red meat per capita—and also stands out as having one of the highest cancer rates in the world.[4] Australia is another example of a country with very high rates of cancer and heart disease; nonetheless, most people in Australia eat meat only from grass-fed animals—more than 70 percent of the meat is from cattle that spend their lives grazing. In fact, the United States imports much of its supply of grass-fed meat from Australia.

The point is this: Natural animal products may be a touch safer than products from animals raised differently, and certainly it makes sense to eat cleaner, more natural sources for the smaller amounts of animal products that you might consume. But to achieve optimal health, there is no escaping the fact that you must significantly reduce or eliminate the consumption of animal products, whether naturally raised or not.

Even primitive cultures with diets high in animal products and (obviously) no processed foods, sweets, or *trans* fats show early development of heart disease. For example, in the Horus study, the mummified remains and arteries of four ancient populations were examined, including the Unangan hunters of the Aleutian Islands. The examination of the Unangan remains identified severe atherosclerosis. This was highly significant, especially given the relatively young age of death noted in the remains.[5] Other scientific investigations have documented the fact that evidence does not support the often-touted myth that populations that eat high amounts of fish and meat have a lower rate of heart disease, stroke, and cancer. Facts regarding the Inuit people show that they had an unusually high rate of strokes and typically died young.[6]

The Mongols, another population that eats a large amount of meat, were noted to develop a much higher rate of heart disease compared with people in parts of China. Advanced atherosclerosis showed up at an early age, and researchers also noted increased nervous disorders, hardening of the kidneys, and cholesterol deposits in the eyes, even in the young.[7]

By comparison, populations that based their diets on natural plant foods, such as the Tarahumara Native American people of Mexico and the Africans in Uganda in the first half of the twentieth century, as well as numerous rural societies in Africa, were found to be free of heart disease.[8] The popular Paleo diet craze is wishful thinking for meat lovers. It is a hypothesis that does not hold up to scientific scrutiny.

Even more ominous for meat lovers are more recent studies that looked at large populations and tracked participants for many years—adding to the accuracy of the results. In particular, a landmark study published in 2014 tracked six thousand people in the 50–65 age range for eighteen years. When comparing the highest and lowest quartiles of animal protein consumption, researchers found that participants consuming the higher amount had a 75 percent increased risk of death and a fourfold increased risk of cancer.[9]

Let's stop for a moment and reflect on this finding. This is a life-and-death choice we are discussing.

Thousands of studies have now documented health risks from meat-heavy diets. These risks cannot be ignored—a point made by scientists from the World Cancer Research Fund (WCRF) and the American Institute for Cancer Research (AICR). These organizations systematically analyzed more than one thousand studies and confirmed that *diets low in fibrous plant foods and high in meat were linked to bowel cancer.* As a result, the WCRF/AICR Continuous Update Project (CUP) came out with firm recommendations for people to consume a whole-food, plant-rich diet.[10]

Vegetables Repair, Restore, and Heal the Body

The more vegetables eaten as a percentage of total calories, the more the protection against heart disease and strokes. Hundreds of studies document this effect, and I focus on a few here that show this strong relationship.

One such study followed a random sample of more than sixty-five thousand people in England and found that vegetables had the strongest protective effect, with each daily portion reducing overall risk of death by 16 percent. Salad contributed to a 13 percent risk reduction per portion, and each portion of fresh fruit was associated with a smaller, but still significant, 4 percent reduction. "We all know that eating fruit and vegetables is healthy, but the size of the effect is staggering," wrote Dr. Oyinlola Oyebode, lead author of the study.[11]

The clear message here is that the more fruit and vegetables you eat, the less likely you are to die prematurely at any age. Vegetables have a larger effect than fruit, but fruit still makes a substantial difference.

Other studies have repeatedly shown the same thing: The higher the percentage of vegetables in the diet (and to a lesser degree, fruit), the lower the risk of death and the more life span is enhanced. Three relevant meta-analyses reviewed the protection available against heart attacks, strokes, cancers, and overall life span with this dietary emphasis.[12]

Collectively, these meta-analyses reviewed a large number of other studies, which contain hundreds of thousands of individual cases and almost a hundred thousand deaths, to conclusively document the *inverse association between cardiovascular death and vegetable consumption*. However, they also showed that consumption of a large amount of these foods is required for substantive benefits. Three servings a day of fruits and vegetables is inadequate, but five or more servings a day can powerfully reduce the high prevalence of cardiovascular illness in the modern world.

Obviously, as portions of fruits, vegetables, beans, mushrooms, whole grains, nuts, and seeds increase in a person's diet, portions of animal products decrease accordingly. It is the *combination* of increased plants and decreased animal products that synergistically offers the highest degree of protection. Predictable reversal of disease requires nutritional excellence, so when you are going for reversal, you have to go almost all the way to see consistent benefits. You will see what this looks like in the coming chapters.

Animal Products as a Percentage of Total Calories and as a Factor in Disease Promotion

Assume for a minute that all plant foods you eat are unrefined, whole foods. Then we can use the scientific data to devise a relationship between the percentage of plant food versus animal food you eat and your risk of developing cardiovascular disease. Higher amounts of animal products equate to higher risk.

You can use your personal food preferences and aversion to risk to choose a preferred level. Although I may think it is foolish to take a risk with the one body we are given, I nevertheless recognize that this is a personal choice. Keep in mind that you need to keep animal product intake to levels below 5 percent of total calories to assure the reversal of disease.

Percent Animal Product + Percent Plant Product = 100% of Calories

RISK LEVEL	PERCENT ANIMAL PRODUCT	PERCENT PLANT PRODUCT
Disease reversal	0–5	95–100
Disease prevention	6–15	94–85
Moderate risk	16–25	84–75
High risk	26+	74 or less

The information in the chart and graph (next page) reflects my decades of clinical experience in this field and my review of hundreds of studies that demonstrate this relationship. Most of the supportive studies are referenced in this book.

Of course, not all unrefined plant foods are created equal or are of equal benefit, and not all animal products are of equal detriment.

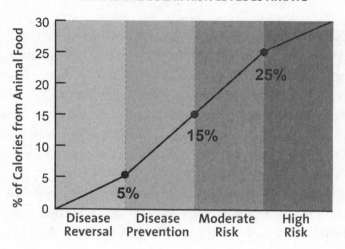

CARDIOVASCULAR RISK LEVEL ESTIMATE

For example, green vegetables have features that reduce inflammation and accelerate disease reversal.[13] And certain animal products, such as commercial beef and processed meats, are more disease-promoting in our diets than others, such as frogs, salamanders, sardines, snakes, and wild salmon.

What this graph demonstrates visually is the opportunity of choice. People who want to ensure the highest probability of excellent results can remain within the most favorable range. Those with a higher degree of genetic risk or who have already developed signs of cardiovascular compromise can make the right choice, recognizing that consuming animal products is only one variable of risk (and of course this graph is based on an assumption of average genetic risk).

This is a graphic representation of the continuum of gradually increasing risk with a higher percentage of calories from animal food in the diet, even within each stratification. This means that a person with a higher genetic risk may need to stay in the lower range within the category to achieve that degree of protection or risk. Intake of all animal products is included here because diets higher in animal protein are linked to higher degrees of inflammation,[14] and some of these potentially negative effects result from high consumption of all types of animal foods, including fish, dairy, and eggs.

Wild fish would be a good choice if you want to use a small amount of animal products in your diet; however, the issue of contamination and mercury in fish is still a concern. Fish and nonfat dairy are generally lower in calories per ounce than other animal products. But because of the contamination factor in fish and the promotion of IGF-1 from egg whites and dairy, I still recommend that all animal products be limited to these low levels in the diet. (See Chapter 10 for further discussion of fish and seafood.)

I still believe that if you suffer from serious cardiovascular disease, you will need to eat a completely vegan diet or something close to it to maximize the metabolic benefits of this eating style. However, most healthy people with reasonably favorable genetics and without life-threatening, vulnerable plaque can achieve excellent cardiovascular health throughout life and still be able to eat a small amount of animal products in their diet. Five percent of animal products for a 2,000-calorie diet is about 8 to 10 ounces a week, and 10 percent of calories is about 16 to 18 ounces per week. So you can keep your intake within the lowest range by not exceeding about one small 2- to 3-ounce serving three or four days a week.

Red meats have about 100 calories per ounce, and lean white meats and fish have about 50 calories per ounce. So you can eat a bit more of white meats.

I generally instruct patients that if they are using a small amount of meat, poultry, or seafood to flavor a dish one evening, they should make the next day completely vegan. Also, if they use a nonfat dairy product, such as an unsweetened yogurt or ricotta filling in a dish, they should not have any other animal product that day and should eat a completely vegan diet the next day. All animal products, including dairy and fish, can be treated the same way, if held to these limitations.

And yes, you must *eliminate* refined carbohydrates from your diet.

I chose animal products as the negative variable in the graph above rather than refined carbohydrates because the link between disease and high-glycemic, refined carbohydrates and commercial baked goods is so strong that it is not a source of controversy or debate. To put it bluntly, you would have to be insane to eat such foods regularly, or to include them in this discussion of healthy eating for cardiovascular disease reversal.

Refined carbohydrates, such as commercial baked goods made with white flour and sugar, need to be 100 percent *gone* from your world. This is just something that you have to accept if you want to prevent and reverse heart disease. I don't think anyone can argue that cakes, cookies, pancakes, and white bread can ever be health-promoting foods.

As we have already seen, agave nectar, honey, maple syrup, rice syrup, raw sugar, and fruit juices all contain a glycemic load or fructose concentration that is metabolically unfavorable. Fruit should be the only sweetener you use, but you should still limit its use. You should have a maximum of one or two fruits with meals, and unsulfured dried fruit used as sweetener should be limited to 2 tablespoons a day. I have developed hundreds of fantastic desserts that meet these criteria, some of which are featured in Chapter 9. They are delicious and not as sweet as conventional desserts.

Of course, there are always those nutritional skeptics who deny that anything we eat causes heart disease. To them, bad health is just fate—not salt, not butter, not cheese, meat, eggs, or sweets. They can always find some inconsistency in the data to explain away these confounding and complicated relationships, so they are able to deny everything in order to justify the diet they want to eat.

These nutritional skeptics deny the validity of any trial result that disagrees with their preferred way of eating, despite careful studies being done by thousands of dedicated nutritional scientists and the advancements that have been made in study design and the control of confounding variables. The same arguments were used for decades to deny the danger of cigarette smoking; the studies were never good enough for some people to establish with certainty the causative relationship between smoking and lung cancer and other diseases. I guess we have to accept the reality that not everyone can be—or wants to be—helped, so we'll still need lots of cardiologists to treat those people.

Now let's examine some of the most popular "heart healthy" diets.

The DASH Diet—Dietary Approaches
to Stop Hypertension

The Dietary Approaches to Stop Hypertension, or DASH, diet has been sponsored, promoted, and tested by the U.S. National Heart, Lung, and Blood Institute. Wow—it's the only diet officially recommended by the U.S. government, so it must be one of the best, right? It is said to be a flexible and balanced eating plan based on research studies that show that it lowers blood pressure. As a result, it is the diet program most recommended by physicians and cardiologists.

Much like the Mediterranean diet, which has also been demonstrated to have cardiovascular benefits, the so-called advantages of the DASH diet are shown when it is compared with the SAD. However, you don't buy a dilapidated old car because it is a touch better than a junkyard wreck.

Just because a program is better than the dangerous way most Americans eat does not mean it is effective at reversing heart disease or offers maximum protection against cardiovascular death. Certainly, this diet is much better than the one that most Americans eat, but that does not make it ideal. Many people following the DASH diet still are needlessly at risk of heart attacks and strokes that will never happen if they are advised to alter their diet even more. If you are currently on the DASH diet, please read the following closely.

The DASH diet is a compromise diet in the right direction, and could have population-wide benefits to reduce disease incidence somewhat. But its limitations exclude it from being able to reverse atherosclerosis in most people with advanced heart disease. The DASH diet is lower in sodium, sugar, and animal products than most Americans are presently eating, but it still permits the following:

> Up to 6 ounces of animal products per day
>
> 3 ounces of dairy products per day
>
> 1 tablespoon of white sugar a day

And, "if you have trouble digesting dairy products," proponents advise, "try taking lactase enzyme pills with these foods. These pills are available at drug stores and grocery stores. You also can buy lactose-free or lactose-reduced milk at the grocery store."

In other words, DASH diet proponents strongly promote the consumption of these foods that have been linked to disease. Dairy products have been closely linked with a higher occurrence of prostate cancer and ovarian cancer in numerous studies.[15] This relationship is difficult to deny. The strong influence that the dairy industry has on government dietary guidelines seems evident in the development of this diet.

The "Dietary Guidelines for Americans, 2010" recommends that everyone keep sodium intake below 2,300 milligrams of sodium a day, and those with high blood pressure reduce it further, to 1,500 mg/day.[16] The DASH-sodium study showed that participants who kept their sodium below 1,500 mg/day were able to reduce their blood pressure by an average of 8.9 mmHg.[17] It is only this low-sodium version of the DASH diet that showed these benefits, compared with the control diet that had a high sodium level. The low-sodium (1,500 mg/day or less) DASH diet led to a mean systolic blood pressure that was 7.1 mmHg lower in participants without hypertension and 11.5 mmHg lower in participants with hypertension. This is a significant benefit if expanded to societal proportions and could save millions of life years and billions of dollars in needless medical costs. But this still does not make the DASH diet the gold standard.

The DASH diet may lower cholesterol a bit and reduce blood pressure about 10 points in people who had been eating a much worse diet, but it is a far cry from excellence. The too-liberal use of animal products limits the potential benefits of this diet. To my knowledge, not even one case of heart disease reversal has ever been recorded with this program. By comparison, the Nutritarian approach has been shown to lower blood pressure an average of 25 points, not 7 to 10 points, and that 25-point drop was accompanied by a 60 percent reduction in medication use.[18] And there are hundreds of documented cases of heart disease reversal as well.

The common feature of all diets that are effective in lowering blood pressure, lowering cholesterol, and reversing heart disease is that each one is composed (predominantly) of unrefined plant foods. When the glycemic effect of the plant choices and the micronutrient density, food diversity, and caloric density are all considered, and adjusted to be favorable, the benefits can be maximized.

Some of you might be asking at this point: How do I eat if I already have high blood pressure, high cholesterol, and maybe even a significant burden of atherosclerosis and chest pain?

The answer is this: Moderation does not work and will not reverse your condition; therefore, moderation can kill. Although a few servings of animal products a week, or a few servings of white rice or white bread may not significantly increase the risk of premature death in a healthy individual, if you have a significant disease burden, these minor deviations from an optimal diet could retard the reversal that is possible. You want to take no chances and accept no compromises. Why gamble with your life?

A few other well-known diet-styles have been shown to prevent and reverse heart disease and are far more effective than the DASH diet. They have been documented to be effective and excellent choices, and they are all rich in unrefined plant foods.

Reviewing the details of each approach and examining their similarities and minor differences is a useful exercise in understanding the important principles, pros, and cons of each. Remember: All of these dietary approaches are dramatically more effective than standard medical care, which emphasizes the use of drugs and medical interventions. These nutritional approaches are also significantly more effective than the watered-down DASH diet. The best part is that the physicians using these approaches have routinely seen their patients recover from serious CAD.

The Dean Ornish Dietary Approach

Dr. Dean Ornish takes the DASH diet a big step farther with the message that eating fat makes you fat and can hinder the results you want to achieve through diet. He reduces animal products more significantly and therefore is able to incorporate more plant foods. Even though Ornish permits one serving of nonfat milk or yogurt and one serving of egg whites daily, many of his devotees find it just simpler to go all the way to a vegan or near-vegan diet.

I consider Dr. Ornish's scientific accomplishments to be revolutionary and historical. He was the first to demonstrate that lifestyle medicine can be much more powerful than drugs and surgery and that heart disease was not just preventable, but reversible. Ornish demonstrated effectiveness even with the sickest patients. Dr. Ornish and his team then went on to show that dietary excellence can affect the progression of early-stage prostate cancer, which in some cases may be reversed.[19]

In his book *The Spectrum: A Scientifically Proven Program to Feel Better, Live Longer, Lose Weight, and Gain Health*, Ornish describes the sickest heart patients, those waiting for a heart transplant, who improved so much by following his diet plan that they no longer needed a transplant. Ornish says that within a year of starting his program of lifestyle changes, "even severely blocked arteries became less blocked," and after five years "there was even more reversal." Remember, under the care of a conventional cardiologist, all patients with advanced disease get slowly worse and worse. Undoubtedly, Ornish's program works, and its efficacy to reverse coronary atherosclerosis has been proven in randomized, controlled trials.

The Lifestyle Heart Trial studied the effects of the Ornish diet in combination with stress-reduction support groups, meditation, and mild exercise such as walking and yoga. On average, Ornish's patients lost 24 pounds in a year and their LDL cholesterol levels were reduced 37 percent (HDL cholesterol levels did not change). Additionally, there was a 91 percent reduction in angina frequency and a significant regression of angiographically measured coronary stenosis.[20]

It is unclear to what degree the other lifestyle modifications, such as exercise and stress reduction, which are integral parts of the Ornish program, play a part in these results. Ornish has said that he believes the support groups and meditation help participants stay on the diet.

The Ornish reversal program is stricter and less flexible than the program he describes in *The Spectrum*. In his early heart disease reversal protocol, Ornish strove to keep the fat content of the diet to less than 10 percent of calories, which necessitated omitting nuts and seeds. However, recently, given the preponderance of evidence showing the health benefits of nuts and seeds, Dr. Ornish modified his dietary guidelines for his reverse heart disease program to include moderate amounts of these foods.

Ornish advises avoiding all meats (including chicken and fish); all oils and oil-containing products (including margarines and most salad dressings); avocados, olives, and high-fat and "low-fat" dairy (including whole milk, yogurt, butter, cheese, egg yolks, cream); and sugar and simple sugar derivatives (honey, molasses, corn syrup, high-fructose corn syrup).

Ornish does not recommend the regular consumption of fish because of its pollutants, but he does recommend 1 to 3 grams of a purified fish oil or DHA-EPA algae supplement. He notes that these beneficial fatty acids offer significant protection against sudden cardiac death in heart patients.

The Ornish program is vegetarian, but as mentioned, it does allow a limited amount of egg whites and nonfat milk or yogurt daily. His heart disease program has always restricted the intake of sugar, concentrated sweeteners, and refined carbohydrates.

Where my interpretation of the evidence had differed somewhat from Ornish over the past twenty years was his restriction of nuts and seeds. However, it is commendable that he has been convinced by accumulating research to modify his stance, which includes a meta-analysis specifically examining this issue of cardiovascular mortality and nuts, including 354,933 individuals, which clearly demonstrated that the regular consumption of nuts and seeds dramatically reduced heart disease deaths.[21] Clearly, our recommendations are now in much closer alignment

My experience with thousands of patients, many with very advanced disease, over the past twenty-five years has also demonstrated that completely avoiding nuts and seeds, which are beneficial high-fat foods, is simply not necessary to reverse heart disease.

Like Ornish, I recommend omega-3 supplements, and we have both recommended algae-derived DHA-EPA, though I use a lower dose than he specifies. My view on DHA and EPA supplementation is a bit more conservative, as I am concerned that the relatively high dose of DHA-EPA (especially fish oils) may give less health benefit compared with lower doses. It's important to consider the risks of higher dosages of fish oil (see Chapter 4 for details on this controversy).

It is clear that the Ornish approach is far superior to standard medical care and the typical watered-down nutritional advice given to heart patients for years and years. He has been a trailblazer in the field of lifestyle medicine. The fact that Medicare now covers the Ornish program is indicative that lifestyle medicine is effectively infiltrating mainstream medicine.

The Caldwell Esselstyn Dietary Approach

In 1995, Dr. Caldwell Esselstyn first published his long-term nutritional research demonstrating the arrest and reversal of CAD in seventeen severely ill patients followed for five years. That same study was updated at twelve years in his book *Prevent and Reverse Heart Disease: The Revolutionary, Scientifically Proven, Nutrition-Based Cure.* He has since reviewed the findings beyond twenty years, making it one of the longest longitudinal studies of its type. Esselstyn's patients were instructed to follow a whole-food, vegan diet with no added oils. Exercise was encouraged but not required. The plan also did not require the practice of meditation, relaxation, yoga, or other psychosocial support approaches, such as Ornish's program.

A recently published article of his reports on 198 consecutive patients counseled on plant-based nutrition.[22] The patients had established cardiovascular disease and wanted to switch to plant-based nutrition in addition to their usual cardiovascular care.

Participants were considered compliant if they eliminated dairy, fish, meat, and added oil from their diets; 177 adhered to the diet program. They were followed for an average of 3.7 years, but some were followed for more than 13 years. Almost all of the compliant participants had no further cardiovascular issues. In the compliant group, the researchers observed only a few cardiac events of questionable etiology, possibly (as was claimed) resulting from the side effects of medical care, and one fatal stroke due to disease progression. The twenty-one people who were not adherent fared much worse, as expected, with just routine cardiology care; thirteen of them suffered another cardiac event.

Esselstyn and his team explained why they thought this program was so effective:

> No other nutrition study has completely eliminated oils (including food products that may contain even small quantities of added oil of any kind), and all animal, fish, and dairy products, which would avoid foods known to injure endothelial cells, as well as all food-derived cholesterol and saturated fat. In avoiding exposure to lecithin and carnitine contained in eggs, milk and dairy products, liver, red meat, poultry, shellfish and fish, participants in our study were unlikely to have intestinal flora capable of producing trimethylamine oxide (TMAO), a recently identified atherogenic compound produced by the intestinal flora unique to omnivores that ingest animal products.

The point is this: If you are looking for maximal health results, there are likely advantages to avoiding oil and animal products in your diet.

Esselstyn's work is unique and impressive because he was able to demonstrate the arrest and reversal of CAD with careful, long-term follow-up of enrolled patients. He also demonstrated that these patients were able to follow his dietary model with excellent adherence; only a very small number dropped out despite the rigorousness of the diet.

Patient education was key to compliance, as the researchers note: "[Participants] were educated to fully comprehend which foods injure endothelial cells and how transitioning to a whole-food, plant-based diet empowers them as the locus of control to halt and potentially reverse their disease." The information provided and effort taken to thoroughly educate the patients about the benefits of this approach paid off.

> *Important Note:* The success of an individual following any diet is proportional to the knowledge and expertise in nutritional science that person gains. A nutritional approach is rarely effective if it is just handed out to people without a thorough education regarding its benefits, how to do it, and how to make foods taste good.

It is important to note that, like Ornish's earlier program, Esselstyn's recommends getting less than 10 percent of calories from fat. His diet excludes oils and all nuts and allows only 1–2 tablespoons of flaxseeds or chia seeds. A multivitamin with B12 is recommended, but he does not advise any DHA-EPA supplement. The assumption made is that the small amount of alpha-linolenic acid from the flax or chia is enough to meet everyone's need for EPA and DHA and that there is no benefit from such supplementation.

This raises the question: Can all people's needs for essential fats be met, with no negative outcomes created, from a diet that does not include nuts and seeds (except the 1 tablespoon of flaxseed) and without EPA and DHA supplementation? Can this severe a restriction in fat create other, unintended consequences?

In Chapter 5 I laid out the evidence that vegan diets that exclude nuts and seeds have been linked to a significant reduction in overall life span. Added to Esselstyn's recommendation of this extreme degree of fat restriction is his opinion that vegans do not need to supplement with DHA fat. I have presented the evidence that the potential for DHA-EPA deficiency in vegans is real and potentially dangerous. It increases the risk of brain shrinkage with aging, and depression, especially in women.

Numerous studies (mentioned above) have also demonstrated that the lack of nuts and seeds in the diet increases cardiovascular mortality. So there could be a small subset of Esselstyn's adherent followers whose pay a severe price for this fat radicalism, and it would most likely be those with heart disease and lower body fat reserves.

Clearly, Esselstyn's program is effective for the prevention and reversal of heart disease in the vast majority of cases. But the combination of extreme fat avoidance, with the exclusion of nuts and seeds, and the lack of recommendation for DHA consumption may place some of his followers (a minority) at risk for other life-altering negative consequences.

I recommend Esselstyn's program with a caution to include a small amount of walnuts (or other nuts) and to take a low-dose EPA-DHA supplement. With those minor modifications, it would be very close to the Nutritarian approach that I recommend.

The Pritikin Diet

In the early 1970s, Nathan Pritikin, an inventor with a passion for nutrition and fitness, began testing his theory that heart disease could be treated with lifestyle changes. Many alternative health professionals at that time were voicing the opinion that heart disease was reversible through excellent nutrition, though the medical profession generally ignored this chatter or considered it quackery. There was no Internet back then, and it was more difficult for people to find these alternative viewpoints.

At the time, I was a teenager and already eating a whole-food, flexitarian diet. I had started this after reading the nutritional writings of Herbert Shelton, a chiropractor and naturopath from Texas. Shelton started his in-patient "health school" in San Antonio and began accepting heart patients in 1928. Twenty years later, he founded the American Natural Hygiene Society.

I also read books by other leaders and historical figures in the natural food movement, visited health retreats, and observed, met, and read about many people who had recovered from advanced heart disease with natural food, vegan, and almost-vegan diet programs. My point is that nutritional reversal from heart disease has been practiced and observed for more than one hundred years. Pritikin's work was instrumental and brought more attention to these methods after he became ill with heart disease at a relatively young age.

Pritikin was only forty-one years old when he was diagnosed with severe obstructive CAD in 1957. He used nutrition to treat his own

heart disease even though his doctor told him that nutritional interventions could not reverse his condition. By 1959, Pritikin had become
a vegetarian, and within a few years, his heart problems had disappeared. By 1975, he had opened a health resort and soon developed a
loyal following, including some medical doctors.

Much of what Pritikin advocated forty years ago is mainstream
today. Since then, many studies in medical journals have documented
that people who adopt a vegetable-rich diet, such as the Pritikin diet,
achieve dramatic results, lowering cholesterol and blood pressure in
just a few weeks, which results in long-term cardiac benefits.

In 1983 the *Journal of Cardiac Rehabilitation* published a five-year
follow-up on sixty-four people who went to the Pritikin Longevity Center.
These people had angina and had been told they needed coronary bypass
surgery. Eighty percent were able to avoid surgical intervention, and only
32 percent still had angina five years later.[23] Most of the people were able
to reverse their disease, and it is most likely that those who still had symptomatic disease had not carefully followed the center's recommendations.

Years later, when health scientists realized LDL oxidation and LDL
particle density, and not merely LDL numbers, were more accurate determinants of cardiovascular risk, eighty participants in the Pritikin
program were demonstrated to have significant improvements in these
parameters after a three-week stay.[24] Diets rich in vegetables don't
merely lower LDL—they lower body weight, lower blood pressure, and
increase vascular elasticity. Such diets also reduce inflammation and
change the chemical structure of the LDL molecule to remove its risks.
Evidence has accumulated for many years showing that food is the best
medicine for heart disease.

The Pritikin diet is healthier than the more popular DASH diet. It
is made up predominantly of natural plant foods, with only one serving of nonfat dairy and one serving of other animal products per day.
The Pritikin program limits the size of the animal product serving to
3–4 ounces and recommends fish, white meats, or wild meats, not red
and processed meats. It is similar to my Nutritarian diet, except that I
restrict animal products more (closer to Ornish and Esselstyn). In addition, I pay extra attention to the nutritional density of foods and to

the anticancer effects of a portfolio of specific natural foods with additional proven benefits.

However, the modern Pritikin approach has moved even closer to my Nutritarian approach. That's because now, for those with cardiovascular disease, the program recommends limiting poultry to only one serving a week and red meat to one serving a month. And to maximize the benefits, the modern Pritikin diet recommends legumes such as beans, peas, lentils, and tofu instead of lean fish or poultry. This puts it even more in line with my recommendations.

The CHIP Program

Another well-researched like-minded intervention over the past twenty years has been the CHIP, a program founded by Dr. Hans Diehl. Over 75,000 people have graduated from the Complete Health Improvement Program (CHIP), an educationally intensive, community-based lifestyle intervention program designed to facilitate reversal of chronic diseases. The twelve-week "boot camp" program involving eighteen group sessions (forty-five-minute video lectures, forty-five-minute class discussion), encourages participants to move toward a plant-based whole food diet emphasizing foods-as-grown: vegetables and fruits, whole grains, plenty of legumes, nuts and seeds.

Participants' biometrics are assessed at the start, middle, and end of the twelve-week intensive program with optional retesting during the nine-month "ClubCHIP" maintenance phase. The clinical results (including two randomized controlled trials) can be found in more than 30 peer-reviewed professional publications.[25]

The Nutritarian Diet

I prefer not to call the diet-style I recommend a "Fuhrman" diet; instead, I call the nutrient-dense, plant-rich (NDPR) diet that I recommend a *Nutritarian diet*. Eating healthy, natural foods is not the prerogative or invention of one individual; as I pointed out above, similar diets have been prescribed to the sick for more than one hundred years. I am merely reviewing the world's scientific literature to inform, explain, and motivate people. I use my broad patient experience and extensive knowledge in this subject to maximize the benefits of eating healthfully and to make it tasty and easy to do for more people.

The word *nutritarian* means rich in nutrients, and that is the Nutritarian diet's defining feature. Yet a broad range of food preferences still can be considered Nutritarian. A *vegetarian diet* has the defining feature of not containing animal-flesh foods, but that alone doesn't necessarily make it a healthful diet. A *vegan diet* contains no animal products; that is, it excludes dairy and eggs, too. A *plant-based diet* has no specific meaning, since the word "based" (one would assume) refers to the majority of calories. The unhealthy SAD is "plant-based," with 70 percent of its calories being derived from plant foods. So the term "plant-based" does not properly articulate the healthful, beneficial meaning it is meant to convey.

The Nutritarian diet-style is vegetable-based but also includes whole grains, fruits, beans, nuts, and seeds. It allows significant leeway in the proportional amounts of healthy, whole plant foods, deriving about 15–25 percent of calories from fat (mostly from nuts and seeds). Processed foods such as oils, white flour, and sweeteners are excluded or considered compromises for occasional use.

I recommend 1–2 tablespoons of flaxseeds and/or chia seeds daily, plus 1–3 ounces of raw seeds and nuts (depending on caloric needs), plus about 200–300 milligrams of DHA-EPA, preferably not fish oil. My dietary and supplemental recommendations are designed for effectiveness and long-term safety, alleviating concerns about nutritional completeness.[26]

All of the diets with documented cardiovascular benefits have more similarities than differences. By now, you should be able to understand the science, the logic, and the reasoning behind designing the right diet-style to protect against and even reverse heart disease. The main point to remember is that if our population would move a big step in the right direction with any of these diets, heart disease would be rare.

When you compare these four effective plant-rich diets, you'll see that the main difference is the use of nuts and seeds and whether a DHA-EPA supplement is recommended.

Summary of the Pros and Cons of Heart Disease–Reversing Diets

DASH

ASSETS: Heightened awareness due to its support by the U.S. government and medical authorities for many years. It is an option for people who aren't willing to accept more radical, effective changes in their diets.

WHAT COULD MAKE IT BETTER? Remove the acceptance of white sugar, cut out the oil, and reduce the permitted and recommended animal products by at least half.

Ornish

ASSETS: Not just a diet program, but also uses meditation, exercise, and support groups to enhance compliance and perhaps efficacy. It has many years of proven efficacy and significant support from both medical authorities and medical insurance companies.

WHAT COULD MAKE IT BETTER? A reduction in the permitted amount of nonfat dairy and egg whites and switching those calories for at least 1 ounce of walnuts, chia seed, flaxseeds, or hemp seeds. More caution may be indicated regarding the amount of supplemental DHA-EPA advised.

Esselstyn

ASSETS: The fact that it is totally vegan (and oil-free) likely offers additional benefits, and it is pure in its simplicity. Compliance and efficacy are enhanced when people have clear limits that are not ambiguous.

WHAT COULD MAKE IT BETTER? It needs a classification of high-carbohydrate plant foods based on glycemic effect and nutrient content to direct participants to the healthiest plant choices. It may be considerably safer if 1 ounce of walnuts and a low-dose DHA-EPA supplement were added.

Pritikin

ASSETS: It has almost forty years of experience, proven results, and the availability of a health resort that offers a complete getaway package. Being immersed in a resort hotel with a learning program and all food supplied can make it easier for people to learn and adapt to the program.

WHAT COULD MAKE IT BETTER? It should have less-ambiguous recommendations for people with heart disease. It also needs clear-cut supplemental recommendations and clear limits on animal products for the public.

Nutritarian (Fuhrman)

ASSETS: The attention to nutrient density and the anticancer effects of "superfoods" such as cruciferous greens, onions, and mushrooms adds a degree of dietary refinement, thereby enhancing benefits.

WHAT COULD MAKE IT BETTER? Reduce sweet fruits and remove dried fruits for people who are glucose intolerant or diabetic, adjusting the glycemic effect of the diet, as discussed in my book *The End of Diabetes*. Some critics of my approach also point out that some people may overeat nuts and seeds and therefore consume too many calories (because these foods are calorically dense), inhibiting their weight loss and thus the full potential of cardiovascular disease reversal. This could be a legitimate concern for those people who have problems with emotional overeating and self-control. But my twenty-five years of clinical experience, with thousands of people adopting this protocol, have demonstrated that individuals who cannot control their consumption of nuts and seeds are relatively rare. We shouldn't have to restrict, and even hurt, the longevity potential of ninety-nine people for the one person who has trouble following the recommendations to not eat too many nuts and seeds.

The foundation of the Nutritarian approach is to eat when hungry and to not snack between meals. Use seeds and nuts as part of the meal, such as in dressings or recipes, and be aware of their caloric density. Obviously, a person can eat too many nuts and seeds and remain

overweight because of that, but that would be an example of someone who did not understand or follow this program accurately. That
means eating some nuts and seeds, instead of—not in addition to—
eating oil and high-glycemic carbs. In other words, eat more greens,
more beans, more nuts and seeds, and less high-glycemic foods, such
as bread, potatoes, raisins, and dates. The seeds and nuts should take
the place of those carbohydrate calories and are not to be eaten in addition to them.

The Most Effective
Nutritional Programs Are Similar

It is easy to see the similarities among the diets with documented cardiovascular benefits. All of them are very cautious with the use of oils
because of their caloric density. More olive oil in the diet is associated
with more weight gain and obesity.[27] Even back in 1965, a study demonstrated that heart patients given olive oil and corn oil had a higher
risk of heart attack and death rate than the control group with a lower-
fat diet.[28]

Modern studies have confirmed that more of these (omega-6) oils
in the diet is associated with higher mortality from heart disease.[29] Is
there a level of oil that may be permissible and still allow disease reversal to occur to the 90th percentile level? Maybe, but that level likely
needs to be very small, such as less than 1 teaspoon a day (40 calories),
not likely a tablespoon, as allowed in the standard DASH diet. And if
you want more security that reversal will be most effective and offer
the most protection, then eliminate all the oils and limit fat exposure
to whole foods, such as seeds and walnuts.

There should be no controversy that reducing animal products and
increasing the amount of natural plant foods in the diet can revolution-
ize our health-care system, end the expensive and invasive coronary
artery treatments of stenting and bypass surgery, and save millions of
life years.

The common denominators of all diets shown to reduce heart disease deaths are clear. I might not be right about everything, but I study this emerging science every day. In addition, the accumulated evidence of the past one hundred years attests to what is now an avalanche of information supporting the conclusions given here.

A Nutritarian diet has been shown to dramatically reverse diabetes, eliminate high blood pressure, solve the problem of food addiction and overeating, and help people take back control of their health destiny. It has enabled thousands of people to restore their failing health after facing the most serious, life-threatening illnesses possible, and this has not been limited to heart disease. Superior nutrition prevents cancer, and I have used it for more than two decades to reverse headaches, asthma, allergies, frequent infections, diabetes, and serious autoimmune diseases that conventional medical authorities consider irreversible.

In my twenty-five years of medical practice as a family physician advocating superior nutrition, I even have seen cardiac patients who could barely walk go back to living a full, vibrant life. Nutritional excellence is not just powerful medicine; it restores and saves lives where conventional cardiology cannot.

Of the many hundreds of cases demonstrating dramatic reversal from the most serious degree of heart disease, I have observed many people whose plaque burden was undetectable within a few years. Generally, the numerous people who have followed my recommendations to the letter, and have had their plaque measured, have seen massive reductions in plaque even within year one.

I doubt that most people, even health-care professionals, will stop going to fast-food restaurants, swear off white flour products and soda, or cut their animal product consumption by 80–90 percent. But even if the junk food–addicted mass of people insist on marching off to an early grave, this doesn't mean that *you* have to follow the crowd.

My chosen role is to present the options to you, describe what is best without compromise, make food taste great, and then let you choose to either control your health destiny or not. At least you have the opportunity. If you decide not to, that is your choice. I revel in the fact that those people who have embraced my guidance have received spectacular results and will continue to enjoy the healthiest lives possible.

I take a different approach from the many nutritional leaders who try to accommodate everyone's desire to water down the recommendations, to make changes that they are comfortable with, to try to improve their health just a bit, to slow the progression of disease or lower their blood pressure or cholesterol a bit. To me, that is not enough.

I want to make sure that those people who follow my advice are optimally and dramatically protected against cancer, that they push the envelope of human longevity, and that they eliminate their dependence on doctors' surgical procedures and risky medications. This is not only the most sensible way to live, but it is a highly pleasurable way, too. Especially when you give yourself a chance to change your food preferences, end your food addictions, learn the recipes, and readjust your taste preferences. Thousands have done so and have reaped the rewards. *I know you can do it, too.*

CHAPTER EIGHT

The Nutritarian Plan

As anyone who's ever been on a diet knows, relying on willpower alone to help you stick to a plan sets you up for failure. That's why the Nutritarian diet-style has been successful for thousands of people over the past two decades: It's not about deprivation. It's about eating natural, nutrient-dense foods and preparing them so that they taste delicious. Make use of the sample menus and recipes in this book to kick-start your voyage to optimal health—and then create some tasty and healthful combinations of your own. For those with serious health problems or an urgent need to lose weight quickly, I have included my Radical Weight Reduction Menu (page 247). Above all, remember that your taste buds will adjust to your new way of eating, and you will soon find yourself wondering how you ever settled for the SAD, or DAD (deadly American diet).

To convince yourself that this diet-style isn't about deprivation, take a look at the menus in this chapter and the sample recipes in the next chapter. My specialty is making healthy eating taste great. I have been preparing natural foods since I was 15 years old, giving me more than forty-five years of experience with Nutritarian cooking. Try as many of these recipes as possible, and mark the ones you like the best.

I have shared almost two thousand more recipes in my books and on my website, www.DrFuhrman.com. Most of them have been rated by people who have tried them, so you can see the favorites. I recommend my *Eat to Live Cookbook* for more terrific recipe ideas.

Pick out the ones you think you will like best. Make them and discover your ten favorites (please don't include desserts in this list). Over the next three months, identify the four main dishes you enjoy the most, the three salad dressings you prefer, and the three soups that are your favorites.

Gradually, as you learn to prepare and cook healthy foods in creative and delicious ways, you will begin to understand that this way of eating can be very satisfying and delicious. Remember, it takes time—up to six months—to really retrain and strengthen your taste buds to prefer a different way of eating. But most people find that within the first six weeks, they have made tremendous progress in learning all the interesting ways they can make fruits and veggies, beans, nuts, seeds, and whole grains taste great. Many people report that their taste sensitivities and preferences change significantly even during this first six-week period.

Think about retraining your palate in the same way you start going to the gym. You may not appreciate and enjoy it right away, because you get sore and can't comfortably do very much at first. But, with time, it gets much easier—you no longer get sore, and you actually enjoy pushing your body and seeing the changes in your muscles and frame. The same thing is true with food. Be patient. You may not like these foods as much as I do at first. But just as thousands of others who are eating this way, you will come to enjoy this diet-style more and more, the longer you do it.

One of the secrets to success is to avoid empty-calorie foods such as sugar, sweeteners, white flour, processed foods, and fast foods. They fuel addictive food behaviors and have no nutritional value. The adaptation and strengthening of your taste muscles and appreciation of subtle natural flavors will only happen if you eat healthfully and cut out all sweets and salt. The overuse of sweets and salt has weakened the ability of the taste buds; sweets and salt mask the great natural flavors of food and make you think that foods need more salt or sugar.

If you continue to eat highly salted foods, all vegetables will taste flat unless heavily salted. If you continue to add sweetening agents, whether natural or artificial, in and on whatever you eat, you will never appreciate the subtle sweetness and flavors in berries or the sweetness in a leaf of romaine lettuce. Six weeks off the sugar, salt, and oil, and your taste buds will awaken. You will experience new flavor profiles that you will love.

I want to maximize both your success and your enjoyment of food. I am advising you to let me control your food choices and menus for now. *Don't make eating decisions and choices on your own right now; don't mess with an approach that has been proven to work for thousands of people.*

In other words, most of you have not succeeded in losing your excess weight. You have not succeeded in achieving great health, free of diseases and medications. Your decisions so far have been based on your instinctual drives, which were conditioned by the foods you were accustomed to eating. In order to undo and retrain those ingrained preferences, you need to suspend eating what you want for now and just eat what I want you to. Don't worry, you will get your eating free-will back—but first you have to (as Nike says) "just do it."

The first thing you have to do is get out a marker and make a sign to put on your fridge that reads: *The Salad Is the Main Dish.* You have to make the promise to eat a large salad as the main dish of a meal at least once a day. Did you put the book down and do that? This is the most important thing you can do. Did you make the promise?

I PROMISE TO EAT A LARGE SALAD, AS THE MAIN DISH OF THE MEAL, AT LEAST ONCE A DAY.

_____

YOUR NAME RIGHT HERE

Remember to put some cruciferous vegetables into that raw green salad: shredded red or green cabbage, baby kale, arugula, watercress, Chinese cabbage, or baby bok choy. Also, add some thinly sliced red onion or scallion, maybe some tomato or pomegranate kernels, and then top it off with one of the dressings you will learn about, made by blending whole nuts and seeds (instead of oil) with other savory ingredients. I use the Russian Fig Dressing made with almonds, tomato sauce, and fig vinegar the most. I include it with many of my other favorite dressings in Chapter 9. Since salad is so important in this program, it is important that you learn to make a few healthy salad dressings that you love.

After salad dressings, the next most important food is a hearty bean soup or stew. One basic technique we use frequently in my house is to use carrot juice, celery juice, tomato juice, with water as the soup base and then add beans, veggies, and herbs we have on hand. Make a giant pot of soup on the weekend and use the leftovers stored in the fridge for the next few days. A salad and bowl of bean soup for lunch should be your standard.

Eat Large Portions

Yes, you read that right: Eat bigger portions than you likely have in the past. In fact, you "crowd out" your desire for unhealthy foods by eating larger amounts of healthy food to occupy the space in your stomach. I want you to especially eat large portions of cooked green vegetables. I love artichokes, asparagus, Brussels sprouts, zucchini, and string beans and eat huge amounts of them. See how many cooked, low-starch vegetables you can comfortably eat. The amount you can eat of these is almost unlimited because they are so low in calories.

Memorize this list of foods that you should eat liberally:

1. All green vegetables, both raw and cooked, including frozen. If it is green, you get the green light. Don't forget raw peas, snow pea pods, kohlrabi, okra, and frozen artichoke hearts.

2. Non-green, non-starchy vegetables, including tomatoes, peppers, eggplant, mushrooms, onions, garlic, leeks, cauliflower, water chestnuts, hearts of palm, and roasted garlic cloves.

3. Raw starchy vegetables, such as raw carrots, raw beets, jicama, radish, and parsnips. They are all great, shredded raw, in your salad.

4. Beans/legumes, including split peas, lima beans, lentils, soybeans, black beans, and all red, white, and blue beans. Soak them over-

night, then rinse and cook them, add them to salads and soups, make bean burgers, sprout them, and eat bean pasta.

5. Low-sugar fruits, one or two with breakfast and about one more each meal.

6. Try to have berries or pomegranate at least once a day. Frozen berries are the most cost effective.

You need to rethink portion sizes and learn to consume large amounts of the right foods. The more vegetables you eat, the better. It is almost impossible to overeat when you eat the right foods. Still, you should never eat until you are uncomfortable or full. You can always eat more in a few hours when you are hungry again.

The Lowdown on Beans, Nuts, Seeds, Grains, and Animal Products

Try to include a daily cup of cooked beans, either in soup, in a chili or bean stew, or added to your salad. Make sure you also get at least 1 ounce (¼ cup) of raw seeds and nuts every day. In addition to that, add a heaping tablespoon of ground flaxseeds or chia seeds, too; these are superfoods that can transform your health. If you are overweight, do not eat more than 2 ounces of nuts and seeds per day. Most of this nut and seed allotment will be used to make delicious salad dressings and dips.

Grain products are lower on the nutrient density scale, so limit yourself to one serving per day of whole grain products such as steel cut oats, wild or black rice, quinoa, farro, cornmeal, or 100 percent whole grain bread. Remember, an intact grain has a lower glycemic index than one ground into a flour, so steel cut oats are better than oatmeal flakes, which are better than oat flour. Soaked or sprouted grains and seeds can also be made into a delicious cracker using a dehydrator or your oven set on the lowest setting. I like to add lots of onion and dried tomato to my crackers.

If you currently are dealing with moderate or severe heart disease, I suggest that you do not eat any animal products; do the vegan version of this diet-style. By eliminating animal products, you eliminate any excess risk and can make this health transition much more smoothly. It also makes things simpler. You don't have to measure portions or be concerned if you are perhaps eating too much, which could slow or inhibit disease reversal.

If you are otherwise in good health and you desire animal products, you can chop a small amount into small pieces and add it to any soup, vegetable, or bean dish to enhance flavor. Don't eat more than 1–2 ounces per day. If you decide to use small amounts of animal products in your diet, then your animal product consumption should be a mix of fish and wild fowl. You should avoid eating red meats and cheese, or only consume these very rarely. I generally advise that the intake of all animal products combined should not exceed 8–10 ounces a week for a woman and 10–12 ounces a week for a man. Avoid all processed, cured, and barbecued meats and full-fat dairy.

The Cornerstone of Your New Heart-Protecting Diet

With time, you will feel like I do, that this is the most emotionally satisfying way to eat, because you like the food and intellectually you know it is good for the future you, too. Making this change may be difficult for you at first and your taste preferences may not change overnight, because developing new habits and tastes takes time. You first must develop a new and different mind-set.

The first step is to learn which foods are richest in lifesaving nutrients and how to make these foods enjoyable so that they become the foundation of what you eat. The cornerstone of your new diet is the list of foods below. Memorize them, because these are the foods with the highest nutrient density. The secret to your success is to eat primarily the natural foods in this list that contain high nutrient levels. Eat less of everything else that is not on this list.

At least 90 percent of your diet should be from whole plant foods such as the following:

Green vegetables—including kale, Swiss chard, broccoli, artichokes, string beans, asparagus, spinach, cabbage, lettuce, snow peas, and peas

Yellow/orange vegetables—including carrots, butternut squash, winter squash, spaghetti squash, sweet potato, and corn

Beans/legumes—including chickpeas, red kidney beans, lentils, and adzuki beans

Fresh fruits—including blueberries, strawberries, kiwis, apples, oranges, grapes, pears, watermelon, and pomegranates (Eat dried fruits, including raisins and dates, only in small amounts.)

Nonstarchy vegetables—including eggplant, mushrooms, peppers, tomatoes, and onions

Raw nuts and seeds—including pistachios, filberts, almonds, sunflower seeds, sesame seeds, walnuts, cashews, pecans, chia seeds, and flaxseeds

Intact grains—including steel cut oats, millet, wild rice, buckwheat groats, and hulled barley

Minimally processed grain or bean products—including sprouted breads, flaked or rolled grains (oatmeal), bean pasta, tofu, tempeh, unsweetened soy or nut milks in moderate quantities

You should also eliminate two things from your diet:

Eliminate or severely limit animal products. If using animal products (strive to keep to less than 10 ounces a week), use only wild, low-mercury seafood or naturally raised fowl. Animal products are best used in very small amounts as flavor enhancers or as a condiment, not as a main dish.

Eliminate all refined grains and sweeteners. Avoid all white flour products, white rice, processed/cold breakfast cereals, sugar, and other sweetening agents.

THE NUTRITARIAN DIET VERSUS
THE STANDARD AMERICAN DIET

NUTRITARIAN DIET	SAD
Vegetable-based	Grain-based
Lots of fruit, beans, seeds, nuts	Lots of dairy and meat
Oil used sparingly	Oils comprise major caloric load
Animal products 0 to 3 times a week	Animal products 2 to 4 times a day
Nutrient-dense calories	Nutrient-poor calories

Keep It Simple

In this chapter, I provide you with two weeks of menus, and in the next chapter you'll find lots of great recipes. But you do not have to prepare lots of recipes; if you want to stick to basic foods prepared simply, no problem. Eating this way can fit into any lifestyle, no matter how much or how little time you have for food preparation. Just use these guidelines to structure your meals.

For Breakfast

Intact grain, such as steel cut oats, hulled barley, or buckwheat groats (cooked by boiling in water on a low flame). If you soak the grain overnight, the cooking time will be much shorter in the morning. Add ground flaxseeds, hemp seeds, or chia seeds to this hot cereal, along with fresh or frozen fruit. Use mostly berries, with shredded apple and cinnamon.

Or a serving of coarsely ground, 100 percent whole grain bread with raw nut butter.

Or as a quick and portable alternative, have a green smoothie, such as my Green Berry Blended Salad.

For Lunch

A big (*really, really* big!) salad with a nut/seed-based dressing (see Chapter 9 for some great choices)

Vegetable bean soup

One fresh fruit

For Dinner

Raw vegetables with a healthful dip

A cooked green vegetable that is simply and quickly prepared: steamed broccoli florets; sautéed leafy greens such as kale, collard greens, or Swiss chard; asparagus, frozen artichoke hearts, or frozen peas.

A vegetable dish that has some starchy component or intact grain with it, such as a bean/oat/mushroom burger on a whole wheat pita or a stir-fried dish with onions, cabbage, mushrooms, and water chestnuts with wild rice or other intact grain and a sauce such as Thai peanut sauce.

A small amount of fruit for dessert, such as frozen cherries or apple slices with nut butter.

What Is an Intact Grain?

Whole grains are higher in nutrients than refined grains, but they are not necessarily *intact grains*. To meet the definition of a whole grain, all the parts of the grain should be there, but it can be ground up into a fine powder like pastry flour, which has a high glycemic load. The word "intact" refers to a whole grain that still retains the shape and appearance of the way it was grown and harvested. It has not been ground into a powder (flour). As you would expect, because they are not ground and contain the full fibrous shell, intact grains are digested slowly and have a more favorable glycemic index.

Examples of intact whole grains are oat groats and steel cut oats. Grains have a continuum of wholesomeness and glycemic effects. From most wholesome to least, for oats it would go oat groats → steel cut oats → oatmeal → quick cook oats → oat flour. All of these are whole grains, but only the first two are intact whole grains. The oats in oatmeal are cut and rolled, and the quick cook oats are cut even more finely and then cooked and rolled.

It is always best to eat your grains mostly in the form of intact whole grains and not made into flour and then bread. Some breads are made from intact sprouted grains or coarsely ground grain and therefore are more favorable than others. Manna Organics bread, Ezekiel bread, and Alvarado Street Bakery bread are examples of national brands, available in the frozen section of health food stores, whose grains are more intact (not finely ground) and therefore more nutritionally favorable.

Here are some common grains that can be eaten in their intact form:

Amaranth: A gluten-free grain that is particularly high in protein compared with other grains, and even higher in lysine. It maintains its crunchiness after cooking in water. Be sure to use lots of water when you cook it because it thickens the water.

Barley: Hulled or dehulled barley is considered intact because just the inedible hull is removed. Pearled barley is not a whole grain. Barley is high in beta-glucan, which helps lower cholesterol. Soak barley overnight before cooking. It is great cooked like rice; mixed with beans, onions, herbs, and spices; used in soup; eaten as a breakfast cereal; or used in dehydrated crackers.

Brown rice: Brown rice has gotten bad press lately since *Consumer Reports* published a story on arsenic levels in brown rice secondary to fertilizers used and the increased uptake of arsenic in the bran of the rice. At this point, I do not recommend consumption of brown rice on a regular basis, as there are lots of other better options, including wild rice.

Buckwheat: Buckwheat is not related to wheat, so it is a favorable grain for wheat-sensitive people. It is also rich in protein and fiber and has been shown to lower cholesterol. Buckwheat groats can be soaked in advance and then used to make porridge, a seasoned side dish, or crackers. Kasha is toasted buckwheat.

Millet: This versatile, gluten-free grain is a staple crop in India and Africa. Mildly sweet and nutty, it can be used in both main dishes and desserts. Depending on the length of time it is cooked, it can be slightly crunchy or soft and creamy. Serve it with stir-fried dishes, add it to salads, or make a breakfast porridge with cooked millet, nuts, seeds, and fruit.

Quinoa: Although quinoa is usually considered a whole grain, it is actually a seed. It is a good protein source and cooks in just ten to fifteen minutes. Rinse quinoa before cooking because it is coated with a bitter compound called saponin. Quinoa tastes great by itself, or for a substantial salad, toss it with veggies, nuts, and a flavored vinegar or light dressing. It makes a great addition to veggie burgers and even works well in breakfast or dessert puddings.

Rye: A cereal grain with less gluten than wheat, the rye berry can be boiled whole or used in cereals in the rolled form, like oats. You can coarsely grind it in a blender and then soak it and use it to give a nice flavor to coarse breads and crackers.

Sorghum: Hearty, chewy sorghum doesn't have an inedible hull so you can eat it with all its outer layers, thereby retaining the majority of its nutrients. Use it in its whole grain form as an addition to vegetable salads or cooked dishes. It has a mild flavor that won't compete with the delicate flavors of other food ingredients. For best results, soak it in water overnight, then cook it for about an hour.

Teff: Tiny, whole grain teff has been a staple of Ethiopian cooking for thousands of years. It is the smallest grain in the world; about 100 grains are the size of a kernel of wheat. It has a mild, nutty flavor, cooks quickly, and is a good source of calcium and iron. Serve it with fruit and cinnamon for a hot breakfast cereal or add it to stews, baked goods, or veggie burgers.

Wheat berries: A wheat berry is the entire wheat kernel, the intact whole grain, composed of the bran, germ, and endosperm. The chewy texture of wheat berries makes them an interesting, hearty addition to a variety of salads. They can also be used as an alternative to rice. Cook in boiling water for about fifty minutes or until tender.

Wild rice: This is not actually rice but the seed of a semi-aquatic grass that is native to North America. Wild rice is rich in antioxidants and is a good alternative to brown rice, especially since it is not contaminated with arsenic. Wild rice bursts open when cooked, so it is easy to tell when it is done. Combine with mushrooms, onions, and your favorite herbs for a simple side dish or add to soups and stuffing.

Obviously, people with celiac disease or those who are gluten or wheat intolerant should avoid wheat and other gluten-containing grains, including spelt, Kamut, triticale, barley, and rye.

Tips and Tricks for Nutritarian-Style Cooking

Eating the way I am recommending can be a big change from what you are used to, but you will quickly learn the tricks of the trade and come up with lots of creative ideas for making healthy recipes and meals. Invariably, if you stick with this diet-style, you will get well and even prefer to eat this way. You will learn to enjoy the simple flavors of real food and to appreciate how much better you feel.

During the first week of your transformation, try to accomplish these four tasks (see Chapter 9 for recipes):

1. Make the Garlic Nutter Spread because you can use it as a spread or a dip.

2. Make another dressing or dip you love.

Once you have some salad dressings and dips that you like, it becomes easy to eat any vegetable raw: Just dip it in a great dressing or delicious sauce. Remember, the sauce makes the food special.

3. Make a healthy cracker.

4. Make a veggie bean soup.

Blending

A durable, high-powered blender is well worth the investment. I make many of my smoothies, dressings, soups, and desserts with a blender. Since I use whole-food ingredients such as vegetables, fruits, nuts, seeds, and dried fruit, it is important that the machine have enough power and speed to efficiently process these ingredients to the desired smooth consistency. Inexpensive models will not provide a smooth, creamy texture, and their motors tend to burn out after a month or two of daily use. If you have only a standard, moderately priced blender, add a bit more water to make a thinner dip or dressing. You can use a thick carrot, wide end down, or a thick rib of celery like a plunger to push the food down into the blades to aid in blending.

I make smoothies and blended salads by blending together raw leafy green vegetables, fruit, and seeds or nuts. This is an effective way to increase nutrient absorption, because a blender crushes the cell walls of the plants more efficiently than chewing, making it easier for our bodies to absorb the beneficial phytochemicals contained inside the plants' cells. But, the main advantage of blending a salad, instead of chewing one, is that you can consume it more quickly when you don't have much time to eat.

As I've already mentioned, refined oils are devoid of nutrients, so I use nuts, seeds, and avocados to make my Nutritarian dressings. These ingredients provide fatty acids that are essential to our well-being. The right high-powered blender, such as the Vitamix brand, will be able to process these ingredients into a creamy, delicious salad dressing. Similarly, you can make creamy soups by blending raw nuts into the soup to provide a smooth texture and rich flavor. The refreshing fruit sorbets and ice "creams" that I enjoy and recommend also require the ability to smoothly combine frozen fruit, dried fruit, nuts, and seeds.

Steaming Vegetables

Steaming a veggie is quick and easy. You only need a steamer pot with a lid or a steamer basket to place in a pot with a lid. Alternatively, you can improvise a steamer by placing in the bottom of a pot a few stalks of celery or the outer leaves of lettuce or cabbage that you were going to discard. Add a small amount of water and the food you are cooking, cover, and cook for the appropriate length of time.

Don't steam vegetables until they are very soft. By then, the water has turned green and you have washed away half of the water-soluble nutrients. The trick is to stop steaming when the veggies have just started to become tender and still retain some firmness. Boil water in a pot with a tight lid first, then add the vegetables, cover, and start your timer. These are the steaming times that I find work best. (They assume the artichokes have been cut in half and prepped, and cabbage and broccoli stems have been sliced.)

Artichokes	18 minutes
Asparagus	13 minutes
Bok choy	10 minutes
Broccoli	14 minutes
Brussels sprouts	13 minutes
Cabbage	13 minutes
Kale, collards, Swiss chard	10 minutes
Snow peas	10 minutes
String beans	13 minutes
Zucchini	13 minutes

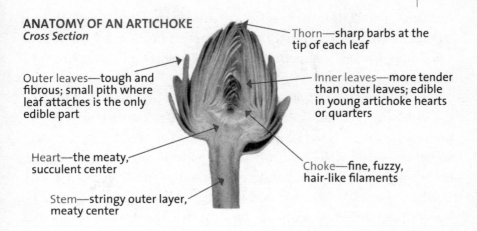

ANATOMY OF AN ARTICHOKE
Cross Section

Thorn—sharp barbs at the tip of each leaf

Outer leaves—tough and fibrous; small pith where leaf attaches is the only edible part

Inner leaves—more tender than outer leaves; edible in young artichoke hearts or quarters

Heart—the meaty, succulent center

Choke—fine, fuzzy, hair-like filaments

Stem—stringy outer layer, meaty center

TIPS FOR PREPARING AN ARTICHOKE

To cook an artichoke, slice 1 inch off the tip. Cut off about ¼ inch or less of the very bottom piece of the stem to expose the fresh green bottom, keeping the remaining stem attached. Then, using a large sharp knife, slice the artichoke in half lengthwise. Once sliced in half, you can see the fuzzy inedible choke part. Use a small pointed knife to cut a deep half-moon-shaped incision where the heart meets the choke. Scoop out and discard the fibrous and hairy choke from the center of each half. Place the artichoke in a steamer basket over several inches of water. Bring the water to a boil, cover, and steam for eighteen minutes. Set the artichoke aside until it's cool enough to handle.

To eat, peel off the outer leaves one at a time. Tightly grip the outer end of the leaf, place the opposite end in your mouth, and pull through your teeth to remove the soft, pulpy, delicious portion of the leaf. You can also scrape off the edible portion with a butter knife. Then you can eat it plain or prepare a healthful dip or dressing. Continue until all the leaves are removed. Cut the remaining heart into pieces and enjoy!

Water-Sautéing and Cooking with a Wok

Since you should avoid or greatly limit oils in your diet, I recommend sautéing vegetables with water or cooking them in a wok. These methods are preferable to boiling, baking, or roasting. When vegetables are boiled, some of the nutrients are lost in the cooking water. Soup is the exception because all the nutrients are retained in the liquid. During baking, roasting, or grilling, the high temperatures cause the formation of *acrylamides,* compounds that can cause genetic mutations and increase the risk of cancer.

To water-sauté, use a small amount of water or other liquid to sauté the vegetables, including onions and garlic. Heat a skillet, wok, or pan on high heat until water sizzles when dropped on the pan. Add a tablespoon or two of water and, when hot, add the vegetables and cook, covering occasionally. Add additional liquid as needed until the vegetables are tender, but don't add too much water or the food will be boiled, not sautéed. To enhance flavor in the onions, garlic, or other vegetables you are cooking, let the pan get dry enough for the food to start to brown just a little before you add more liquid. You can also use low-sodium vegetable broth, coconut water, tomatoes, or wine for sautéing vegetables.

Use a wok or skillet to cook vegetables in a flavorful cooking liquid that contributes a distinctive taste and provides a sauce for the dish. To wok- or stir-fry successfully, you need a large wok or skillet so the ingredients can cook evenly and not be too crowded. Cut ingredients into uniform-size pieces and give hard vegetables such as carrots, broccoli, and cauliflower a head start before adding other, softer vegetables. Add leafy vegetables toward the end of the cooking time since often they only need to wilt a bit, which doesn't take much time.

Do not overcook vegetables, which causes them to lose valuable nutrients.

Cooking with Herbs and Spices—for Flavor and Health

Learn to use flavorful herbs and spices instead of salt to season your foods. As we saw in Chapter 6, salt dulls your taste buds, and soon food begins to taste bland unless it is heavily salted. When you stop using salt, your sense of taste returns and you can learn to appreciate a wide variety of subtle flavors. Add fresh herbs such as dill and basil liberally to your dishes—they add flavor and also have beneficial health effects. Plus, never forget Simon and Garfunkel's cooking tips for using fresh herbs: parsley, sage, rosemary, and thyme.

Use herbs and spices to impart mild or bold flavors to your recipes. International cuisines each have their own characteristic set of seasonings, which add flavor without the use of salt. You can add a moderate level of heat with ingredients such as black pepper, cayenne pepper, or crushed red pepper flakes. Vinegar and citrus ingredients such as lemon, lime, and orange are also terrific flavor enhancers. I love to use raw or roasted garlic to pump up the flavor when I cook.

Unlike salt, which has the potential to increase your risk of developing disease (see Chapter 6), many herbs and spices show promise for having beneficial properties. For instance, studies show that *curcumin,* the active substance in turmeric, may reduce inflammation, help fight infections and some cancers, and treat digestive problems.[1] Turmeric is a popular Indian spice that has a warm, mild flavor that resembles a cross between ginger and orange. It gives Indian curry its flavor and yellow color.

Many cuisines worldwide use gingerroot; it is featured particularly in Asian cooking and pairs well with garlic in savory sauces and dressings. Ginger contributes a zesty, pungent flavor and has been valued since ancient times for its ability to soothe nausea and gastrointestinal distress. Ginger contains *gingerols,* active phytochemicals that are responsible for ginger's characteristic flavor and help to reduce the body's inflammatory response. Some studies show that ginger can alleviate pain and improve mobility in people with osteoarthritis and rheumatoid arthritis.[2]

The sweet-spicy flavor of cinnamon enhances the taste of entrees, breakfasts, and desserts. The two major types of cinnamon used in food preparation are Ceylon cinnamon and cassia cinnamon. Look for Ceylon cinnamon, which has a sweeter, more delicate taste and is known as "true cinnamon." Cassia cinnamon is more commonly found at your grocery store and is less expensive, but it should not be consumed liberally. It contains high levels of coumarin, a naturally occurring substance that has the potential to damage the liver in high doses. Ceylon cinnamon contains only traces of coumarin. For people with diabetes, cinnamon may play a role in regulating blood sugar. Cinnamon contains phytochemicals that enhance insulin signaling and facilitate glucose uptake and storage by the body's cells.[3]

Desserts

I can't say it too often: This diet is not about willpower and sacrifice. You can indulge in satisfying, delicious desserts. As you can see from the dessert recipes in Chapter 9, it is possible to create nutritious and tasty treats using only whole, natural ingredients: fresh, frozen, or unsulfured dried fruit; raw nuts and seeds; and whole grains.

Stick to natural, whole foods as sweeteners. If you are using dried fruit such as dates or raisins, use just enough to make the dish moderately sweet. I do not recommend agave nectar or honey, which are concentrated sweeteners with minimal nutritional value. Avoid artificial sweeteners such as aspartame, saccharine, and sucralose because their safety is questionable.

Many of the desserts in this book have been sweetened with dried fruit or dates. I try not to use more than one date per serving in the dessert recipes, so they may be less sweet than the desserts you are accustomed to eating. With time, your ability to sense sweet will increase, and you will prefer them this way.

My favorite desserts are homemade fruit sorbets and ice creams that you can easily make in minutes. By blending frozen fruit (bananas, berries, peaches, cherries, mango) with some nuts (cashews, almonds, macadamia nuts) or seeds (hemp, chia, flax), maybe some dried fruit (dates, unsulfured apricots, or pineapple) and a splash of nondairy milk, you can make your own refreshing creations. The frozen desserts in Chapter 9 will give you some ideas to get you started.

Reading Labels

In most cases, reading the label of a packaged, processed product will persuade you to put it back on the shelf. Generally, avoid foods in packages, but such information can occasionally be useful. For example, if you are occasionally consuming bread products, make sure that they are 100 percent whole grain. "Enriched wheat flour" is just white flour. Check the list of ingredients to make sure it says "whole wheat flour" and not just "wheat flour," or a combination of whole wheat and white/wheat flour.

Note the sodium content of the packaged food items you purchase— you'll be surprised to see how much sodium is in the products you use every day. Look for foods that are labeled "no salt added" or "low sodium." As you saw in Chapter 6, food that is labeled "low sodium" must have less than 140 milligrams of sodium per serving. Be careful of products labeled "reduced sodium"; all that means is that they contain 25 percent less sodium per serving than the regular version of that food, which could still be very high.

Two Weeks of General Sample Menus

The two weeks of general sample menus that follow will give you great ideas for planning delicious Nutritarian meals. These menus feature recipes designed to taste great while providing maximum nutrient density—without added salt, refined oils, or artificial and processed ingredients.

You can choose to follow these menus to the letter or pick and choose the meals and recipes that work for your lifestyle and preferences. You can switch around the foods and recipes and eat them in different combinations or at different meals.

To reduce the amount of time you spend in the kitchen, make large amounts and then use the leftovers for three to four days. Use a homemade salad dressing for several days. Make a big pot of soup and split it up into small containers so it can provide several dinners and/or lunches. Leftovers from dinner make an easy lunch the next day.

These two weeks of sample menus provide you with enough dishes to last almost twice as long as two weeks. These menus will get you started and show you the pattern of eating that I want you to become comfortable with. I hope that in no time you will be trying new dishes and even thinking up some of your own.

The daily menus are based on approximately 1,700 calories, but you can adjust them depending on your needs. If you need to lose weight, you can modify the menus and reduce calories by eating less dried fruits and nuts, avocado, and bread and cutting back on fruit a bit, too. If you are physically active and require additional calories, increase the portion sizes and add more raw nuts and seeds, avocado, beans, and intact whole grains.

If you have diabetes, reduce or remove dried fruit from
your menu. In general, diabetics should have only one
fruit serving with each meal. I strongly recommend
that people with both type 1 and type 2 diabetes read
my book *The End of Diabetes.*

If you have a serious medical condition such as recurring angina at low
workloads, a recent transient ischemic attack (TIA) or cerebral embolic event,
uncontrolled blood pressure despite medication use, poorly controlled
diabetes, or you are significantly overweight, I suggest you follow the most
aggressive version of this program—the Radical Weight Reduction Menu
(page 247)—to drop body weight quickly over the first six weeks, thereby
dramatically lessening your risk of stroke and heart attack—or even death.
The Radical Weight Reduction Menu is similar to the aggressive menu in
my book *The End of Diabetes,* as it starts out lower in calories and with an
even lower glycemic load to facilitate rapid results and enable the rapid
discontinuation of medication.

Recipes for items marked with an asterisk are included in Chapter
9 of this book.

Week 1

Monday

BREAKFAST

Nutritarian Granola*

Unsweetened soy, almond, or hemp milk

Mixed berries (fresh or use defrosted frozen berries)

LUNCH

Black Bean and Sweet Potato Quesadillas*

DINNER

Broccoli Mushroom Bisque*

Salad with mixed greens, tomatoes, and chopped red onion

Lemon Basil Vinaigrette*

Vanilla Zabaglione with Fresh Fruit*

NUTRITION FACTS FOR THIS MENU: CALORIES 1712; PROTEIN 64g; CARBOHY-
DRATE 257g; TOTAL FAT 61g; SATURATED FAT 9g; SODIUM 667mg; FIBER 51g; BETA-
CAROTENE 35,038ug; VITAMIN C 347mg; CALCIUM 830mg; IRON 22mg; FOLATE
688ug; MAGNESIUM 690mg; ZINC 11mg; SELENIUM 44ug

PROTEIN 14 percent; CARBOHYDRATE 56 percent; TOTAL FAT 30 percent

Tuesday

BREAKFAST

Eat Your Greens Fruit Smoothie*
Granny's Granola Bars*

LUNCH

Raw veggies with Artichoke Hummus*
Broccoli Mushroom Bisque* (leftover)
Watermelon or other fruit

DINNER

Cauliflower, Coconut, and Turmeric Soup* topped with Crispy
Chickpeas* (if desired, add a small amount of chicken or shrimp)
Napa Cabbage Salad with Sesame Peanut Dressing*

NUTRITION FACTS FOR THIS MENU: CALORIES 1701; PROTEIN 64g; CARBOHY-
DRATE 242g; TOTAL FAT 68g; SATURATED FAT 12g; SODIUM 603mg; FIBER 55g; BETA-
CAROTENE 39,876ug; VITAMIN C 519mg; CALCIUM 882mg; IRON 22mg; FOLATE
956ug; MAGNESIUM 725mg; ZINC 13mg; SELENIUM 56ug

PROTEIN 14 percent; CARBOHYDRATE 52.6 percent; TOTAL FAT 33.4 percent

Wednesday

BREAKFAST

    Swiss Cherry Oatmeal*

LUNCH

    Big salad with romaine lettuce, shredded red cabbage, and beans
        (and other assorted vegetables as desired)

    Russian Fig Dressing*

    Strawberries

DINNER

    Raw veggies with Artichoke Hummus* (leftover)

    Creamy Kale and Mushroom Casserole

    Chia Pudding*

NUTRITION FACTS FOR THIS MENU: CALORIES 1779; PROTEIN 69g; CARBOHY-
DRATE 261g; TOTAL FAT 63g; SATURATED FAT 13g; SODIUM 593mg; FIBER 73g; BETA-
CAROTENE 29,730ug; VITAMIN C 429mg; CALCIUM 949mg; IRON 23mg; FOLATE
1053ug; MAGNESIUM 686mg; ZINC 11mg; SELENIUM 53ug

PROTEIN 14.6 percent; CARBOHYDRATE 55.4 percent; TOTAL FAT 30 percent

Thursday

BREAKFAST

Mango, Coconut, and Quinoa Breakfast Pudding*

Almond Hemp Nutri-Milk*

LUNCH

Farro and Kale Salad with White Beans and Walnuts*

Steamed asparagus

Fresh figs or unsulfured dried figs

DINNER

Dr. Fuhrman's Famous Anticancer Soup*

Baked Eggplant Fries*

Berries or other fruit

NUTRITION FACTS FOR THIS MENU: CALORIES 1729; PROTEIN 65g; CARBOHY-DRATE 269g; TOTAL FAT 57g; SATURATED FAT 7g; SODIUM 313mg; FIBER 55g; BETA-CAROTENE 28,536ug; VITAMIN C 257mg; CALCIUM 954mg; IRON 21mg; FOLATE 989ug; MAGNESIUM 725mg; ZINC 13mg; SELENIUM 54ug

PROTEIN 14 percent; CARBOHYDRATE 58 percent; TOTAL FAT 28 percent

Friday

BREAKFAST

Two pieces of fruit

1 ounce (about ¼ cup) raw almonds or walnuts

LUNCH

Dr. Fuhrman's Famous Anticancer Soup* (leftover)

Salad with mixed greens, tomato, and chopped red onion (and
other assorted vegetables as desired)

Italian Dressing with Roasted Garlic*

Defrosted frozen peaches or other fruit

DINNER

Lentil Walnut Burritos with Peppers, Onions, and Salsa*

Steamed broccoli

Seasoned Kale Chips and Popcorn*

NUTRITION FACTS FOR THIS MENU: CALORIES 1703; PROTEIN 62g; CARBOHY-
DRATE 256g; TOTAL FAT 64g; SATURATED FAT 9g; SODIUM 643mg; FIBER 56g; BETA-
CAROTENE 41,414ug; VITAMIN C 614mg; CALCIUM 779mg; IRON 20mg; FOLATE
880ug; MAGNESIUM 581mg; ZINC 11mg; SELENIUM 25ug

PROTEIN 13.3 percent; CARBOHYDRATE 55.4 percent; TOTAL FAT 31.3 percent

Saturday

BREAKFAST

> Turmeric and Ginger Tea*
> Banana Cocoa Muffins*
> Cantaloupe or other fresh fruit

LUNCH

> Big salad with romaine lettuce, arugula, tomatoes, and white beans
> Italian Dressing with Roasted Garlic*
> Grapes or other fruit

DINNER

> Three-Seed Burgers* or Black Bean and Turkey Burgers*
> Seasoned Sweet Potato Fries*
> Cabbage, Apple, and Poppy Seed Slaw*
> Vanilla or Chocolate Nice Cream*

NUTRITION FACTS FOR THIS MENU: CALORIES 1727; PROTEIN 59g; CARBOHY-DRATE 279g; TOTAL FAT 56g; SATURATED FAT 9.5g; SODIUM 850mg; FIBER 47g; BETA-CAROTENE 27,580ug; VITAMIN C 195mg; CALCIUM 758mg; IRON 21mg; FOLATE 743ug; MAGNESIUM 676mg; ZINC 11mg; SELENIUM 58ug

PROTEIN 12.7 percent; CARBOHYDRATE 60.2 percent; TOTAL FAT 27.1 percent

Sunday

BREAKFAST

Chickpea Omelet with Mushrooms, Onions, and Kale*
Blueberries or other berries

LUNCH

Taco Salad Wraps*
Mango or other fruit

DINNER

Asian Vegetables with Batter-Dipped Tofu*
Pinoli Cookies*

NUTRITION FACTS FOR THIS MENU: CALORIES 1748; PROTEIN 77g; CARBOHY-
DRATE 273g; TOTAL FAT 52g; SATURATED FAT 6g; SODIUM 822mg; FIBER 63g; BETA-
CAROTENE 25,235ug; VITAMIN C 394mg; CALCIUM 1205mg; IRON 21mg; FOLATE
1087ug; MAGNESIUM 537mg; ZINC 10mg; SELENIUM 40ug

PROTEIN 16.4 percent; CARBOHYDRATE 58.5 percent; TOTAL FAT 25.1 percent

Week 2

Monday

BREAKFAST

Cherry Smoothie*

1 ounce (¼ cup) sunflower seeds

LUNCH

Edamame Black Bean Salad* served over baby greens

Almond Coconut Macaroons*

DINNER

Salad with mixed greens, watercress, and chopped red onion (and
other assorted vegetables as desired)

Walnut Vinaigrette Dressing*

Nutritarian Goulash*

Rustic Mashed Cauliflower with Roasted Garlic and Spinach*

NUTRITION FACTS FOR THIS MENU: CALORIES 170; PROTEIN 76g; CARBOHYDRATE
222g; TOTAL FAT 73g; SATURATED FAT 13g; SODIUM 438mg; FIBER 58g; BETA-
CAROTENE 20,283ug; VITAMIN C 369mg; CALCIUM 1080mg; IRON 25mg; FOLATE
1327ug; MAGNESIUM 768mg; ZINC 14mg; SELENIUM 71ug

PROTEIN 16.5 percent; CARBOHYDRATE 48 percent; TOTAL FAT 35.5 percent

Tuesday

BREAKFAST

Granny's Granola Bars*

Melon or other fruit

LUNCH

Big salad with romaine lettuce, tomatoes, sliced avocados, and
pumpkin seeds

Walnut Vinaigrette Dressing*

Apple or other fruit

DINNER

Golden Austrian Cauliflower Cream Soup*

Broccoli and Chickpea Salad*

Strawberries with Almond Chocolate Dip*

NUTRITION FACTS FOR THIS MENU: CALORIES 1816; PROTEIN 56g; CARBOHY-
DRATE 262g; TOTAL FAT 78g; SATURATED FAT 9g; SODIUM 477mg; FIBER 59g; BETA-
CAROTENE 42,870ug; VITAMIN C 681mg; CALCIUM 745mg; IRON 20mg; FOLATE
1031ug; MAGNESIUM 698mg; ZINC 12mg; SELENIUM 36ug

PROTEIN 11.5 percent; CARBOHYDRATE 53 percent; TOTAL FAT 35.5 percent

Wednesday

BREAKFAST

Savory Steel Cut Oats*

Defrosted frozen cherries or other fruit

LUNCH

Golden Austrian Cauliflower Cream Soup* (leftover) or whole grain
wrap with turkey or hummus, lettuce, tomato, and avocado

Steamed Broccoli with Fresh Tomato Sauce*

Seeded Crackers with Dried Tomatoes*

DINNER

Lentil and Mushroom Ragù over Polenta with Fresh Tomato Salsa*

Salad with mixed greens and orange sections

Orange Sesame Dressing*

Watermelon or other fruit

NUTRITION FACTS FOR THIS MENU: CALORIES 1825; PROTEIN 75g; CARBOHY-
DRATE 313g; TOTAL FAT 47g; SATURATED FAT 7g; SODIUM 596mg; FIBER 74g; BETA-
CAROTENE 32,615ug; VITAMIN C 682mg; CALCIUM 1075mg; IRON 28mg; FOLATE
1280ug; MAGNESIUM 767mg; ZINC 15mg; SELENIUM 55ug

PROTEIN 15.4 percent; CARBOHYDRATE 63.3 percent; TOTAL FAT 21.3 percent

Thursday

BREAKFAST

> Blueberry and Flaxseed Oatmeal*
>
> V6 Vegetable Cocktail*

LUNCH

> Baba Ghanoush over Mixed Greens*
>
> Sautéed mushrooms
>
> Seeded Crackers with Dried Tomatoes* (leftover)
>
> Melon or other fruit

DINNER

> Broccoli and Shiitake Mushrooms with Thai Curry Wok Sauce*
>
> Black and brown rice
>
> Vanilla or Chocolate Nice Cream*

NUTRITION FACTS FOR THIS MENU: CALORIES 1730; PROTEIN 67g; CARBOHY-
DRATE 290g; TOTAL FAT 50g; SATURATED FAT 8g; SODIUM 441mg; FIBER 67g; BETA-
CAROTENE 23,997ug; VITAMIN C 480mg; CALCIUM 655mg; IRON 20mg; FOLATE
1035ug; MAGNESIUM 704mg; ZINC 14mg; SELENIUM 56ug

PROTEIN 14.3 percent; CARBOHYDRATE 61.7 percent; TOTAL FAT 24 percent

Friday

BREAKFAST

> Two pieces of fruit
>
> 1 ounce (¼ cup) pumpkin seeds

LUNCH

> Chipotle Avocado and White Bean Wraps*
>
> Creamy Cucumber and Onion Salad*
>
> Clementines or other fruit

DINNER

> Baba Ghanoush* (leftover) with raw vegetables
>
> Split Pea and Lentil Soup*
>
> Roasted cauliflower

NUTRITION FACTS FOR THIS MENU: CALORIES 1704; PROTEIN 76g; CARBOHY-
DRATE 263g; TOTAL FAT 54g; SATURATED FAT 8g; SODIUM 461mg; FIBER 69g; BETA-
CAROTENE 13,112ug; VITAMIN C 401mg; CALCIUM 613mg; IRON 20mg; FOLATE
917ug; MAGNESIUM 753mg; ZINC 13mg; SELENIUM 25ug

PROTEIN 16.6 percent; CARBOHYDRATE 57.1 percent; TOTAL FAT 26.3 percent

Saturday

BREAKFAST

> Breakfast Burrito* (with tofu or eggs)
> Mixed berries (fresh or use defrosted frozen berries)

LUNCH

> Chickpea Curry in a Hurry*
> Steamed green beans

DINNER

> Bean Pasta with Brussels Sprouts and "Blue Cheese"*
> Salad with romaine, spinach, and chopped red onion (and other
>   assorted vegetables as desired)
> Almond Vinaigrette Dressing*
> Chocolaty Brownies*

NUTRITION FACTS FOR THIS MENU: CALORIES 1795; PROTEIN 88g; CARBOHY-
DRATE 256g; TOTAL FAT 64g; SATURATED FAT 14g; SODIUM 822mg; FIBER 77g; BETA-
CAROTENE 37,992ug; VITAMIN C 410mg; CALCIUM 1387mg; IRON 31mg; FOLATE
1494ug; MAGNESIUM 855mg; ZINC 13mg; SELENIUM 60ug

PROTEIN 18 percent; CARBOHYDRATE 52.4 percent; TOTAL FAT 29.6 percent

Sunday

BREAKFAST

Turmeric and Ginger Tea*

Nutritarian Granola*

Unsweetened soy, hemp, or almond milk

Strawberries

LUNCH

Big salad with baby greens, chopped kale, sautéed mushrooms,
and black beans

Almond Vinaigrette Dressing*

Apple Oat Flaxseed Bars*

DINNER

Baked Eggplant Parmesan with Fresh Tomato Sauce*

Salad with mixed greens, baby kale, and shredded red cabbage
(and other assorted vegetables as desired)

Sunny Tuscan Dressing*

Banana Pineapple Sorbet*

NUTRITION FACTS FOR THIS MENU: CALORIES 1745; PROTEIN 71g; CARBOHY-
DRATE 269g; TOTAL FAT 60g; SATURATED FAT 9g; SODIUM 433mg; FIBER 75g; BETA-
CAROTENE 22,673ug; VITAMIN C 365mg; CALCIUM 1019mg; IRON 24mg; FOLATE
1231ug; MAGNESIUM 763mg; ZINC 12mg; SELENIUM 48ug

PROTEIN 15 percent; CARBOHYDRATE 56.5 percent; TOTAL FAT 28.5 percent

Radical Weight Reduction Menu

Sometimes, a radical nutritional intervention is needed:

1. To save the life of a person who is at high, short-term risk

2. For psychological reasons, to get some radical results up front

3. Because of intolerable medication side effects

4. For an upcoming surgery or medical procedure that is too dangerous to pursue at the present body weight

For these and other reasons, a dietary design that is nutritionally superior yet more aggressively low in calories and glycemic load is needed. This takes the place of a fast or modified fast, and physicians can use it to achieve short- and long-term goals, as it is safe to maintain for extended periods or until the patient has lost the desired amount of weight. Weight loss of 40 pounds within the first two months can easily be achieved for obese individuals.

Contrary to popular belief, a high-nutrient, low-calorie intake is *not* harmful or dangerous for people who are overweight as long as micronutrient and water intake are adequate. Once a more stable condition is achieved, a person can transition to a mildly higher caloric load while continuing to follow a Nutritarian diet. Weight loss will continue, albeit at a slower rate.

The only documented risk of rapid weight loss is gallstone formation, which I have seen only rarely with this approach. The high fiber and nutrient levels and the use of nuts and seeds all limit bile production and stone formation. At the same time, the formation of gallstones and the possibility of requiring a laparoscopic removal of the gallbladder would not be an unreasonable price to pay for losing 50 to 150 pounds of life-threatening body fat. However, this still would be a very unusual occurrence under these guidelines.

The easiest way to achieve this aggressive goal is to limit eating to two meals a day. That means a late brunch around 10 A.M. and an early dinner around 4 P.M. When you do this, fat burn accelerates because you spend more time in the fat-burning phase of the digestive cycle.

Once postprandial (after the meal) glucose levels have returned to baseline, the body increases its use of fat. So living longer in this stage of the metabolic cycle, with more distance between meals, further accelerates the burning of body fat.

The design of the menus that follow allow for maximum fat burn by limiting the time spent eating and digesting food.

The longer you live in the catabolic phase of the digestive cycle, the longer you live. This means that you are living more hours each day not digesting food. Plus, you are living off stored calories and therefore burning more fat between 6 P.M., when blood glucose starts to return to normal baseline two hours after dinner, and 10 A.M.—a total of sixteen hours straight.

After the first three days, when withdrawal symptoms from unhealthy eating habits lessen considerably, you will not be uncomfortably hungry, even with the smaller number of calories. Remember, the high level of micronutrients supplied here will powerfully lessen your hunger. Drinking a cup of lemon water, green tea, or other herbal tea can help you avoid the desire to eat when you wake up in the morning. Note that this phase has only two fruit servings a day and a limited amount of nuts and seeds for further caloric reduction—usually 1 ounce for women and 1½ ounces for men. Stay with this phase until you and your doctor decide you are out of danger. It is important not to consume more than a very limited amount of caffeine, as it will enhance withdrawal symptoms (toxic hunger), making it much harder to not eat.

Brunch

1. 1 cup fresh or frozen berries or pomegranate kernels, covered with flax, hemp, or chia milk (made by blending 1 tablespoon of flaxseeds, chia seeds, or hemp seeds with 1 cup water and, if desired, some cocoa powder)

2. Raw greens such as romaine lettuce hearts, baby greens, sliced peppers, fennel, or celery

Choose one additional option:

1. Oven-roasted, balsamic-glazed peppers, tomatoes, and onions with defrosted frozen asparagus or artichokes

2. Eggplant baked until soft and served with water-sautéed or diced raw onions and cinnamon

3. Zucchini steamed with dill and onion

4. Edamame and frozen peas with roasted garlic

Or any of these recipes found in Chapter 9:

1. Baked Tempeh in Spicy Tomato Sauce

2. Better Burgers

3. Chickpea Omelet with Mushrooms, Onions, and Kale

4. Creamy Cucumber and Onion Salad

5. Crispy Chickpeas

6. Eat Your Greens Fruit Smoothie

7. Savory Steel Cut Oats

8. V6 Vegetable Cocktail

Early Dinner

1. A big green salad with lettuce, thin-sliced red onion, tomatoes, and other assorted vegetables and a healthy dressing (Try a creamy hemp seed herbal dressing made from hemp milk, seeds, and a fruit-flavored vinegar, or a roasted tomato basil dressing made from tomato paste, soaked dried tomatoes, raw and roasted garlic, vinegar, roasted red pepper, chopped scallions, basil, cumin, and cinnamon. Or use one of the dressings in Chapter 9. Take care to use only 1 ounce of nuts and seeds per serving in the dressing or eat the 1 ounce of nuts separately if you use a straight no-oil vinaigrette. You might prefer to lightly toast the nuts and seeds and then chop and sprinkle them on top of the cooked green vegetables.)

2. Or raw vegetables with a Nutritarian dip such as the following examples from Chapter 9: Artichoke Hummus, Feisty Hummus, Italian Dressing with Roasted Garlic, or Baba Ghanoush over Mixed Greens.

Choose one or more of the following options:

1. A bowl of vegetable bean soup, such as Split Pea and Lentil Soup or Tomato Barley Stew (Chapter 9)

2. Defrosted frozen green vegetable such as broccoli, kale, collard greens, bok choy, string beans, or artichokes, steamed or cooked in a wok. These should be made with steamed or water-sautéed mushrooms and can be flavored with mashed, roasted garlic, dry-pan–sautéed, or diced raw onions. If desired, serve with Home-Style Tomato Sauce (Chapter 9).

3. One serving of a low-sugar fruit, such as a green apple, orange, two kiwis, or strawberries

Or any of these recipes found in Chapter 9:

1. Baked Eggplant Fries

2. Italian-Style Zucchini Spaghetti

3. Kale with Sweet Corn

4. Napa Cabbage Salad with Sesame Peanut Dressing

5. Nutritarian Goulash

6. Rustic Mashed Cauliflower with Roasted Garlic and Spinach (made with only ¼ cup of cashew butter)

7. Slow-Simmered Collard Greens

8. Sweet and Easy Squash Casserole

Remember: You can eat the same dish for more than one meal and use leftovers for a few days. Note that even foods that are moderately glycemic are reduced in this menu and are not included with breakfast because insulin resistance is highest in the morning.

If you are in an emergency situation, the most important advice is: *Do not make choices and decisions about what to eat and what not to eat just yet. For now, allow me to make these decisions for you.* Choose only from the options in the menus above. In order to give this method a chance and see results, you must do it exactly as prescribed, without modifications. You can choose to eat the same foods day after day, and you do not need to have the variety of options listed here. You can eat a brunch choice for dinner or a dinner choice for brunch, but you need to choose food options from those offered on the menus above.

Keep it simple at first. You do not have to eat all the foods listed above if you are not hungry. Eat what you feel comfortable eating, and no more. Try to stop eating before you feel uncomfortably full; you should feel comfortably full or satisfied. It is okay to just have a large salad and some fruit or a salad and some soup. Pay close attention to chewing raw vegetables very, very well. You can also pour hot soup right over some shredded raw vegetables, so you eat your salad and soup mixed together, using the soup as a salad dressing.

The Key to Success

The key is to understand the Nutritarian principles and then be creative in your cooking. Rely on herbs, spices, flavored vinegars, roasted garlic, dried tomatoes, fruits, and toasted seeds to make interesting flavors and dishes without relying on salt and oil, like most people do.

If you don't have time to cook, I have developed a line of boxed soups and salad dressings to make it convenient for even the busiest person to eat the Nutritarian way. Today, more and more healthy options are arising that meet these guidelines, making the Nutritarian diet-style easier than ever before. And if you need to eat on the go, you will find a steadily growing number of food establishments that offer healthy, plant-based options.

After only a short time following this Nutritarian plan, you will discover that you enjoy and appreciate the great flavors of natural, healthy foods. As you savor the flavors, you will be content in the knowledge that you are doing something wonderful to and for your body. I promise that eating a Nutritarian diet will ultimately give you great pleasure and energy like you have never felt before. Depending on your food choices, food can either hurt or heal you. I know you will enjoy the healing.

CHAPTER NINE

The End of Heart Disease Recipes

Salads

Soups and Stews

Main Dishes and Vegetable Side Dishes

Burgers, Wraps, and Fast Food

* Flavored vinegars and seasoning mixes marked with an asterisk are available at www.Dr.Fuhrman.com; however, you can substitute other brands of the similar products.

BEVERAGES AND SMOOTHIES

Almond Hemp Nutri-Milk
Serves: 6

1 cup hulled hemp seeds
1 cup raw almonds, soaked 6 to 8 hours
2 Medjool or 4 regular dates, pitted
4 cups water
½ teaspoon alcohol-free vanilla flavoring

Place all ingredients in a high-powered blender. Blend until smooth. If desired, strain through a nut milk bag or fine mesh strainer. To make chocolate Nutri-Milk, add 2 to 3 tablespoons natural cocoa powder to blender along with other ingredients.

PER SERVING: CALORIES 305; PROTEIN 10g; CARBOHYDRATES 23g; TOTAL FAT 21.5g; SATURATED FAT 1.9g; SODIUM 16mg; FIBER 13.6g; BETA-CAROTENE 15mcg; CALCIUM 246mg; IRON 0.9mg; FOLATE 13mcg; MAGNESIUM 71mg; ZINC 1.8mg; SELENIUM 0.8mcg

Cherry Smoothie
Serves: 2

4 stalks kale, tough stems removed
1 cup unsweetened soy, hemp, or almond milk
⅓ cup carrot juice
1½ cups frozen cherries
1 banana
2 tablespoons ground flaxseeds

Blend ingredients in a high-powered blender.

PER SERVING: CALORIES 251; PROTEIN 10g; CARBOHYDRATE 48g; TOTAL FAT 4.7g; SATURATED FAT 0.6g; SODIUM 134mg; FIBER 7g; BETA-CAROTENE 13,556mcg; VITAMIN C 131mg; CALCIUM 200mg; IRON 3.6mg; FOLATE 73mcg; MAGNESIUM 106mg; ZINC 1mg; SELENIUM 8.2mcg

Eat Your Greens Fruit Smoothie

Serves: 2

   3 ounces baby spinach or kale
   2 ounces romaine lettuce
   1 banana
   1 cup frozen or fresh blueberries
   ½ cup unsweetened soy, hemp, or almond milk
   ½ cup pomegranate juice
   1 tablespoon ground flaxseeds

Blend ingredients in a high-powered blender.

PER SERVING: CALORIES 191; PROTEIN 5g; CARBOHYDRATE 38g; TOTAL FAT 3.7g; SATURATED FAT 0.5g; SODIUM 51mg; FIBER 6.4g; BETA-CAROTENE 5442mcg; VITA-MIN C 59mg; CALCIUM 168mg; IRON 1.8mg; FOLATE 86mcg; MAGNESIUM 66mg; ZINC 0.8mg; SELENIUM 2.2mcg

Green Berry Blended Salad

Serves: 2

   2 ounces kale, tough stems removed
   2 ounces spinach
   1 cup frozen strawberries
   1 cup frozen blueberries
   1 orange, peeled
   1 cup unsweetened soy, hemp, or almond milk
   2 tablespoons ground flaxseeds

Blend ingredients in a high-powered blender.

PER SERVING: CALORIES 224; PROTEIN 8g; CARBOHYDRATE 39g; TOTAL FAT 6g; SATURATED FAT 0.6g; SODIUM 102mg; FIBER 8.9g; BETA-CAROTENE 4316mcg; VITA-MIN C 116mg; CALCIUM 163mg; IRON 3.2mg; FOLATE 133mcg; MAGNESIUM 110mg; ZINC 0.9mg; SELENIUM 8.8mcg

Turmeric and Ginger Tea

Serves: 2

    2 cups water
    1 Medjool date or 2 regular dates, pitted
    1 teaspoon grated turmeric root (or ⅓ teaspoon ground turmeric)
    1 teaspoon grated ginger root (or ⅓ teaspoon ground ginger)

Blend water and dates in a high-powered blender. Place in a small saucepan and bring to a boil. Add turmeric and ginger, reduce heat and simmer 10 to 15 minutes. Strain the tea. Serve with lemon if desired.

Note: If using ground turmeric and ginger, simmer for 7 minutes and do not strain.

PER SERVING: CALORIES 35; CARBOHYDRATE 9g; TOTAL FAT 0.1g; SODIUM 12mg; FIBER 0.9g; BETA-CAROTENE 11mcg; CALCIUM 16mg; IRON 0.3mg; FOLATE 2mcg; MAGNESIUM 10mg; ZINC 0.1mg

V6 Vegetable Cocktail

Serves: 1

    3 Roma tomatoes, roughly chopped
    1 stalk celery
    ½ bell pepper (any color is fine)
    1 green onion
    1 carrot
    2 cups chopped leafy greens (such as lettuce, kale, or spinach)
    1½ teaspoons lemon juice
    ½ teaspoon freshly grated horseradish
    5 ice cubes

Blend ingredients in a high-powered blender.

PER SERVING: CALORIES 115; PROTEIN 6g; CARBOHYDRATE 24g; TOTAL FAT 1.2g; SATURATED FAT 0.2g; SODIUM 147mg; FIBER 8.4g; BETA-CAROTENE 13,864mcg; VITAMIN C 130mg; CALCIUM 164mg; IRON 2.8mg; FOLATE 217mcg; MAGNESIUM 85mg; ZINC 1.4mg; SELENIUM 1.1mcg

BREAKFAST OPTIONS

Banana Cocoa Muffins

Serves: 24

15 Medjool or 30 regular dates, pitted
½ cup coconut water
2 cups garbanzo bean flour
1 teaspoon baking soda
1 teaspoon baking powder
¾ cup natural cocoa powder
1 tablespoon Ceylon cinnamon
1½ cups chopped apple
6 very ripe bananas
2 teaspoons alcohol-free vanilla flavoring
⅓ cup cooked garbanzo beans
2 teaspoons apple cider vinegar
1 cup walnuts, chopped
½ cup unsweetened shredded coconut
9 ounces wilted chopped fresh spinach

Soak the dates in coconut water for 30 minutes. Preheat the oven to 350°F. Line muffin tins with paper liners and wipe them very lightly with olive oil. Whisk together in a small bowl the garbanzo bean flour, baking soda, baking powder, cocoa, and cinnamon. In a high-powered blender, purée the dates and the soaking coconut water, apples, bananas, vanilla, garbanzo beans, and apple cider vinegar until smooth. Pour into a large mixing bowl and stir in the walnuts, coconut, and spinach until evenly distributed. Then fold in the flour mixture until just combined. Do not over mix. Fill the muffin tins almost full and bake for 55 to 65 minutes, rotating in the oven after 35 minutes. They are done when a toothpick inserted into the center comes out clean. Let the muffins cool in the muffin tins on a wire rack for 10 minutes, then remove from the tins to the wire rack and cool completely.

Refrigerate or freeze in resealable plastic bags.

PER SERVING: CALORIES 163; PROTEIN 4g; CARBOHYDRATE 30g; TOTAL FAT 5.1g; SATURATED FAT 1.6g; SODIUM 68mg; FIBER 4.9g; BETA-CAROTENE 622mcg; VITAMIN C 6mg; CALCIUM 46mg; IRON 1.5mg; FOLATE 43mcg; MAGNESIUM 64mg; ZINC 0.8mg; SELENIUM 7.7mcg

Blueberry and Flaxseed Oatmeal

Serves: 4

1¾ cups water
1 cup old-fashioned or steel cut oats (see Note)
3 Medjool or 6 regular dates, pitted and chopped
¼ teaspoon coriander
2 bananas, sliced
1 cup chopped or grated apple
1 cup fresh or frozen blueberries
2 tablespoons ground flaxseeds

In a saucepan, bring the water to a boil and stir in all ingredients except blueberries and ground flaxseeds. Simmer for 5 minutes. Stir in blueberries and flaxseeds before serving.

Note: If using steel cut oats, increase water to 3½ cups and simmer for 20 minutes or until tender.

PER SERVING: CALORIES 206; PROTEIN 4g; CARBOHYDRATE 43g; TOTAL FAT 3.5g; SATURATED FAT 0.5g; SODIUM 6mg; FIBER 6.7g; BETA-CAROTENE 33mcg; VITAMIN C 8mg; CALCIUM 24mg; IRON 5.5mg; FOLATE 19mcg; MAGNESIUM 38mg; ZINC 0.3mg; SELENIUM 1.8mcg

Breakfast Burrito

Serves: 2

½ cup chopped onion
1 cup chopped green bell pepper
1 cup sliced mushrooms
1 cup diced tomatoes
3 cups baby spinach or baby kale
8 ounces (½ block) firm tofu (or 3 eggs whites, see Note)
1 tablespoon nutritional yeast
1 teaspoon MatoZest*, Mrs. Dash, or other no-salt seasoning
    blend to taste
2 (100% whole grain) flour tortillas

Water-sauté onions, peppers, mushrooms, and tomatoes until onion is translucent. Add greens and continue cooking until just wilted. Squeeze out as much water as possible from the tofu, then crumble it over the vegetable mixture and cook until tofu is just starting to turn golden. Stir in nutritional yeast and seasoning. Spread the cooked mixture on the tortillas and roll up to form burritos.

Note: This recipe can be made with egg whites instead of or in addition to the tofu. Blend egg whites with ¼ cup nondairy milk, pour over the vegetable tofu mixture, and cook until eggs are done.

PER SERVING: CALORIES 370; PROTEIN 26g; CARBOHYDRATE 50g; TOTAL FAT 9.6g; SATURATED FAT 1.5g; SODIUM 234mg; FIBER 12.4g; BETA-CAROTENE 9832mcg; VI-TAMIN C 199mg; CALCIUM 377mg; IRON 6.7mg; FOLATE 69mcg; MAGNESIUM 67mg; ZINC 1.8mg; SELENIUM 4.4mcg

Buckwheat Seed Breakfast

Serves: 3

½ cup buckwheat groats
½ cup fresh or frozen blueberries
¼ cup grapes or any other fruit
¼ cup walnuts, chopped
¼ cup goji berries or raisins
1 teaspoon cinnamon (use Ceylon cinnamon if possible)
1 teaspoon alcohol-free vanilla flavoring
¼ cup unsweetened soy, hemp, or almond milk
¼ cup raw sunflower seeds
1 tablespoon chia seeds
1 tablespoon unsweetened, natural cocoa powder, if desired
1 tablespoon hemp seeds
1 banana

Mix all ingredients except hemp seeds and banana in a medium-size bowl and place in an airtight container in the fridge overnight. The next morning, top with hemp seeds and sliced banana and serve.

PER SERVING: CALORIES 343; PROTEIN 10g; CARBOHYDRATE 49g; TOTAL FAT 15g; SATURATED FAT 1.6g; SODIUM 18mg; FIBER 9.5g; BETA-CAROTENE 434mcg; VITA-MIN C 11mg; CALCIUM 90mg; IRON 3.2mg; FOLATE 61mcg; MAGNESIUM 152mg; ZINC 2mg; SELENIUM 12.5mcg

Chickpea Omelet with Mushrooms, Onions, and Kale

Serves: 2

For the Omelet Batter:
  ¾ cup chickpea flour
  ½ cup unsweetened soy, hemp, or almond milk (plus more if needed)
  2 teaspoons apple cider vinegar
  2 teaspoons nutritional yeast
  ½ teaspoon MatoZest* or other no-salt seasoning blend, adjusted
    to taste
  ½ teaspoon turmeric
  ¼ teaspoon baking soda
  ⅛ teaspoon black pepper

For the Vegetables:
  ½ cup chopped onions
  ½ cup chopped red pepper
  2 cloves garlic, chopped
  1 cup sliced mushrooms
  2 cups thinly sliced kale
  ½ cup low-sodium salsa or chopped tomato

In a small bowl, whisk together the omelet batter ingredients. Add an additional 1 to 2 tablespoons nondairy milk if mixture is too thick to pour. In a 10-inch nonstick skillet, heat 2 to 3 tablespoons water and sauté onions, red pepper, and garlic for 2 minutes; add mushrooms and continue to cook until soft and tender, about 3 more minutes. Add kale and stir until wilted. Remove from the pan. Clean the skillet and lightly wipe with olive oil. Pour half of the batter into the pan and swirl to evenly cover the bottom. Place half of the sautéed vegetables on top of one side of the omelet. Cook until the omelet bubbles and starts to firm up along the edges (about 2 minutes). Gently fold over one side and cook for another minute. Cover with a lid, remove from heat and allow to steam for 5 minutes. Repeat to make second omelet. Serve with salsa or chopped tomato.

PER SERVING: CALORIES 251; PROTEIN 16g; CARBOHYDRATE 39g; TOTAL FAT 4.3g; SATURATED FAT 0.5g; SODIUM 241mg; FIBER 8.6g; BETA-CAROTENE 6998mcg; VITAMIN C 139mg; CALCIUM 212mg; IRON 4.1mg; FOLATE 211mcg; MAGNESIUM 114mg; ZINC 2.5mg; SELENIUM 7.5mcg

Granny's Granola Bars

Serves: 10 bars

2 ripe bananas

1 Granny Smith apple, chopped into small pieces

1 cup raisins

1 cup chopped walnuts

½ cup raw sunflower seeds

¼ cup unhulled sesame seeds

1 teaspoon cinnamon or pumpkin pie spice

2 cups old-fashioned rolled oats

Preheat the oven to 300°F. Mash bananas to a soft consistency. Add remaining ingredients. Add a small amount of nondairy milk if needed to ease stirring. Lightly oil a 9 × 9-inch baking pan or glass dish. Pour mixture into baking dish and press to firm consistency. Bake mixture for 40 minutes. Remove from oven and let cool. Cut into bars. Wrap with aluminum foil and place in the fridge or freezer.

PER SERVING: CALORIES 272; PROTEIN 7g; CARBOHYDRATE 34g; TOTAL FAT 14g; SATURATED FAT 1.5g; SODIUM 3mg; FIBER 5g; BETA-CAROTENE 15mcg; VITAMIN C 4mg; CALCIUM 63mg; IRON 5.6mg; FOLATE 37mcg; MAGNESIUM 66mg; ZINC 1mg; SELENIUM 6mcg

Mango, Coconut, and Quinoa Breakfast Pudding
Serves: 5

¾ cup quinoa

1½ cups water

2 Medjool or 4 regular dates, pitted

1½ cups unsweetened soy, hemp, or almond milk

1 teaspoon alcohol-free vanilla flavoring

½ teaspoon cinnamon

1 (10-ounce) package frozen mango or 2 fresh mangoes, peeled and diced, divided

2 tablespoons Mangosteen Fruit Vinegar* or other fruit-flavored vinegar

⅛ cup chopped macadamia nuts

⅛ cup unhulled sesame seeds

1 cup packed chopped kale

1 cup packed chopped spinach

¼ cup dried currants

3 tablespoons unsweetened shredded coconut

Preheat the oven to 350°F. Rinse quinoa and drain in a fine-mesh sieve. In a large saucepan, bring quinoa and water to a boil. Reduce heat and simmer, uncovered, until grains are translucent and the mixture is the consistency of a thick porridge, about 20 minutes. In a high-powered blender, blend dates, nondairy milk, vanilla, cinnamon, half the mangoes, and Mangosteen Fruit Vinegar. In a large bowl, combine cooked quinoa, blended date mixture, nuts, seeds, kale, spinach, the remaining diced mango, and currants. Pour into a lightly oiled baking pan (9 × 9-inch works well), sprinkle with coconut, and bake 30 to 40 minutes. Best made a day ahead and refrigerated.

PER SERVING: CALORIES 330; PROTEIN 9g; CARBOHYDRATE 55g; TOTAL FAT 10g; SATURATED FAT 3.1g; SODIUM 56mg; FIBER 7g; BETA-CAROTENE 2441mcg; VITAMIN C 67mg; CALCIUM 122mg; IRON 3.3mg; FOLATE 139mcg; MAGNESIUM 118mg; ZINC 1.6mg; SELENIUM 9mcg

Nutritarian Granola
Serves: 10

½ cup raw almond or cashew butter
1 medium apple, peeled and quartered
1 ripe banana
1½ teaspoons ground cinnamon
¼ teaspoon ground nutmeg
1½ teaspoons alcohol-free vanilla flavoring
4 cups old-fashioned rolled oats
1 cup chopped raw walnuts or pecans
½ cup raw pumpkin seeds
¼ cup unhulled sesame seeds
⅓ cup unsweetened shredded coconut
1 cup currants

Preheat the oven to 225°F. Place the nut butter, apple, banana, cinnamon, nutmeg, and vanilla flavoring in a high-powered blender and blend until smooth and creamy. In a large bowl, mix the oats, nuts, seeds, and coconut. Add the blended mixture and toss to combine. Transfer the mixture to two parchment-lined baking pans. Do not overcrowd the pans so the granola can bake evenly. Bake for 30 minutes, stirring occasionally. After baking, stir in currants. Allow to cool, then store in an airtight container.

PER SERVING: CALORIES 337; PROTEIN 9g; CARBOHYDRATE 38g; TOTAL FAT 19.1g; SATURATED FAT 4g; SODIUM 5mg; FIBER 6.4g; BETA-CAROTENE 15mcg; VITAMIN C 2mg; CALCIUM 58mg; IRON 8.9mg; FOLATE 19mcg; MAGNESIUM 91mg; ZINC 1.7mg; SELENIUM 3.7mcg

Savory Steel Cut Oats

Serves: 4

  1 small onion, chopped
  1 cup mushrooms
  1 cup steel cut oats
  2 cups water or low-sodium vegetable broth
  1 cup unsweetened soy, hemp, or almond milk
  2 tablespoons nutritional yeast
  2 dashes of turmeric
  1½ teaspoons Cajun, southwest, or spicy no-salt seasoning
      of choice
  Dash of black pepper
  Dash of chipotle chili powder, or to taste
  1 ounce unsulfured, no-salt-added dried tomatoes, soaked until
      softened, and chopped
  3 cups fresh baby spinach

Dry sauté onions in a nonstick pan for 1 to 2 minutes, then add
mushrooms and continue to sauté until vegetables are tender. Add
onion and mushroom mixture and remaining ingredients except
spinach to a pot, heat to boiling, reduce heat, and simmer, stirring
occasionally, until the water is absorbed and the oats are creamy,
about 20 minutes. Stir in the spinach; take off the burner, cover, and
let sit a bit until the spinach is soft. If desired, garnish with chopped
red bell pepper.

PER SERVING: CALORIES 148; PROTEIN 9g; CARBOHYDRATE 23g; TOTAL FAT 3.2g;
SATURATED FAT 0.5g; SODIUM 58mg; FIBER 5g; BETA-CAROTENE 1346mcg; VITAMIN
C 11mg; CALCIUM 127mg; IRON 7.4mg; FOLATE 57mcg; MAGNESIUM 54mg; ZINC
1.6mg; SELENIUM 5mcg

Swiss Cherry Oatmeal

Serves: 3

2 cups water
1 cup old-fashioned or steel cut oats (see Note)
¾ cup frozen cherries or berries
¾ cup unsweetened soy, hemp, or almond milk
2 tablespoons ground flaxseeds
1 Medjool date or 2 regular dates, pitted
½ teaspoon alcohol-free vanilla flavoring
¼ cup raisins
¼ cup chopped almonds

Heat water to boiling. Add oats and cook for 5 minutes. Meanwhile, place frozen cherries, milk, flaxseeds, and dates in a high-powered blender and blend until smooth and creamy. Combine oats, fruit mixture, and vanilla. Cover and chill overnight. Serve topped with raisins and chopped almonds. Can be stored up to three days in the refrigerator.

Note: If using steel cut oats, increase water to 4 cups and simmer for 20 minutes or until tender.

PER SERVING: CALORIES 271; PROTEIN 9g; CARBOHYDRATE 42g; TOTAL FAT 9.1g; SATURATED FAT 1g; SODIUM 41mg; FIBER 7g; BETA-CAROTENE 204mcg; VITAMIN C 1mg; CALCIUM 65mg; IRON 8.1mg; FOLATE 22mcg; MAGNESIUM 65mg; ZINC 0.6mg; SELENIUM 4.5mcg

SALAD DRESSINGS, DIPS, AND SAUCES

Almond Vinaigrette Dressing
Serves: 6

1 cup unsweetened soy, hemp, or almond milk
1 cup raw almonds
¼ cup balsamic vinegar
2 tablespoons fresh lemon juice
¼ cup raisins
2 teaspoons Dijon mustard
1 clove garlic

Blend ingredients in a high-powered blender until creamy and smooth.

PER SERVING: CALORIES 181; PROTEIN 7g; CARBOHYDRATE 13g; TOTAL FAT 12.5g; SATURATED FAT 1g; SODIUM 38mg; FIBER 3.4g; BETA-CAROTENE 1mcg; VITAMIN C 2mg; CALCIUM 122mg; IRON 1.3mg; FOLATE 13mcg; MAGNESIUM 75mg; ZINC 0.9mg; SELENIUM 1.3mcg

Artichoke Hummus

Serves: 6

1 (12-ounce) bag frozen artichoke hearts

1½ cups cooked garbanzo beans or 1 (15-ounce) can no-salt-added garbanzo beans

2 tablespoons raw tahini or unhulled sesame seeds

2 tablespoons MatoZest* or other no-salt seasoning blend, adjusted to taste

2 tablespoons chopped onion

1 bulb roasted garlic, skins removed (see Note)

1 clove raw garlic

1 lemon, juiced

2 tablespoons water

Cook artichoke hearts according to package directions. Drain. Blend all ingredients until smooth. Add additional water if needed to adjust consistency. Use as a dip for raw veggies.

Note: Garlic can be roasted with the entire bulb intact and skin on or it can be roasted using peeled and separated cloves. Roast at 300°F for about 25 minutes or until soft.

PER SERVING: CALORIES 139; PROTEIN 7g; CARBOHYDRATE 22g; TOTAL FAT 3.9g; SATURATED FAT 0.5g; SODIUM 40mg; FIBER 6.3g; BETA-CAROTENE 7mcg; VITAMIN C 11mg; CALCIUM 75mg; IRON 2mg; FOLATE 159mcg; MAGNESIUM 48mg; ZINC 1.2mg; SELENIUM 2.7mcg

Creamy Blueberry Dressing

Serves: 4

  2 cups fresh or frozen (thawed) blueberries
  ½ cup pomegranate juice
  ¼ cup raw cashew butter or ½ cup raw cashews
  3 tablespoons Wild Blueberry Vinegar* or other fruit-flavored
    vinegar

Blend all ingredients in a food processor or high-powered blender
until smooth and creamy.

PER SERVING: CALORIES 106; PROTEIN 2g; CARBOHYDRATE 16g; TOTAL FAT 4.3g;
SATURATED FAT 0.7g; SODIUM 5mg; FIBER 2.4g; BETA-CAROTENE 22mcg; VITAMIN C
2mg; CALCIUM 14mg; IRON 0.8mg; FOLATE 15mcg; MAGNESIUM 31mg; ZINC 0.6mg;
SELENIUM 1.9mcg

Feisty Hummus

Serves: 4 (yields 1½ cups)

  1 cup cooked garbanzo beans or canned, no-salt-added or
    low-sodium, drained
  ¼ cup water
  ¼ cup raw unhulled sesame seeds
  1 tablespoon fresh lemon juice
  1 tablespoon VegiZest* or other no-salt seasoning blend, adjusted
    to taste
  1 teaspoon Bragg Liquid Aminos or low-sodium soy sauce
  1 teaspoon horseradish
  1 clove raw garlic

Blend all ingredients in a high-powered blender until creamy and
smooth. Serve with raw and lightly steamed vegetables or as a filling
ingredient with a whole grain wrap or pita.

PER SERVING: CALORIES 103; PROTEIN 5g; CARBOHYDRATE 12g; TOTAL FAT 4.5g;
SATURATED FAT 0.6g; SODIUM 54mg; FIBER 3.6g; BETA-CAROTENE 6mcg; VITAMIN C
3mg; CALCIUM 95mg; IRON 2.2mg; FOLATE 71mcg; MAGNESIUM 45mg; ZINC 1.1mg;
SELENIUM 3.9mcg

Garlic Nutter Spread

Serves: 4

3 bulbs garlic
1 cup raw cashews
⅓ cup water or nondairy milk
1 tablespoon nutritional yeast

Preheat the oven to 300°F. Roast garlic in a small baking dish for about 25 minutes or until soft. When cool, remove and discard skins. Combine garlic and remaining ingredients in a high-powered blender. Blend until smooth.

Use to season cooked vegetables or add extra flavor to soups and sauces. Spread it on a wrap or pita sandwich. Make a salad dressing by adding tomato sauce, vinegar, and some basil.

PER SERVING: CALORIES 230; PROTEIN 9g; CARBOHYDRATE 18g; TOTAL FAT 15.2g; SATURATED FAT 2.7g; SODIUM 9mg; FIBER 2g; BETA-CAROTENE 1mcg; VITAMIN C 7mg; CALCIUM 55mg; IRON 2.8mg; FOLATE 9mcg; MAGNESIUM 108mg; ZINC 2.6mg; SELENIUM 10mcg

Home-Style Tomato Sauce

Serves: 4

3 cups diced tomatoes
8 unsulfured, unsalted dried tomatoes, finely diced
1 small yellow onion, diced
8 cloves garlic, minced
1 tablespoon MatoZest* or other no-salt Italian seasoning blend,
    adjusted to taste
Freshly ground black pepper, to taste
2 tablespoons fresh basil, chopped

In a saucepan, cook tomatoes and dried tomatoes over medium-low heat until soft, about 10 minutes. Place in a food processor or blender and purée. Heat 2 to 3 tablespoons water in a medium skillet and sauté the onion and garlic for 2 minutes or until tender. Add the puréed tomato mixture, MatoZest, and pepper. Bring to a gentle boil, reduce heat to low, cover, and simmer for 1 hour. Add basil and adjust seasonings to taste, adding a little more MatoZest if you wish.

PER SERVING: CALORIES 53; PROTEIN 3g; CARBOHYDRATE 11g; TOTAL FAT 0.5g; SATURATED FAT 0.1g; SODIUM 15mg; FIBER 2.6g; BETA-CAROTENE 666mcg; VITAMIN C 24mg; CALCIUM 41mg; IRON 1mg; FOLATE 34mcg; MAGNESIUM 27mg; ZINC 0.4mg; SELENIUM 1.1mcg

Italian Dressing with Roasted Garlic
Serves: 4

4 to 8 cloves garlic, roasted (see Note)
1 cup unsweetened soy, hemp, or almond milk
½ cup raw cashew butter
2 tablespoons nutritional yeast
2 tablespoons fresh lemon juice
1 tablespoon white wine vinegar or more to taste
2 tablespoons Dijon mustard
2 tablespoons fresh parsley
1 teaspoon dried basil
¼ teaspoon crushed red pepper flakes
Pinch of dried oregano
⅛ teaspoon black pepper or to taste

Blend ingredients together in a high-powered blender or food processor. Adjust seasonings if necessary.

Note: Garlic can be roasted with the entire bulb intact and skin on, or it can be roasted using peeled and separated cloves. Roast at 300°F for about 25 minutes or until soft.

PER SERVING: CALORIES 239; PROTEIN 10g; CARBOHYDRATE 14g; TOTAL FAT 17.4g; SATURATED FAT 3.3g; SODIUM 119mg; FIBER 2.3g; BETA-CAROTENE 131mcg; VITAMIN C 7mg; CALCIUM 112mg; IRON 2.4mg; FOLATE 27mcg; MAGNESIUM 105mg; ZINC 2.8mg; SELENIUM 6.9mcg

Lemon Basil Vinaigrette

Serves: 4

2 tablespoons fresh lemon juice
2 tablespoons balsamic vinegar
½ cup water
¼ cup raw almonds or ⅛ cup raw almond butter
¼ cup raisins
⅓ cup fresh basil leaves
1 teaspoon Dijon mustard
1 clove garlic

Blend ingredients in a high-powered blender until smooth.

PER SERVING: CALORIES 86; PROTEIN 2g; CARBOHYDRATE 11g; TOTAL FAT 4.5g; SATURATED FAT 0.3g; SODIUM 21mg; FIBER 1.5g; BETA-CAROTENE 84mcg; VITAMIN C 4mg; CALCIUM 40mg; IRON 0.7mg; FOLATE 8mcg; MAGNESIUM 29mg; ZINC 0.3mg; SELENIUM 0.8mcg

Maui Luau Wok Sauce

Serves: 4

⅓ cup unsweetened, shredded coconut
½ cup water
1½ cups pineapple chunks
1 teaspoon Bragg Liquid Aminos or low-sodium soy sauce
1 scallion, sliced (2 tablespoons)
2 cloves garlic
½ teaspoon minced ginger
3 unsulfured dried apricots, soaked in ¼ cup water for 30 minutes
½ teaspoon no-salt seasoning blend such as Mrs. Dash
1 tablespoon Passion Fruit Vinegar* or rice vinegar

Place all ingredients in a blender and blend until smooth.

To use as a cooking sauce for your favorite vegetables, heat ¼ cup water in a large nonstick wok or skillet, add your choice of vegetables, cover, and cook until crisp-tender, about 4 to 8 minutes, depending on the vegetable, stirring occasionally and adding additional water as needed. Uncover, add desired amount of Maui Luau Wok Sauce, and continue cooking until mixture is heated through.

PER SERVING: CALORIES 89; PROTEIN 1g; CARBOHYDRATE 12g; TOTAL FAT 5g; SATURATED FAT 4.3g; SODIUM 61mg; FIBER 1.6g; BETA-CAROTENE 96mcg; VITAMIN C 12mg; CALCIUM 21mg; IRON 0.6mg; FOLATE 3mcg; MAGNESIUM 17mg; ZINC 0.3mg; SELENIUM 1.7mcg

Orange Sesame Dressing

Serves: 3

> 4 tablespoons unhulled sesame seeds, divided
> ¼ cup raw cashew nuts or ⅛ cup raw cashew butter
> 2 navel oranges, peeled
> 2 tablespoons Blood Orange Vinegar*, Riesling Reserve Vinegar*,
>   or white wine vinegar

Toast the sesame seeds in a dry skillet over medium-high heat for 3 minutes, mixing with a wooden spoon and shaking the pan frequently. In a high-powered blender, combine 2 tablespoons of the sesame seeds, cashews, oranges, and vinegar. If needed, add orange juice for a thinner consistency. Sprinkle remaining sesame seeds on top of the salad.

Serving Suggestion: Toss with mixed greens, tomatoes, red onions, and additional diced oranges or kiwi.

PER SERVING: CALORIES 162; PROTEIN 5g; CARBOHYDRATE 17g; TOTAL FAT 9.6g; SATURATED FAT 1.5g; SODIUM 4mg; FIBER 3.5g; BETA-CAROTENE 82mcg; VITAMIN C 55mg; CALCIUM 133mg; IRON 2.2mg; FOLATE 43mcg; MAGNESIUM 76mg; ZINC 1.4mg; SELENIUM 5.4mcg

Pistachio Mustard Dressing

Serves: 4

¾ cup unsweetened soy, hemp, or almond milk
⅓ cup raw shelled pistachio nuts
2 tablespoons VegiZest* or other no-salt seasoning blend,
   adjusted to taste
1 tablespoon Dijon mustard
¼ teaspoon garlic powder

Blend all ingredients in a high-powered blender until smooth.

PER SERVING: CALORIES 90; PROTEIN 5g; CARBOHYDRATE 7g; TOTAL FAT 5.7g; SAT-URATED FAT 0.7g; SODIUM 69mg; FIBER 2g; BETA-CAROTENE 27mcg; VITAMIN C 3mg; CALCIUM 86mg; IRON 1.2mg; FOLATE 21mcg; MAGNESIUM 30mg; ZINC 0.5mg; SELENIUM 2.3mcg

Russian Fig Dressing

Serves: 4

⅔ cup no-salt-added or low-sodium pasta sauce
⅔ cup raw almonds or 6 tablespoons raw almond butter
¼ cup raw sunflower seeds
6 tablespoons Black Fig Vinegar* or balsamic vinegar
2 tablespoons raisins or dried currants

Blend ingredients in a food processor or high-powered blender until smooth.

PER SERVING: CALORIES 243; PROTEIN 8g; CARBOHYDRATE 18g; TOTAL FAT 16.9g; SATURATED FAT 1.4g; CHOLESTEROL 0.9mg; SODIUM 20mg; FIBER 4.6g; BETA-CAROTENE 170mcg; VITAMIN C 1mg; CALCIUM 90mg; IRON 1.9mg; FOLATE 38mcg; MAGNESIUM 104mg; ZINC 1.3mg; SELENIUM 5.7mcg

Sunny Tuscan Dressing

Serves: 4

¼ cup dried, unsulfured apricots
1 navel orange, peeled
2 tablespoons unhulled sesame seeds or tahini
¼ cup raw cashews
2 tablespoons Lemon Basil Vinegar* or balsamic vinegar
1 teaspoon dried basil
½ teaspoon dried oregano
2 scallions (white part only)

Soak apricots in ½ cup water for 30 minutes. Add apricots and soaking water to a high-powered blender along with remaining ingredients and blend until smooth.

PER SERVING: CALORIES 120; PROTEIN 3g; CARBOHYDRATE 15g; TOTAL FAT 6.1g; SATURATED FAT 1g; SODIUM 6mg; FIBER 2.5g; BETA-CAROTENE 354mcg; VITAMIN C 22mg; CALCIUM 86mg; IRON 2.1mg; FOLATE 23mcg; MAGNESIUM 53mg; ZINC 1mg; SELENIUM 3.5mcg

Walnut Vinaigrette Dressing

Serves: 4

¼ cup balsamic vinegar
½ cup water
¼ cup walnuts
¼ cup raisins
1 teaspoon Dijon mustard
1 clove garlic
¼ teaspoon dried thyme

Blend ingredients in a high-powered blender until smooth.

PER SERVING: CALORIES 84; PROTEIN 1g; CARBOHYDRATE 11g; TOTAL FAT 4.2g; SATURATED FAT 0.4g; SODIUM 21mg; FIBER 0.8g; BETA-CAROTENE 3mcg; VITAMIN C 1mg; CALCIUM 20mg; IRON 0.6mg; FOLATE 7mcg; MAGNESIUM 16mg; ZINC 0.3mg; SELENIUM 0.9mcg

SALADS

Baba Ghanoush over Mixed Greens

Serves: 4

1 (1½-pound) eggplant
1 cup cooked garbanzo beans or low-sodium or no-salt-added
   canned garbanzo beans
2 tablespoons raw tahini or unhulled sesame seeds
2 tablespoons fresh lemon juice
2 cloves garlic, finely chopped
⅓ cup water
1 teaspoon Bragg Liquid Aminos
5 ounces romaine lettuce, chopped
5 ounces mixed baby greens

Preheat the oven to 350°F. Prick eggplant, place on baking sheet, and
bake for 45 minutes, turning occasionally, until soft. Let it cool and
then peel. In a high-powered blender, combine eggplant, garbanzo
beans, tahini, lemon juice, garlic, water, and Bragg Liquid Aminos.
Blend until smooth. Combine romaine and mixed baby greens and
serve baba ghanoush on a bed of greens. Baba ghanoush and greens
can also be served in a whole wheat pita or wrap.

PER SERVING: CALORIES 155; PROTEIN 8g; CARBOHYDRATE 23g; TOTAL FAT 5.1g;
SATURATED FAT 0.7g; SODIUM 83mg; FIBER 9.2g; BETA-CAROTENE 3954mcg; VITA-
MIN C 13mg; CALCIUM 104mg; IRON 2.5mg; FOLATE 190mcg; MAGNESIUM 61mg;
ZINC 1.4mg; SELENIUM 2.4mcg

Broccoli and Chickpea Salad

Serves: 4

For the Salad:
> 6 cups broccoli, cut into small florets
> 1½ cups cooked chickpeas or 1 (15-ounce) can no-salt-added or low-sodium chickpeas, drained
> ¼ cup chopped red onion
> 1½ cups halved cherry tomatoes
> ¼ cup pine nuts or walnuts, toasted

For the Dressing:
> ¼ cup fresh lemon juice
> ½ cup water
> ¼ cup walnuts
> ¼ cup pitted and chopped dates
> 1 teaspoon Dijon mustard
> 1 clove garlic

Steam broccoli until just tender, 5 to 7 minutes. Once cool, combine with chickpeas, onion, cherry tomatoes, and nuts. Blend dressing ingredients in a high-powered blender. Toss salad with desired amount of dressing. Leftover dressing may be reserved for another use.

PER SERVING: CALORIES 298; PROTEIN 13g; CARBOHYDRATE 40g; TOTAL FAT 12.9g; SATURATED FAT 1.1g; SODIUM 70mg; FIBER 8.9g; BETA-CAROTENE 809mcg; VITAMIN C 139mg; CALCIUM 119mg; IRON 3.8mg; FOLATE 218mcg; MAGNESIUM 105mg; ZINC 2.5mg; SELENIUM 7mcg

Cabbage, Apple, and Poppy Seed Slaw
Serves: 8

For the Slaw:

    3 medium Granny Smith apples, coarsely grated
    2 tablespoons lemon juice
    8 cups shredded green cabbage (1 small head)
    3 medium carrots, coarsely grated
    4 green onions, thinly sliced
    2 tablespoons poppy seeds

For the Dressing:

    1 cup soft tofu
    ½ cup unsweetened soy, hemp, or almond milk
    ¼ cup Spicy Pecan Vinegar* or apple cider vinegar
    3 Medjool or 6 regular dates, pitted
    Black pepper, to taste

Toss grated apples with lemon juice. Combine with remaining slaw ingredients. Blend dressing ingredients in a high-powered blender until smooth and creamy. Toss with slaw.

PER SERVING: CALORIES 128; PROTEIN 4g; CARBOHYDRATE 25g; TOTAL FAT 2.7g; SATURATED FAT 0.4g; SODIUM 39mg; FIBER 5.3g; BETA-CAROTENE 2096mcg; VITAMIN C 32mg; CALCIUM 136mg; IRON 1.3mg; FOLATE 57mcg; MAGNESIUM 40mg; ZINC 0.7mg; SELENIUM 3.5mcg

Creamy Cucumber and Onion Salad

Serves: 4

½ cup unsweetened soy, hemp, or almond milk
½ cup raw cashews or ¼ cup raw cashew butter
¼ cup white vinegar
1 teaspoon low-sodium mustard
1 small clove garlic, peeled
4 large cucumbers, thinly sliced
1 medium white sweet onion, thinly sliced
1 tablespoon fresh dill or 1 teaspoon dried dill

Combine nondairy milk, cashews, vinegar, mustard, and garlic in a high-powered blender and blend until smooth and creamy. Combine cucumbers, onion, and dill and toss with desired amount of dressing. Refrigerate for at least 1 hour before serving.

PER SERVING: CALORIES 170; PROTEIN 6g; CARBOHYDRATE 19g; TOTAL FAT 8.5g; SATURATED FAT 1.4g; SODIUM 42mg; FIBER 3.5g; BETA-CAROTENE 88mcg; VITAMIN C 13mg; CALCIUM 108mg; IRON 2.3mg; FOLATE 44mcg; MAGNESIUM 98mg; ZINC 1.7mg; SELENIUM 4.6mcg

Edamame Black Bean Salad

Serves: 4

12 ounces frozen shelled edamame
1½ cups cooked black beans or 1 (15-ounce) can low-sodium or
    no-salt-added black beans, drained
1 medium tomato, chopped
½ medium green bell pepper, chopped
¼ cup chopped red onion
¼ cup chopped cilantro
1 ripe avocado
1 tablespoon lime juice
1 cup unsweetened soy, hemp, or almond milk
¼ cup raw cashews
1 Medjool or 2 regular dates, pitted

Bring a saucepan of water to a boil, add edamame, and boil for two
minutes. Drain and rinse with cold water. In a large bowl, combine
the edamame, beans, tomato, bell pepper, onion, and cilantro. Blend
avocado, lime juice, nondairy milk, cashews, and dates in a high-
powered blender. Add half of the dressing to the edamame and black
bean mixture and toss. Add additional dressing to adjust to desired
consistency.

PER SERVING: CALORIES 339; PROTEIN 19g; CARBOHYDRATE 38g; TOTAL FAT 14.5g;
SATURATED FAT 1.6g; SODIUM 44mg; FIBER 13.7g; BETA-CAROTENE 232mcg; VITA-
MIN C 30mg; CALCIUM 101mg; IRON 4.5mg; FOLATE 407mcg; MAGNESIUM 155mg;
ZINC 2.7mg; SELENIUM 5.7mcg

Farro and Kale Salad with White Beans and Walnuts

Serves: 4

>   1 cup farro (see Note)
>   3¼ cups low-sodium or no-salt-added vegetable broth, divided
>   2 cups whole baby kale leaves or chopped kale
>   ¼ cup unsulfured dried blueberries or currants
>   1 cup cooked white beans
>   ¼ cup walnut pieces or lightly toasted pine nuts
>   1 teaspoon chia seeds
>   2 tablespoons balsamic vinegar
>   1 tablespoon fresh lemon juice
>   1 teaspoon Dijon mustard
>   Ground black pepper, to taste

Place farro in a pot with 3 cups of the vegetable broth and bring to a boil. Reduce heat to a simmer, cover the pot, and cook for 30 to 45 minutes, until grains are tender but not split and have absorbed all of the liquid (or cook according to package instructions). Remove from heat and transfer to a large bowl. Add the kale, dried blueberries, white beans, and walnuts to the farro. Stir to allow the warm farro to wilt the kale. To make the dressing, whisk together the chia seeds, the remaining ¼ cup vegetable broth, vinegar, lemon juice, mustard, and pepper in a small bowl. Allow to stand for 15 minutes to thicken. Toss farro salad with enough dressing to moisten it but not make it too wet.

Note: Look for whole grain or semi-pearled farro, which are higher in nutrient density. Pearled farro cooks faster, but the nutritious germ and bran have been removed.

PER SERVING: CALORIES 306; PROTEIN 9g; CARBOHYDRATE 57g; TOTAL FAT 6.2g; SATURATED FAT 0.7g; SODIUM 183mg; FIBER 9.9g; BETA-CAROTENE 3102mcg; VITAMIN C 47mg; CALCIUM 113mg; IRON 3.3mg; FOLATE 51mcg; MAGNESIUM 84mg; ZINC 1.7mg; SELENIUM 20.9mcg

Napa Cabbage Salad with Sesame Peanut Dressing

Serves: 4

For the Dressing:

¼ cup no-salt-added, natural peanut butter
2 tablespoons unhulled sesame seeds
¼ cup unsweetened soy, hemp, or almond milk
¼ cup water
¼ cup rice vinegar
3 regular dates or 1½ Medjool dates, pitted
1 clove garlic, chopped
1 tablespoon chopped fresh ginger
1 teaspoon Bragg Liquid Aminos

For the Salad:

6 cups shredded napa cabbage
1 small red bell pepper, thinly sliced
1 cup thinly sliced snow peas
6 green onions, sliced

Blend dressing ingredients in a high-powered blender until smooth. Combine salad ingredients in a large bowl and toss with desired amount of dressing.

Note: For your convenience, I make a line of healthful bottled salad dressings. Try Dr. Fuhrman's Sesame Ginger Dressing (about ¾ cup) in place of the dressing listed in this recipe.

PER SERVING: CALORIES 175; PROTEIN 7g; CARBOHYDRATE 16g; TOTAL FAT 10.5g; SATURATED FAT 1.5g; SODIUM 85mg; FIBER 4g; BETA-CAROTENE 1052mcg; VITAMIN C 65mg; CALCIUM 143mg; IRON 2mg; FOLATE 142mcg; MAGNESIUM 74mg; ZINC 1.3mg; SELENIUM 3.6mcg

SOUPS AND STEWS

Broccoli Mushroom Bisque

Serves: 4

1 head broccoli, cut into florets
8 ounces mushrooms, sliced
3 carrots, coarsely chopped
1 cup coarsely chopped celery
1 onion, chopped
2 cloves garlic, minced
2 tablespoons VegiZest* or 2 teaspoons Mrs. Dash no-salt
    seasoning blend
2 cups carrot juice
4 cups water
½ teaspoon nutmeg
½ cup raw pecans

Place all the ingredients except the pecans in a soup pot. Cover and simmer for 20 minutes or until the vegetables are just tender. In a food processor or high-powered blender, blend two-thirds of the soup liquid and vegetables with the nuts until smooth and creamy. Return to the pot and reheat before serving.

PER SERVING: CALORIES 221; PROTEIN 9g; CARBOHYDRATE 31g; TOTAL FAT 9.8g; SATURATED FAT 0.9g; SODIUM 168mg; FIBER 6.4g; BETA-CAROTENE 14,968mcg; VI-TAMIN C 49mg; CALCIUM 133mg; IRON 2.5mg; FOLATE 101mcg; MAGNESIUM 73mg; ZINC 2.8mg; SELENIUM 40.1mcg

Butternut Breakfast Soup

Serves: 6

4 cups frozen butternut squash
2 medium apples, peeled, seeded, and chopped
4 cups (packed) kale, tough stems and center ribs removed and
    leaves chopped, or frozen kale, chopped
1 cup chopped onion
2 tablespoons Pomegranate Balsamic Vinegar* or other fruit-
    flavored vinegar
5 cups carrot juice, fresh (5 pounds of carrots, juiced) or store-
    bought refrigerated
½ cup unsweetened soy, almond, or hemp milk
½ cup raw cashews
¼ cup hemp seeds
1 teaspoon cinnamon
½ teaspoon nutmeg

Place squash, apples, kale, onion, vinegar, and carrot juice in a soup
pot. Bring to a boil, lower heat, cover, and simmer for 30 minutes or
until kale is tender. Purée half of the soup with the nondairy milk,
cashews, and hemp seeds in a high-powered blender. Return blended
mixture to soup pot. Add cinnamon and nutmeg.

PER SERVING: CALORIES 314; PROTEIN 9g; CARBOHYDRATE 58g; TOTAL FAT 8.3g;
SATURATED FAT 1.3g; SODIUM 167mg; FIBER 9.7g; BETA-CAROTENE 28,816mcg;
VITAMIN C 106mg; CALCIUM 267mg; IRON 4.3mg; FOLATE 70mcg; MAGNESIUM
159mg; ZINC 1.9mg; SELENIUM 8.4mcg

Cauliflower, Coconut, and Turmeric Soup

Serves: 4

½ cup unsweetened shredded coconut
1 teaspoon chopped fresh ginger
1 cup water
1 medium onion, chopped
4 cloves garlic, chopped
3 cups sliced shiitake mushrooms
1 head cauliflower, cut into pieces
4½ cups low-sodium or no-salt-added vegetable broth
½ teaspoon turmeric
½ teaspoon ground coriander
¼ cup raw macadamia nuts
¼ cup raw walnuts
1 bunch kale, tough stems removed, chopped
½ cup shredded cooked chicken or ½ cup raw chopped shrimp,
   optional (see Note)

Blend coconut, ginger, and water in a high-powered blender until smooth and creamy. In a soup pot, heat 2 to 3 tablespoons water and water-sauté onion and garlic for 2 minutes, then add mushrooms and sauté until onions and mushrooms are tender. Add blended coconut mixture, cauliflower, vegetable broth, turmeric, and coriander. Bring to a boil, reduce heat, cover, and simmer for 15 minutes or until the cauliflower is tender. In a high-powered blender, blend two-thirds of the soup liquid and vegetables with the macadamia nuts and walnuts until smooth and creamy. Return to the pot and reheat. Steam the kale until wilted and just tender, about 6 to 8 minutes. Divide steamed kale into four soup bowls and serve the soup on top. For added crunch, top with Crispy Chickpeas (page 328).

Note: If desired, add chicken or shrimp after soup is blended and returned to the soup pot. Add ½ cup cooked shredded chicken and reheat or add ½ cup chopped raw shrimp and simmer for 3 to 4 minutes or until shrimp turns pink.

PER SERVING: CALORIES 305; PROTEIN 9.3g; CARBOHYDRATE 29g; TOTAL FAT 19.7g; SATURATED FAT 8.1g; SODIUM 246mg; FIBER 9.1g; BETA-CAROTENE 7728mcg; VITAMIN C 175mg; CALCIUM 205mg; IRON 3.8mg; FOLATE 123mcg; MAGNESIUM 94mg; ZINC 1.7mg; SELENIUM 6.6mcg

Chickpea Mulligatawny Stew

Serves: 6

¾ cup unsweetened flaked coconut
4 cups low-sodium or no-salt-added vegetable broth, divided
3 Medjool dates or 6 regular dates, pitted
1 onion, chopped
¼ cup garlic cloves, chopped
1 carrot, peeled and diced
1 stalk celery, chopped
2 tablespoons white wine
4 ounces cremini mushrooms, chopped
1 Granny Smith apple, peeled and diced
2 tablespoons curry powder
3 cups cooked chickpeas or 2 (15-ounce) cans low-sodium
   or no-salt-added chickpeas, drained
3 cups no-salt-added diced tomatoes, in BPA-free packaging
Cayenne pepper, to taste
1 pound chopped fresh or frozen spinach (or greens of your
   choice)
½ pound steamed broccoli florets
½ pound steamed cauliflower florets

Purée the flaked coconut, 2 cups of the broth, and the dates in a high-powered blender until smooth. Set aside.

In a large soup pot, sauté the onion, garlic, carrot, and celery in the white wine until the onions are translucent and lightly browned. Add the mushrooms and apple and continue to cook until the mushrooms release their juices. Add the curry powder and sauté for another minute. Add the chickpeas, tomatoes, coconut purée, and the remaining broth and bring to a boil. Simmer for 10 minutes, taste and adjust with more curry powder and cayenne if desired. Then, stir in the spinach, broccoli, and cauliflower and continue cooking until the spinach is wilted.

PER SERVING: CALORIES 362; PROTEIN 15g; CARBOHYDRATE 57g; TOTAL FAT 10.8g; SATURATED FAT 6.9g; SODIUM 202mg; FIBER 16.2g; BETA-CAROTENE 6771mcg; VITAMIN C 75mg; CALCIUM 232mg; IRON 6.2mg; FOLATE 328mcg; MAGNESIUM 150mg; ZINC 2.7mg; SELENIUM 13.9mcg

Cuban Black Bean Soup with Garlic "Mashed Potatoes"

Serves: 5

For the Soup:
   1 small onion, chopped
   3 cloves garlic, minced
   1 tablespoon chili powder
   2 teaspoons ground cumin
   3 cups cooked black beans or 2 (15-ounce) cans low-sodium black
       beans, drained and rinsed
   3 cups low-sodium or no-salt-added vegetable broth
   ⅔ cup low-sodium all-natural salsa
   1 tablespoon lime juice
   A few dashes of chipotle hot sauce
   ½ bunch cilantro, chopped
   4 green onions, chopped

For the "Mashed Potatoes":
   1 large head cauliflower, chopped
   1 small clove garlic, minced
   ½ to 1 cup soy, hemp, or almond milk (to desired consistency)
   ¼ teaspoon pepper, or to taste
   ¼ cup nutritional yeast
   2 stalks green onions, chopped

Sauté onion and garlic in a splash of low-sodium vegetable broth
until tender. Add chili and cumin, stir until combined. Add beans,
vegetable broth, salsa, lime juice, and hot sauce. Bring to a boil, then
cover and simmer about 45 minutes. Remove from heat and purée
about half of the soup in a high-powered blender. Stir in cilantro and
green onions. Cover and set aside until ready to serve.

Steam cauliflower until tender. Place into high-powered blender along
with remaining ingredients except for green onions and blend until
smooth (add nondairy milk until desired consistency). Serve soup
topped with "mashed potatoes" and garnish with green onions.

PER SERVING: CALORIES 259; PROTEIN 20g; CARBOHYDRATE 42g; TOTAL FAT 3.1g;
SATURATED FAT 0.7g; SODIUM 138mg; FIBER 15.2g; BETA-CAROTENE 503mcg; VITA-
MIN C 88mg; CALCIUM 134mg; IRON 4.6mg; FOLATE 260mcg; MAGNESIUM 123mg;
ZINC 3.3mg; SELENIUM 3.1mcg

Dr. Fuhrman's Famous Anticancer Soup

Serves: 10

1 cup dried split peas
½ cup dried adzuki or cannellini beans
4 cups water
6 to 10 medium zucchini
5 pounds large organic carrots, juiced (6 cups juice; see Note)
2 bunches celery, juiced (2 cups juice; see Note)
2 tablespoons VegiZest* or other no-salt seasoning blend, adjusted to taste
1 teaspoon Mrs. Dash no-salt seasoning
4 medium onions, chopped
3 leek stalks, cut lengthwise and cleaned carefully, then coarsely chopped
2 bunches kale, collard greens, or other greens, tough stems and center ribs removed and leaves chopped
1 cup raw cashews
2½ cups chopped fresh mushrooms (shiitake, cremini, and/or white)

Place the peas and beans and water in a very large pot over low heat. Bring to a boil, and reduce heat. Add the zucchini whole to the pot. Add the carrot juice, celery juice, VegiZest, and Mrs. Dash. Put the onions, leeks, and kale in a blender and blend with a little bit of the soup liquid. Pour this mixture into the soup pot. After at least 10 minutes, remove the softened zucchini with tongs and blend them in the blender with the cashews until creamy. Pour this mixture back into the soup pot. Add the mushrooms and continue to simmer until the beans are soft, about 2 hours total cooking time.

Note: Freshly juiced organic carrots and celery will maximize the flavor of this soup.

PER SERVING: CALORIES 296; PROTEIN 14g; CARBOHYDRATE 49g; TOTAL FAT 7.5g; SATURATED FAT 1.4g; SODIUM 172mg; FIBER 10.2g; BETA-CAROTENE 16,410mcg; VITAMIN C 90mg; CALCIUM 178mg; IRON 4.8mg; FOLATE 203mcg; MAGNESIUM 151mg; ZINC 3mg; SELENIUM 10.1mcg

French Minted Pea Soup

Serves: 3

10 ounces frozen green peas
1 small onion, chopped
1 clove garlic, chopped
3 tablespoons VegiZest*, or other no-salt seasoning, adjusted to
　　taste
3 cups water
1 bunch fresh mint leaves (save a few leaves for garnish)
3 regular dates, pitted
½ cup raw cashews
½ tablespoon Spike no-salt seasoning, or other no-salt seasoning,
　　to taste
4 teaspoons fresh lemon juice
4 cups shredded romaine lettuce or chopped baby spinach
2 tablespoons fresh snipped chives

Simmer peas, onions, garlic, and seasonings in water for about 7
minutes. Pour pea mixture into a high-powered blender or food
processor. Add remaining ingredients except for the lettuce and
chives. Blend until smooth and creamy. Add lettuce or spinach and
let it wilt in hot liquid. Pour into bowls and garnish with chives and
mint leaves.

PER SERVING: CALORIES 313; PROTEIN 14g; CARBOHYDRATE 45g; TOTAL FAT 11.4g;
SATURATED FAT 1.9g; SODIUM 153mg; FIBER 11.6g; BETA-CAROTENE 4496mcg; VI-
TAMIN C 39mg; CALCIUM 192mg; IRON 9mg; FOLATE 210mcg; MAGNESIUM 156mg;
ZINC 3mg; SELENIUM 8.1mcg

Golden Austrian Cauliflower Cream Soup

Serves: 4

1 head cauliflower, cut into pieces
3 carrots, coarsely chopped
1 cup coarsely chopped celery
2 leeks, coarsely chopped
2 cloves garlic, minced
2 tablespoons VegiZest* or other no-salt seasoning blend,
    adjusted to taste
2 cups carrot juice
4 cups water
½ teaspoon nutmeg
1 cup raw cashews
5 cups chopped kale leaves or baby spinach

Place all ingredients except cashews and kale in a pot. Cover and
simmer for 15 minutes or until the vegetables are just tender. In
a food processor or high-powered blender, blend half of the soup
liquid and vegetables with the cashews until smooth and creamy and
return to the pot. Finely chop the kale or spinach and add to the pot;
simmer for 10 more minutes.

PER SERVING: CALORIES 369; PROTEIN 15g; CARBOHYDRATE 48g; TOTAL FAT 16.7g;
SATURATED FAT 1.6g; SODIUM 238mg; FIBER 18.1g; BETA-CAROTENE 17,409mcg;
VITAMIN C 104mg; CALCIUM 359mg; IRON 4.5mg; FOLATE 233mcg; MAGNESIUM
149mg; ZINC 2.4mg; SELENIUM 3.5mcg

Split Pea and Lentil Soup

Serves: 6

1½ cups split peas, rinsed
½ cup lentils, rinsed
¼ cup pine nuts, lightly toasted, plus additional if desired
  for garnish
2 large onions, chopped
3 cloves garlic, chopped
4 stalks celery, chopped
3 cups coarsely chopped mushrooms
5 carrots, diced
1 cup carrot juice
3 cups low-sodium or no-salt-added vegetable broth
3 tablespoons fresh, chopped dill
2 tablespoons salt-free Italian seasoning blend
½ teaspoon dried marjoram
¼ teaspoon ground black pepper

Bring 3 cups of water to a boil, add split peas and lentils and return
to a boil. Reduce heat, partially cover the pot, and simmer for 40
minutes or until split peas and lentils are tender. Place cooked lentils
and split peas and toasted pine nuts in a high-powered blender or
food processor and blend until smooth. While split peas and lentils
are cooking, add remaining ingredients to a large soup pot and
cook over low heat until vegetables are tender, about 15 minutes.
Add blended split pea mixture to soup pot and mix well. If desired,
garnish with additional toasted pine nuts.

PER SERVING: CALORIES 342; PROTEIN 20g; CARBOHYDRATE 57g; TOTAL FAT 5g;
SATURATED FAT 0.5g; SODIUM 163mg; FIBER 21.4g; BETA-CAROTENE 8001mcg; VITA-
MIN C 14mg; CALCIUM 112mg; IRON 4.9mg; FOLATE 252mcg; MAGNESIUM 115mg;
ZINC 3.1mg; SELENIUM 6.3mcg

Tomato Barley Stew
Serves: 2

> 2 cups no-salt-added or low-sodium vegetable broth
> 1 medium onion, chopped
> 2 carrots, diced
> 1 zucchini, chopped
> 1 sweet potato, peeled and chopped
> ¼ cup hulled barley (barley groats)
> 6 tomatoes, chopped
> ⅓ cup unsulfured, no-salt-added sun-dried tomatoes, soaked in
>   warm water to cover for 30 minutes, then finely chopped
> 8 ounces shiitake, oyster, or cremini mushrooms, stems removed
>   and caps chopped

Bring vegetable broth to a simmer; add the onion, carrots, zucchini, and potato. Let simmer about 1 hour and then blend in a high-powered blender. Return puréed mixture to the pot and add the barley, tomatoes, dried tomatoes, and mushrooms and simmer for another 45 minutes.

PER SERVING: CALORIES 326; PROTEIN 12g; CARBOHYDRATE 70g; TOTAL FAT 2.4g; SATURATED FAT 0.4g; SODIUM 273mg; FIBER 16.8g; BETA-CAROTENE 11,979mcg; VITAMIN C 68mg; CALCIUM 139mg; IRON 4.3mg; FOLATE 104mcg; MAGNESIUM 147mg; ZINC 3.2mg; SELENIUM 16.6mcg

MAIN DISHES AND VEGETABLE SIDE DISHES

Asian Vegetables with Batter-Dipped Tofu
Serves: 4

For the Batter-Dipped Tofu:
>   1 (14-ounce) block firm tofu, drained
>   1 cup chickpea flour
>   ¼ cup nutritional yeast
>   1 teaspoon kelp granules
>   1 teaspoon salt-free seasoning blend (such as Mrs. Dash)
>   ½ teaspoon paprika (or cayenne pepper to taste)
>   ⅓ to ½ cup water
>   1 tablespoon Dijon mustard

For the Vegetables:
>   6 cups water
>   5 sprigs cilantro
>   10 scallions, divided
>   1 (3-inch) piece ginger, sliced
>   1 stalk lemongrass, trimmed, tough outer layer removed,
>   thinly sliced
>   2 teaspoons lemon zest
>   3 cloves garlic, crushed
>   2 tablespoons tahini or puréed unhulled sesame seeds
>   5 stalks celery, thinly sliced
>   5 carrots, thinly sliced
>   6 baby bok choy, halved
>   6 napa cabbage leaves, sliced
>   2 cups shiitake mushrooms, larger ones sliced, smaller ones
>   left whole
>   2 teaspoons Bragg Liquid Aminos
>   2 tablespoons arrowroot powder mixed with 2 tablespoons
>   cold water
>   1 Medjool or 2 regular dates, pitted and chopped

Preheat the oven to 350°F. Gently squeeze tofu to remove excess water. Wrap in paper towels, place something heavy on top, and press for 10 minutes to remove additional moisture. Combine flour, nutritional yeast, kelp, salt-free seasoning, and paprika in a bowl. Using a whisk, mix while adding water gradually. Mixture should resemble a thick batter. Stir in mustard. Crumble tofu into pieces and combine with the coating. Place on a parchment-lined baking sheet and bake for 20 to 25 minutes, until batter is dry.

While tofu is cooking, prepare the vegetables. In the bottom of a steamer pot, combine water, cilantro, four of the scallions (cut in 2-inch pieces), ginger, lemongrass, lemon zest, garlic, and tahini. Bring to a boil. Place celery, carrots, baby bok choy, napa cabbage, remaining scallions (sliced lengthwise), and shiitake mushrooms in the steamer basket. Steam until crisp-tender, about 8 minutes. Reserve 3 cups of the liquid from the steamer pot.

Place reserved liquid in a saucepan and bring to a boil. Add Bragg Liquid Aminos and arrowroot/water mixture. Whisk until thickened, about 5 to 8 minutes. Add chopped date and cook for 3 minutes. Cool slightly, add sauce to a blender, and blend until smooth. Portion the steamed vegetables onto four plates. Drizzle with sauce and top with batter-dipped tofu. Garnish with toasted sesame seeds if desired.

PER SERVING: CALORIES 349; PROTEIN 24g; CARBOHYDRATE 50g; TOTAL FAT 7.5g; SATURATED FAT 0.9g; SODIUM 315mg; FIBER 13.7g; BETA-CAROTENE 7033mcg; VITA-MIN C 51mg; CALCIUM 342mg; IRON 4.8mg; FOLATE 269mcg; MAGNESIUM 121mg; ZINC 4.1mg; SELENIUM 10.2mcg

Baked Eggplant Parmesan with Fresh Tomato Sauce

Serves: 6

2 large eggplants, sliced ¼ inch thick
½ cup raw almonds
½ cup nutritional yeast
1 cup 100% whole wheat bread crumbs
Fresh basil, for garnish

For the Tomato Sauce (see Note):
6 cups diced tomatoes
8 unsulfured, unsalted dried tomatoes, finely diced
1 small onion, diced
8 cloves garlic, minced
1 tablespoon MatoZest* or other no-salt Italian seasoning blend, adjusted to taste
¼ teaspoon freshly ground black pepper
¼ cup fresh chopped basil

For the Filling:
1 (14-ounce) package soft tofu
2 tablespoons lemon juice
¼ cup nutritional yeast
1 teaspoon onion powder
1 teaspoon garlic powder
¼ teaspoon black pepper
1 teaspoon dried oregano
1 teaspoon dried basil

Preheat the oven to 350°F. Lightly oil two nonstick baking pans. Arrange eggplant in a single layer and bake about 20 minutes or until eggplant is tender. Set aside. Place raw almonds and nutritional yeast in a food processor and pulse until the texture of grated Parmesan cheese is reached. Remove from food processor and mix with bread crumbs.

To prepare the tomato sauce, cook tomatoes and dried tomatoes in a saucepan over medium-low heat until soft, about 10 minutes. Place in a food processor or blender and purée. Heat 2 to 3 tablespoons water in a medium skillet and sauté the onion and garlic for 2 minutes or until tender. Add the puréed tomato mixture, MatoZest, and pepper. Bring to a gentle boil, reduce heat to low, cover, and simmer for 30 minutes. Stir in basil.

To prepare the filling, place all of the filling ingredients in a food processor or blender and blend until smooth.

To assemble, lightly oil a 13 × 9-inch baking dish. Place a thin layer of tomato sauce on the bottom of the dish, then a layer of eggplant slices. Sprinkle with one-third of the almond mixture. Top with one-third of the tomato sauce and half of the filling. Repeat, then top with a final layer of eggplant, sauce, and almond mixture. Bake uncovered for about 20 minutes, until heated through and lightly browned. Sprinkle with fresh basil just before serving.

Note: If pressed for time, substitute low-sodium jarred tomato sauce.

PER SERVING: CALORIES 326; PROTEIN 20g; CARBOHYDRATE 46g; TOTAL FAT 8.1g; SATURATED FAT 1g; SODIUM 163mg; FIBER 14.6g; BETA-CAROTENE 936mcg; VITA-MIN C 37mg; CALCIUM 156mg; IRON 4.1mg; FOLATE 111mcg; MAGNESIUM 130mg; ZINC 4.8mg; SELENIUM 6.4mcg

Baked Tempeh in Spicy Tomato Sauce
Serves: 4

> 6 tomatoes, cut in quarters
> 1 medium onion, halved
> 4 cloves garlic
> 1 tablespoon fennel seeds
> 1 teaspoon dried basil
> 1 teaspoon dried oregano
> 2 to 3 jalapeño or serrano chili peppers, seeded, or to taste
> 1 cup chopped mushrooms
> 8 ounces tempeh, cut into thin slices

Preheat the oven to 350°F. Blend tomatoes, onion, garlic, fennel, basil, oregano, and chili peppers in a blender or food processor until smooth. Place in a pot and bring to a boil. Add mushrooms, cover, and simmer for at least 30 minutes. Place tempeh in a baking dish and cover with tomato sauce. (Save leftover sauce for another use.) Cover and bake for 30 minutes.

PER SERVING: CALORIES 169; PROTEIN 14g; CARBOHYDRATE 18g; TOTAL FAT 6.8g; SATURATED FAT 1.4g; SODIUM 19mg; FIBER 3.8g; BETA-CAROTENE 849mcg; VITAMIN C 30mg; CALCIUM 123mg; IRON 2.9mg; FOLATE 52mcg; MAGNESIUM 81mg; ZINC 1.2mg; SELENIUM 2.2mcg

Bean Enchilada Bake

Serves: 12

1 large onion, chopped
1 Anaheim pepper, chopped
1 jalapeño pepper, chopped
1 yellow, red, or green bell pepper, chopped
1 large sweet potato or yam, peeled and chopped in small cubes
3 tomatillos (omit if unavailable)
1 tablespoon ground cumin
2 tablespoons chili powder
3 cups cooked black beans or 2 (15-ounce) cans low-sodium
   black beans, drained
3 cups diced tomatoes
1½ cups frozen sweet corn kernels
¼ cup fresh cilantro, chopped
12 sprouted corn tortillas
¼ cup pepitas (shelled pumpkin seeds) as a garnish
½ cup nondairy cheese, optional
½ cup guacamole and/or salsa when serving, optional

Preheat the oven to 350°F. Water-sauté onions and peppers, add sweet
potato, tomatillos, spices, beans, tomatoes, corn, and cilantro. Cover
and simmer, stirring occasionally, for 30 minutes or until potatoes are
cooked through. Add a small amount of water if mixture gets too dry.
Spray a 13 × 9 × 2-inch pan lightly with cooking spray if not nonstick.
Place a small amount of chili mixture on the bottom, then layer six
tortillas, chili mixture, remaining tortillas, and remaining chili mixture.
Sprinkle with pepitas and bake for 20 to 30 minutes. Sprinkle with
nondairy cheese before baking if desired. Serve with guacamole and
salsa if desired.

PER SERVING: CALORIES 318; PROTEIN 15g; CARBOHYDRATE 47g; TOTAL FAT 9.1g;
SATURATED FAT 1.5g; CHOLESTEROL 1.6mg; SODIUM 246mg; FIBER 11.5g; BETA-
CAROTENE 1411mcg; VITAMIN C 41mg; CALCIUM 153mg; IRON 4.2mg; FOLATE
92mcg; MAGNESIUM 68mg; ZINC 1.3mg; SELENIUM 3mcg

Bean Pasta with Brussels Sprouts and "Blue Cheese"

Serves: 6

> 8 ounces bean pasta (see Note), cooked according to package directions, rinsed under cold water and drained
> 2 red onions, chopped
> 1 pound Brussels sprouts, cleaned and left whole if small or cut in half if large
> Freshly ground black pepper, to taste
> ¼ cup chopped parsley, plus more for garnish

For the "Blue Cheese" Sauce:
> ½ cup raw cashews
> ¼ cup unhulled sesame seeds
> 1 (12.3-ounce) package firm tofu
> 4 cloves garlic, peeled
> ½ cup unsweetened soy, hemp, or almond milk
> 3 tablespoons lemon juice
> 1 tablespoon white low-sodium miso
> 6 tablespoons nutritional yeast
> 4 teaspoons apple cider vinegar
> 1 teaspoon onion powder
> 1 tablespoon Dijon mustard

While the pasta is cooking, purée all of the "blue cheese" sauce ingredients in a high-powered blender until smooth.

In a large pan, sauté the onions and Brussels sprouts in a little water or white wine until the onions are translucent and the sprouts are tender, about 10 minutes (if desired, add some chopped apples when you are sautéing the Brussels sprouts). Add pasta and parsley to the pan; pour in the "blue cheese" sauce, and cook until heated through, stirring to coat everything with the sauce. Divide among six plates and sprinkle with additional parsley. Serve immediately.

Note: Several varieties of bean pasta are available at www.DrFuhrman.com.

PER SERVING: CALORIES 379; PROTEIN 25g; CARBOHYDRATE 47g; TOTAL FAT 11.5g; SATURATED FAT 1.8g; SODIUM 195mg; FIBER 13.5g; BETA-CAROTENE 472mcg; VITA-MIN C 74mg; CALCIUM 256mg; IRON 7.8mg; FOLATE 90mcg; MAGNESIUM 112mg; ZINC 5.3mg; SELENIUM 8.1mcg

Black Bean Chili with Cilantro Pesto
Serves: 5

2 cups water or low-sodium or no-salt-added vegetable broth, divided
1 onion, chopped
½ cup celery, chopped
4 garlic cloves, pressed
6 ounces tomato paste, in BPA-free packaging
1½ cups canned diced tomatoes, in BPA-free packaging
1½ tablespoons chili powder
1 teaspoon cumin
2 cups frozen kale, thawed
4½ cups cooked black beans or 3 (15-ounce) cans low-sodium or no-salt-added black beans, drained
¾ cup (packed) cilantro leaves
½ cup raw pecans
½ cup soft tofu
2 teaspoons fresh lemon juice

Heat 2 to 3 tablespoons water or low-sodium vegetable broth in a large pot and sauté onions, celery, and garlic until softened. Add tomato paste, tomatoes, chili powder, cumin, and water or vegetable broth. Mix well, cover, and cook for 30 minutes. Add kale and black beans and simmer for an additional 20 minutes. Adjust seasonings to taste.

To prepare cilantro pesto, place cilantro, pecans, tofu, and lemon juice in a food processor or blender. Process until smooth, scraping down sides of container as necessary. Serve chili with a dollop of cilantro pesto on top.

PER SERVING: CALORIES 377; PROTEIN 21g; CARBOHYDRATE 56g; TOTAL FAT 10.3g; SATURATED FAT 1.1g; SODIUM 148mg; FIBER 19.3g; BETA-CAROTENE 1042mcg; VITAMIN C 42mg; CALCIUM 189mg; IRON 6.5mg; FOLATE 266mcg; MAGNESIUM 168mg; ZINC 3mg; SELENIUM 5.6mcg

Broccoli and Shiitake Mushrooms with Thai Curry Wok Sauce

Serves: 4

For the Thai Curry Wok Sauce:
  1½ cups water
  7 regular dates or 3½ Medjool dates, pitted
  ⅓ cup natural, unsalted peanut butter
  2 tablespoons unsweetened shredded coconut
  1 tablespoon lime juice
  2 tablespoons lemongrass (tough outer layer removed), minced
  1 teaspoon red curry powder
  ½ teaspoon chili powder
  ½ teaspoon ground cumin
  ¼ teaspoon ground turmeric

For the Vegetables:
  1 cup chopped onions
  6 cups broccoli florets
  1 cup thinly sliced red bell pepper strips
  2 cups sliced shiitake mushrooms
  2 cups trimmed snow peas

Blend water and dates in a high-powered blender. Add peanut butter, coconut, lime juice, lemongrass, and spices and blend again until smooth and well combined. Heat ¼ cup water in a large nonstick wok or skillet. Add chopped onions and broccoli, cover and cook for 4 minutes, stirring occasionally and adding additional water as needed to prevent sticking. Remove cover and add red bell pepper strips, shiitake mushrooms, and snow peas and cook for an additional 4 minutes or until vegetables are crisp-tender. Add desired amount of sauce and continue to stir-fry for 1 to 2 minutes to heat through. Serve with wild or black rice, if desired.

PER SERVING: CALORIES 295; PROTEIN 13g; CARBOHYDRATE 38g; TOTAL FAT 13.5g; SATURATED FAT 3.2g; SODIUM 70mg; FIBER 11.4g; BETA-CAROTENE 1123mcg; VITAMIN C 174mg; CALCIUM 117mg; IRON 3.4mg; FOLATE 151mcg; MAGNESIUM 110mg; ZINC 2.6mg; SELENIUM 11.9mcg

California Creamed Kale

Serves: 4

2 bunches kale, leaves removed from tough stems and chopped
1 cup raw cashews
¾ cup unsweetened soy, hemp, or almond milk
4 tablespoons onion flakes
1 tablespoon VegiZest* or nutritional yeast (or other no-salt
   seasoning blend, adjusted to taste)

Place kale in a large steamer pot. Steam 10 to 13 minutes until soft. Meanwhile, place remaining ingredients in a high-powered blender and blend until smooth. Place kale in a colander and press to remove some of the excess water. Coarsely chop the kale and mix with the cream sauce in a bowl.

Note: Use this sauce with broccoli, spinach, or other steamed vegetables too.

PER SERVING: CALORIES 265; PROTEIN 11g; CARBOHYDRATE 24g; TOTAL FAT 16.4g; SATURATED FAT 2.8g; SODIUM 56mg; FIBER 3.5g; BETA-CAROTENE 6539mcg; VITA-MIN C 90mg; CALCIUM 186mg; IRON 4.1mg; FOLATE 45mcg; MAGNESIUM 140mg; ZINC 2.6mg; SELENIUM 7.8mcg

Chickpea Curry in a Hurry

Serves: 2

> 1½ cups cooked chickpeas or 1 (15-ounce) can no-salt-added or
>   low-sodium chickpeas, drained
> ½ cup no-salt-added or low-sodium vegetable broth
> 1½ cups diced tomatoes
> 1 teaspoon garlic powder
> 2 teaspoons curry powder
> ⅓ cup unsweetened dried coconut
> 1 10-ounce box or bag frozen chopped spinach

In a large saucepan, add all ingredients except spinach. Bring to a boil
over high heat, cover, and cook over medium heat for 5 minutes. Add
frozen spinach, break up blocks of spinach with a fork, cover, and
continue cooking until the spinach is cooked, about 5 more minutes.
Stir well before serving.

PER SERVING: CALORIES 340; PROTEIN 22g; CARBOHYDRATE 51g; TOTAL FAT 9.7g;
SATURATED FAT 4.9g; SODIUM 125mg; FIBER 17.7g; BETA-CAROTENE 10,610mcg;
VITAMIN C 54mg; CALCIUM 308mg; IRON 7.8mg; FOLATE 420mcg; MAGNESIUM
192mg; ZINC 3.1mg; SELENIUM 17.1mcg

Chili Pie with Cornbread Topping
Serves: 8

For the Chili:
- 2 cups low-sodium or no-salt-added vegetable broth
- 1 onion, chopped
- 4 cloves garlic, chopped
- 3 tablespoons tomato paste, in BPA-free packaging
- 1½ cups diced tomatoes
- 2 tablespoons chili powder
- 2 teaspoons cumin
- 3 cups frozen chopped broccoli, thawed
- 4½ cups cooked red kidney beans or 3 (15-ounce) cans low-sodium or no-salt-added kidney beans, drained

For the Cornbread Topping:
- 1 cup cornmeal
- 1 cup oat flour
- 1 tablespoon baking powder
- 5 Medjool or 10 regular dates, pitted
- 1 cup unsweetened soy, hemp, or almond milk
- 2 tablespoons ground flaxseeds
- 1 cup frozen corn kernels, thawed

To make the chili, heat 2 to 3 tablespoons water or low-sodium vegetable broth in a large pot and sauté onions and garlic until softened. Add tomato paste, tomatoes, chili powder, cumin, vegetable broth, broccoli, and beans. Bring to a boil, reduce heat, and cook uncovered for 30 minutes until chili has thickened.

To make the cornbread, combine cornmeal, oat flour, and baking powder in a large bowl. Stir well and set aside. In a high-powered blender, combine dates, nondairy milk, and ground flaxseeds. Combine with the dry ingredients, stirring just until well combined. Mixture will be thick.

To assemble the pie, preheat oven to 350°F. Lightly oil a 13 × 9-inch baking dish. Transfer the chili to the baking dish. Sprinkle corn kernels on top. Drop cornbread batter, by the spoonful, on top of the chili until the batter forms an even layer on top, using a fork to lightly spread the batter. It is okay if it is not a perfect layer; sections of the chili may still be visible. Bake for 20 minutes.

PER SERVING: CALORIES 371; PROTEIN 16g; CARBOHYDRATE 73g; TOTAL FAT 3.7g; SATURATED FAT 0.5g; SODIUM 110mg; FIBER 14.8g; BETA-CAROTENE 912mcg; VITA-MIN C 43mg; CALCIUM 194mg; IRON 8mg; FOLATE 201mcg; MAGNESIUM 104mg; ZINC 2.1mg; SELENIUM 8mcg

Chinese Apricot Stir-Fry

Serves: 4

¼ cup white wine
¼ cup unsulfured dried apricots
4 tablespoons water, divided
2 (14-ounce) blocks of extra firm tofu, drained and cubed into bite-size pieces
1 teaspoon garlic powder
2 tablespoons VegiZest* or other no-salt seasoning blend, adjusted to taste
1 teaspoon Bragg Liquid Aminos or low-sodium soy sauce
3 (12-ounce) packages of frozen mixed oriental vegetables
½ teaspoon five-spice powder (see Note)

Note: A blend of five aromatic spices, five-spice powder is commonly used in Chinese and Indian cuisine. It adds a spicy-sweet flavor to a variety of dishes. If you can't find five-spice powder you can make your own.

Five-Spice Powder
1 teaspoon ground cinnamon
1 teaspoon ground cloves
1 teaspoon ground fennel seed
1 teaspoon ground star anise
1 teaspoon ground Szechuan or black peppercorns

Mix the spices together and store in an airtight container.

Pour the wine on top of the apricots and let soak for at least 30 minutes. Heat 2 tablespoons of the water in a large pan and add the tofu. Sprinkle garlic powder over tofu. Sauté the tofu over medium-low heat, turning frequently at first to prevent sticking. In a small bowl, combine the remaining 2 tablespoons of water, VegiZest, apricots, wine, and Bragg Liquid Aminos. Sprinkle half of this mixture over the tofu and continue to simmer. Defrost the frozen vegetables in a microwave or steam on the stovetop. Once defrosted, add the vegetables to the tofu. Sprinkle the remaining sauce over tofu-vegetable mix and add the five-spice powder. Continue to simmer until the liquid is largely cooked off.

PER SERVING: CALORIES 278; PROTEIN 34g; CARBOHYDRATE 31g; TOTAL FAT 15.2g; SATURATED FAT 1.9g; SODIUM 168mg; FIBER 6.4g; BETA-CAROTENE 9mcg; VITAMIN C 19mg; CALCIUM 365mg; IRON 5.2mg; FOLATE 95mcg; MAGNESIUM 119mg; ZINC 2.4mg; SELENIUM 20.9mcg

Italian-Style Zucchini Spaghetti
Serves: 4

   3 medium zucchini, cut to resemble spaghetti (see Note)
   ½ large sweet onion, chopped
   5 garlic cloves, chopped
   4 ounces mushrooms, sliced
   4 medium tomatoes, chopped
   4 basil leaves, chopped

After cutting the zucchini, let it drain in a colander. While zucchini is draining, heat 2 tablespoons water in a sauté pan and sauté onion until tender, about 5 minutes. Add garlic and cook for 30 seconds or until fragrant. Add the mushrooms and cook until softened, then add the tomatoes and basil and cook for another 5 minutes. Serve zucchini topped with the tomato sauce.

Note: Use a vegetable spiralizer for cutting the zucchini so it looks like spaghetti noodles. You can also use a mandolin slicer fitted with a julienne attachment or a vegetable peeler.

PER SERVING: CALORIES 72; PROTEIN 4g; CARBOHYDRATE 15g; TOTAL FAT 0.9g; SATURATED FAT 0.2g; SODIUM 23mg; FIBER 3.7g; BETA-CAROTENE 745mcg; VITAMIN C 47mg; CALCIUM 53mg; IRON 1.2mg; FOLATE 59mcg; MAGNESIUM 48mg; ZINC 0.9mg; SELENIUM 3.7mcg

Kale with Sweet Corn

Serves: 4

> 1 cup fresh corn kernels (about 2 ears) or thawed frozen corn
> 1 bunch kale, tough stems and center ribs removed and leaves
>   chopped
> ½ cup finely chopped onion
> 1 clove garlic, chopped
> ¼ cup no-salt-added or low-sodium vegetable broth
> ¼ cup chopped walnuts and/or slivered almonds, very lightly
>   toasted (see Note)
> ⅛ teaspoon black pepper, if desired
> 2 tablespoons finely chopped scallions

If using fresh corn, boil ears of corn until tender, about 4 minutes.
Cut kernels from cobs with a sharp knife. Set aside. Steam the kale
for 15 minutes or until tender. When the kale is done, place in a
colander and press to remove excess liquid. Heat 2 tablespoons water
in a skillet over medium-high heat. Sauté onion and garlic until soft,
about 2 minutes; add the corn, kale, and vegetable broth. Reduce
heat to low and cook until kale and corn are heated through, stirring
frequently. Toss in the lightly toasted nuts and season with black
pepper if desired. Top with finely chopped scallions.

Note: Toast walnuts and almonds in a preheated oven at 300°F for
3 minutes, stirring frequently.

PER SERVING: CALORIES 109; PROTEIN 4g; CARBOHYDRATE 14g; TOTAL FAT 5.5g;
SATURATED FAT 0.6g; SODIUM 23mg; FIBER 2.7g; BETA-CAROTENE 3289mcg; VITA-
MIN C 48mg; CALCIUM 64mg; IRON 1.1mg; FOLATE 41mcg; MAGNESIUM 41mg;
ZINC 0.6mg; SELENIUM 1.1mcg

Lentil and Mushroom Ragù over Polenta with Fresh Tomato Salsa

Serves: 4

For the Lentil and Mushroom Ragù:
   ½ medium onion, chopped
   2 large carrots, diced
   ½ green bell pepper, chopped
   12 ounces mushrooms, sliced
   4 garlic cloves, minced
   ¼ cup red wine or vegetable broth
   ¼ cup dried porcini mushrooms, rehydrated in enough water
      to cover, then sliced (reserve soaking water)
   28 ounces diced tomatoes
   1 tablespoon tomato paste, in BPA-free packaging
   2 cups water
   1 cup brown lentils
   2 teaspoons dried oregano
   ¼ teaspoon ground black pepper
   ⅛ teaspoon red pepper flakes or more to taste

For the Polenta:
   3 cups water
   ¾ cup cornmeal

For the Salsa:
   2 fresh tomatoes, chopped
   1 small onion, minced
   1 clove garlic, minced
   ½ jalapeño chili pepper, seeded and minced
   3 tablespoons chopped cilantro
   3 tablespoons fresh lime juice

In a large Dutch oven or pot, heat 2 to 3 tablespoons water and water-sauté onions for 3 minutes. Add carrots, green pepper, mushrooms, and garlic and sauté for another 7 minutes or until vegetables are tender. Add wine and cook for 1 minute, stirring constantly. Stir in porcini mushrooms and their soaking water, tomatoes, tomato paste, water, lentils, oregano, black pepper, and red pepper flakes. Heat to boiling; reduce heat to medium-low, and simmer until lentils are tender, about 25 minutes, stirring occasionally. Add more water as needed if the mixture gets too thick.

Meanwhile, to make polenta, bring 3 cups water to a boil over high heat. When water is boiling, slowly whisk cornmeal into the boiling water. When all the cornmeal is added, reduce heat to a very low simmer, cover, and continue cooking until the polenta is smooth and thick, about 10 to 20 minutes, stirring every 5 minutes. To prepare salsa, stir ingredients together in a mixing bowl. Serve ragù over polenta. Top with a generous spoonful of salsa.

PER SERVING: CALORIES 392; PROTEIN 21g; CARBOHYDRATE 77g; TOTAL FAT 2.5g; SATURATED FAT 0.4g; SODIUM 80mg; FIBER 14.4g; BETA-CAROTENE 4315mcg; VITAMIN C 64mg; CALCIUM 114mg; IRON 6.5mg; FOLATE 324mcg; MAGNESIUM 155mg; ZINC 4.6mg; SELENIUM 20.8mcg

Lentil Walnut Burritos with Peppers, Onions, and Salsa
Serves: 6

For the Lentil Filling:
1 cup walnuts, toasted
1¾ cups cooked brown lentils (see Note)
1½ teaspoons dried oregano
1½ teaspoons ground cumin
1½ teaspoons chili powder
2 tablespoons nutritional yeast
1 teaspoon Bragg Liquid Aminos
1–2 tablespoons water or as needed

For the Salsa:
2 fresh tomatoes, chopped
1 small red onion, finely chopped
1 clove garlic, finely chopped
½ jalapeño chili pepper, seeded and minced
3 tablespoons fresh lime juice
1 tablespoon chopped cilantro

To Finish:
   1 large green bell pepper, thinly sliced
   1 large onion, thinly sliced
   6 (100% whole grain) tortillas

Place walnuts in a food processor and pulse several times to chop them. Add the cooked lentils, oregano, cumin, chili powder, nutritional yeast, and Bragg Liquid Aminos and pulse until mixture is thoroughly combined and crumbly. Add 1 to 2 tablespoons water as needed.

Stir together salsa ingredients. Set aside. Heat 2 to 3 tablespoons water in a large skillet and water-sauté pepper and onion until tender. To assemble burritos, spread lentil/walnut mixture on tortillas, top with sautéed peppers, onions, and salsa and roll up.

Note: To cook dry lentils, bring 1 cup lentils and 2 cups water to a boil in a large saucepan. Reduce heat, cover and cook for 25 minutes or until tender. Drain.

PER SERVING: CALORIES 371; PROTEIN 16g; CARBOHYDRATE 47g; TOTAL FAT 15.1g; SATURATED FAT 1.7g; SODIUM 196mg; FIBER 13.4g; BETA-CAROTENE 371mcg; VITAMIN C 35mg; CALCIUM 101mg; IRON 5.5mg; FOLATE 139mcg; MAGNESIUM 67mg; ZINC 2mg; SELENIUM 2.9mcg

Nutritarian Goulash

Serves: 3

1 large onion, chopped
1 large red or green bell pepper, chopped
1 carrot, diced
No-salt-added vegetable stock, as needed
4 to 5 large portobello mushroom caps, sliced
½ cup tomatoes, chopped
1½ cups cooked cannellini beans or 1 (15-ounce) can no-salt-
    added or low-sodium, drained
1 tablespoon minced garlic
1 tablespoon tomato paste, in BPA-free packaging
2 tablespoons balsamic vinegar
2 tablespoons Hungarian sweet paprika, or to taste
1 tablespoon paprika, or to taste
½ teaspoon thyme, fresh or dry
Pinch of dried marjoram
½ teaspoon caraway seeds

In a large flat-bottom pan, sauté the onions, peppers, and carrots with the vegetable stock until soft, about 5 minutes. Add the remaining ingredients and continue to cook for an additional 10 minutes or until the vegetables are tender, adding vegetable stock as needed to avoid sticking. Cover the pot about halfway through the cooking time. Serve over bean pasta, if desired.

Note: Use frozen chopped onions and peppers to reduce prep time.

PER SERVING: CALORIES 226; PROTEIN 13g; CARBOHYDRATE 44g; TOTAL FAT 1.8g; SATURATED FAT 0.4g; SODIUM 54mg; FIBER 12.7g; BETA-CAROTENE 3768mcg; VITA-MIN C 55mg; CALCIUM 144mg; IRON 6.1mg; FOLATE 122mcg; MAGNESIUM 90mg; ZINC 2.3mg; SELENIUM 16.7mcg

Pistachio-Crusted Tempeh with Balsamic-Glazed Shiitakes

Serves: 4

    8 ounces tempeh, diagonally sliced, as thinly as possible
    1 pound shiitake mushrooms, stemmed, thinly sliced

For the Marinade:
    2 cloves garlic, minced
    1 tablespoon chopped fresh basil
    1 tablespoon chopped fresh cilantro
    Pinch of hot pepper flakes
    1 cup low-sodium or no-salt-added vegetable broth
    2 tablespoons balsamic vinegar
    1 teaspoon Bragg Liquid Aminos or low-sodium soy sauce

For the Crust:
    1 cup pistachios, shelled
    4 tablespoons cornmeal
    2 tablespoons nutritional yeast
    1 teaspoon onion powder
    1 teaspoon garlic powder

Place tempeh in a saucepan with water to cover and simmer for 10 minutes. Combine ingredients for marinade. Remove tempeh from water and add to marinade. Marinate for at least 1 hour.

Preheat the oven to 375°F. Process pistachios in food processor until finely chopped. Add remaining crust ingredients and pulse until thoroughly mixed. Place in a large shallow bowl. Remove tempeh from marinade and drain. Reserve marinade. Dip tempeh in crust mixture to coat. Place crusted tempeh and sliced mushrooms side by side on a rimmed baking sheet. Spoon 2 to 3 tablespoons of marinade over the mushrooms. Bake for 13 minutes or until the mushrooms are soft, turning occasionally. Simmer remaining marinade for 2 minutes. Drizzle tempeh and mushrooms with marinade before serving.

PER SERVING: CALORIES 378; PROTEIN 23g; CARBOHYDRATE 31g; TOTAL FAT 21.2g; SATURATED FAT 3.1g; SODIUM 78mg; FIBER 7.7g; BETA-CAROTENE 91mcg; VITAMIN C 2mg; CALCIUM 109mg; IRON 3.8mg; FOLATE 34mcg; MAGNESIUM 119mg; ZINC 3.7mg; SELENIUM 10.5mcg

Rustic Mashed Cauliflower with Roasted Garlic and Spinach

Serves: 4

    1 bulb garlic
    1 medium onion, sliced
    1 medium head cauliflower, cut into chunks
    10 ounces fresh spinach
    ½ cup raw cashew butter
    2 tablespoons nutritional yeast
    2 tablespoons chopped fresh chives
    ⅛ teaspoon black pepper or to taste

Preheat the oven to 350°F. Roast unpeeled garlic in a small baking dish for about 25 minutes or until soft. When cool, squeeze out the soft cooked garlic, removing and discarding the skins. Heat a nonstick skillet and dry-sauté the onion until lightly browned, about 5 minutes, stirring constantly. Steam cauliflower for about 8 to 10 minutes or until tender. Remove and place in a food processor. Add spinach to the steamer and steam until just wilted. Set aside.

Process cauliflower, roasted garlic, cashew butter, and nutritional yeast in a food processor by pulsing to a chunky-smooth consistency. Stir in sautéed onions, wilted spinach, chives, and black pepper. Place in a baking dish and bake for 15 to 20 minutes or until heated through, then broil until just starting to turn golden.

PER SERVING: CALORIES 297; PROTEIN 15g; CARBOHYDRATE 29g; TOTAL FAT 16.9g; SATURATED FAT 3.4g; SODIUM 131mg; FIBER 8.1g; BETA-CAROTENE 4027mcg; VITAMIN C 131mg; CALCIUM 157mg; IRON 4.8mg; FOLATE 292mcg; MAGNESIUM 182mg; ZINC 3.6mg; SELENIUM 6.9mcg

Slow-Simmered Collard Greens

Serves: 6

1 large red onion, sliced

4 cloves garlic, chopped

2 pounds collard greens, tough stems removed and leaves
chopped

2 medium tomatoes, chopped, or 1 cup low-sodium salsa

2 cups water

1 cup dry white wine or low-sodium vegetable broth

½ teaspoon black pepper

Heat ⅛ cup water in a deep skillet or large pot. Water-sauté red onion
and garlic until almost tender. Add collard greens gradually and cook
until slightly wilted. Add tomatoes or salsa, water, wine or vegetable
broth, and black pepper. Bring to a boil, reduce heat to a simmer and
cover. Cook until collards are tender, about 30 minutes, adding more
water as necessary.

PER SERVING: CALORIES 98; PROTEIN 5g; CARBOHYDRATE 14g; TOTAL FAT 0.8g; SAT-
URATED FAT 0.1g; SODIUM 39mg; FIBER 6.5g; BETA-CAROTENE 5994mcg; VITAMIN
C 61mg; CALCIUM 239mg; IRON 0.6mg; FOLATE 262mcg; MAGNESIUM 26mg; ZINC
0.4mg; SELENIUM 2.4mcg

Spinach-Stuffed Mushrooms

Serves: 3

    1 small onion, chopped
    12 large mushrooms, stems separated and chopped, caps left
        whole
    1 clove garlic, minced
    ½ teaspoon dried thyme
    ¼ cup low-sodium or no-salt-added vegetable broth
    5 ounces fresh spinach
    2 tablespoons raw almond butter
    1 tablespoon nutritional yeast
    ¼ teaspoon black pepper, or to taste

Preheat the oven to 350°F. In a large pan, heat 2 to 3 tablespoons of water and water-sauté chopped onion for 2 minutes; add mushroom stems, garlic, and thyme and continue to sauté until onions and mushrooms are tender, about 3 minutes. Add mushroom caps to pan, along with vegetable broth; bring to a simmer and cook for 5 minutes.

Remove mushroom caps from the pan and place them on a lightly oiled baking sheet. Add spinach to onion mixture remaining in the pan and heat until wilted. Remove from heat and stir in almond butter, nutritional yeast, and black pepper. Fill mushroom caps with spinach/onion mixture and bake for 15 to 20 minutes or until golden brown.

Note: If desired, add ½ cup of whole grain bread crumbs to the stuffing mixture.

PER SERVING: CALORIES 117; PROTEIN 7g; CARBOHYDRATE 11g; TOTAL FAT 6.3g; SATURATED FAT 0.5g; SODIUM 56mg; FIBER 3.7g; BETA-CAROTENE 2665mcg; VITA-MIN C 15mg; CALCIUM 114mg; IRON 2.5mg; FOLATE 123mcg; MAGNESIUM 81mg; ZINC 2.1mg; SELENIUM 21.8mcg

Sweet and Easy Squash Casserole

Serves: 4

1 medium butternut squash, cubed (see Note)
½ cup low-sodium or no-salt-added vegetable broth
¼ cup currants or raisins
Juice and zest of 1 lemon
¼ cup sliced almonds, lightly toasted
½ teaspoon cinnamon
¼ teaspoon cardamom
Pinch of black pepper

Preheat the oven to 350°F. Lightly wipe a glass or ceramic cooking dish with olive oil. Add squash and pour vegetable broth on top. Sprinkle with currants, lemon juice, lemon zest, almonds, and spices. Bake for 20 minutes covered. Uncover and bake for an additional 10 minutes or until squash is tender.

Note: To save time, use 4 cups frozen cubed butternut squash.

PER SERVING: CALORIES 127; PROTEIN 3g; CARBOHYDRATE 26g; TOTAL FAT 3g; SATURATED FAT 0.3g; SODIUM 24mg; FIBER 4.4g; BETA-CAROTENE 5921mcg; VITAMIN C 35mg; CALCIUM 97mg; IRON 1.6mg; FOLATE 44mcg; MAGNESIUM 68mg; ZINC 0.5mg; SELENIUM 0.9mcg

BURGERS, WRAPS, AND FAST FOOD

Baked Eggplant Fries
Serves: 4

- ½ cup raw almonds, toasted
- 1 tablespoon cornmeal
- 1 tablespoon nutritional yeast
- 2 teaspoons chia seeds
- ½ teaspoon onion powder
- ½ teaspoon garlic powder
- ½ teaspoon no-salt Italian seasoning
- 1 medium eggplant, peeled and cut into ¼-inch-thick "fries"
- ½ cup chickpea flour
- 1 cup no-salt-added or low-sodium vegetable broth
- 1 cup no-salt-added or low-sodium marinara sauce

Preheat the oven to 400°F. Place almonds in a food processor and pulse until chopped to the consistency of coarse bread crumbs. Remove from food processor and in a shallow bowl, combine with cornmeal, nutritional yeast, chia seeds, onion and garlic powders, and Italian seasoning. Dredge eggplant "fries" in chickpea flour; dip them in the vegetable broth and then into the almond mixture. Place on a wire rack on a baking sheet and bake for 10 minutes; turn and bake an additional 5 to 10 minutes until golden. Serve with marinara sauce for dipping.

PER SERVING: CALORIES 221; PROTEIN 10g; CARBOHYDRATE 25g; TOTAL FAT 10.6g; SATURATED FAT 0.9g; SODIUM 53mg; FIBER 9.5g; BETA-CAROTENE 183mcg; VITAMIN C 7mg; CALCIUM 92mg; IRON 2.6mg; FOLATE 92mcg; MAGNESIUM 105mg; ZINC 1.7mg; SELENIUM 3.2mcg

Better Burgers
Serves: 8

1½ cups old-fashioned rolled oats
1 cup ground walnuts
1 cup water
¼ cup tomato paste, in BPA-free packaging
¼ cup MatoZest* or other no-salt seasoning blend, adjusted to taste
1 cup diced onion
3 cloves garlic, minced
6 cups finely minced mushrooms
2 teaspoons dried basil
½ teaspoon dried oregano
2 tablespoons minced fresh parsley
Freshly ground black pepper, to taste
⅔ cup frozen chopped spinach, thawed

Preheat the oven to 350°F. Combine rolled oats and ground walnuts in a bowl. Set aside. In a small saucepan, whisk together water, tomato paste, and MatoZest. Heat over medium-high heat until boiling. Pour over rolled oats and walnuts. Stir well and set aside. Heat 2 tablespoons water in a sauté pan and add onion and garlic. Sauté until onion is translucent. Add mushrooms, basil, oregano, parsley, and black pepper and additional water if needed to prevent sticking. Cover and cook for 5 minutes or until mushrooms are tender.

In a large bowl, combine sautéed onions and mushrooms, rolled oat and walnut mixture, and spinach. Stir well to combine. With wet hands, shape ⅓ cup of mixture into a patty. Place on a lightly oiled baking sheet and repeat with remaining mixture. Bake patties for 15 minutes; turn them and bake for another 15 minutes.

Remove from oven and cool slightly. Serve on small whole grain hamburger buns or whole grain pita bread halves. Top with thinly sliced raw red onion and sliced tomato.

PER SERVING: CALORIES 200; PROTEIN 9g; CARBOHYDRATE 21g; TOTAL FAT 11.1g; SATURATED FAT 1.1g; SODIUM 44mg; FIBER 4.5g; BETA-CAROTENE 1661mcg; VITA-MIN C 12mg; CALCIUM 57mg; IRON 2.6mg; FOLATE 56mcg; MAGNESIUM 88mg; ZINC 1.5mg; SELENIUM 14.1mcg

Black Bean and Sweet Potato Quesadillas

Serves: 4

1 sweet potato, shredded

2 carrots, shredded

1 small onion, diced

1½ cups cooked black beans or 1 (15-ounce) can no-salt-added or low-sodium, drained

1 teaspoon cumin

1 teaspoon chili powder

1 teaspoon oregano

½ teaspoon paprika

½ bunch kale or other greens, tough stems removed, chopped

8 (100% whole grain) flour tortillas

¼ cup shredded nondairy cheese

1 cup low-sodium salsa

Preheat the oven to 350°F. Heat 2 tablespoons water in a skillet and water-sauté the sweet potato, carrots, and onion together for 5 minutes. Add the black beans and spices, cover and simmer over low heat for another 5 minutes, then add the kale and simmer another 10 minutes or until greens are wilted and tender. Divide the veggie mixture evenly onto four tortillas. Sprinkle with nondairy cheese and top with the remaining four tortillas. Place on a baking pan and bake for 20 minutes. Cut into wedges and serve with salsa.

PER SERVING: CALORIES 404; PROTEIN 15g; CARBOHYDRATE 70g; TOTAL FAT 7.5g; SATURATED FAT 1.9g; SODIUM 480mg; FIBER 11.3g; BETA-CAROTENE 7314mcg; VITAMIN C 31mg; CALCIUM 209mg; IRON 5mg; FOLATE 252mcg; MAGNESIUM 98mg; ZINC 1.9mg; SELENIUM 19.5mcg

Black Bean and Turkey Burgers
Serves: 7

2 cups chopped mushrooms
½ cup old-fashioned rolled oats
¼ cup raw pumpkin seeds
2 carrots, grated
1½ cups cooked black beans or 1 (15-ounce) can low-sodium
  or no-salt-added black beans, drained
½ teaspoon cumin
½ teaspoon coriander
½ teaspoon chili powder
½ teaspoon onion powder
¼ teaspoon black pepper
⅛ teaspoon cayenne pepper
6 ounces (about 1 cup) ground organic turkey (see Note for
  vegan option)

Preheat the oven to 300°F. Heat 1 to 2 tablespoons water in a small
pan and sauté mushrooms until tender and moisture has evaporated,
about 5 minutes. Set aside. Grind oats and pumpkin seeds in a food
processor. Add grated carrots, three-quarters of the beans, and all of
the spices and process until blended. Spoon mixture into a mixing
bowl and stir in sautéed mushrooms, remaining whole beans, and
ground turkey. Form into seven medium-size patties. Place patties
on a baking sheet lined with parchment paper or lightly wiped with
olive oil. Bake for 40 minutes, turning once after 20 minutes. Serve
on a small 100% whole grain roll or pita with sliced red onion, sliced
tomato, lettuce, and low-sodium ketchup.

Note: To make without ground turkey, add an additional 1½ cups
beans.

PER SERVING: CALORIES 137; PROTEIN 12g; CARBOHYDRATE 16g; TOTAL FAT 3.5g;
SATURATED FAT 0.7g; CHOLESTEROL 13.4mg; SODIUM 30mg; FIBER 4.8g; BETA-
CAROTENE 1482mcg; VITAMIN C 1mg; CALCIUM 26mg; IRON 3.1mg; FOLATE 68mcg;
MAGNESIUM 66mg; ZINC 1.5mg; SELENIUM 11.7mcg

Chipotle Avocado and White Bean Wraps
Serves: 4

½ cup raw pumpkin seeds
¼ cup apple cider vinegar
½ cup unsweetened soy, hemp, or almond milk
¼ cup raisins
4 cups shredded red cabbage
1 medium carrot, peeled and shredded
¼ cup chopped fresh cilantro
1½ cups cooked white beans or 1 (15-ounce can) no-salt-added or
    low-sodium white beans, drained
1 ripe avocado
2 tablespoons minced red onion
¼ teaspoon chipotle chili powder or more to taste
4 (100% whole grain) flour tortillas

In a high-powered blender, blend pumpkin seeds to a fine powder.
Add vinegar, nondairy milk, and raisins and process until smooth.
Combine cabbage, carrot, and cilantro and toss with desired amount
of dressing. Save any leftover dressing for another use. Mash beans
and avocado together with a fork or potato masher. Stir in red onion
and chipotle chili powder. To assemble the wraps, spread about ½
cup bean/avocado mixture onto each tortilla and top with cabbage
mixture. Roll up. If desired, cut in half to serve.

PER SERVING: CALORIES 392; PROTEIN 17g; CARBOHYDRATE 55g; TOTAL FAT 13.6g;
SATURATED FAT 2.1g; SODIUM 196mg; FIBER 13g; BETA-CAROTENE 1815mcg; VITA-
MIN C 44mg; CALCIUM 141mg; IRON 5.9mg; FOLATE 88mcg; MAGNESIUM 125mg;
ZINC 1.9mg; SELENIUM 3.7mcg

Corn and Buckwheat Crackers

Serves: 10

½ cup buckwheat or oat groats
1 cup corn kernels, fresh or frozen
2 cups kale, tough stems removed and leaves chopped
1 medium onion, coarsely chopped
2 cloves garlic
Juice of ½ lime
½ cup ground flaxseed
½ cup ground almonds
½ cup cornmeal
1 teaspoon dried thyme
1 teaspoon dried rosemary
¼ teaspoon black pepper

Soak groats for 2 hours in just enough water to cover. Drain excess water. Preheat the oven to the lowest setting (such as 175°F). Place corn kernels, kale, onions, garlic, and lime juice in a food processor and pulse until uniformly chopped. Combine ground flaxseeds, ground almonds, cornmeal, thyme, rosemary, black pepper, and groats. Mix in corn and kale mixture. Spread onto a parchment-lined baking sheet to about ⅛ inch thickness. It is easier to spread if you keep your hands wet. Bake for about 5 hours or until desired crispness, stirring occasionally. If using a dehydrator, dry at 105°F for 6 hours, turn and continue to dry for an additional 3 to 4 hours or until desired crispness. Break into pieces.

PER SERVING: CALORIES 147; PROTEIN 5g; CARBOHYDRATE 20g; TOTAL FAT 6.6g; SATURATED FAT 0.6g; SODIUM 12mg; FIBER 5g; BETA-CAROTENE 1252mcg; VITAMIN C 19mg; CALCIUM 60mg; IRON 1.5mg; FOLATE 26mcg; MAGNESIUM 80mg; ZINC 1mg; SELENIUM 4.2mcg

Crispy Chickpeas

Serves: 4

>   1½ cups cooked chickpeas or 1 (15-ounce) can low-sodium
>   or no-salt-added chickpeas, drained
>   2 teaspoons olive oil
>   ½ teaspoon no-salt seasoning blend or cayenne pepper

Preheat the oven to 350°F. Line a baking sheet with parchment paper.
Place chickpeas, oil, and seasoning in a small bowl. Stir to completely
coat chickpeas. Arrange chickpeas in an even layer on a baking sheet.
Bake until crispy, about 40 to 45 minutes, stirring two to three times
during baking. Serve alone or as a topping for soups or salads.

PER SERVING: CALORIES 81; PROTEIN 4g; CARBOHYDRATE 11g; TOTAL FAT 2.6g;
SATURATED FAT 0.3g; SODIUM 3mg; FIBER 3.2g; BETA-CAROTENE 39mcg; VITAMIN C
1mg; CALCIUM 20mg; IRON 1.2mg; FOLATE 71mcg; MAGNESIUM 20mg; ZINC 0.6mg;
SELENIUM 1.5mcg

Roasted Vegetable Pizza

Serves: 2

>2 cups broccoli florets
>1 large red bell pepper, sliced 1 inch thick
>1 large portobello mushroom, cut into ½-inch slices
>1 teaspoon garlic powder
>1 tablespoon balsamic vinegar
>1 teaspoon Mrs. Dash seasoning or Spike no-salt seasoning
>5 ounces baby spinach
>2 (100% whole grain) tortillas or pita bread
>½ cup no-salt-added or low-sodium pasta sauce
>Nutritarian Parmesan (see Note) or 1 to 2 ounces nondairy
>   mozzarella cheese

Preheat the oven to 350°F. Toss broccoli, bell peppers, and mushrooms with garlic powder, balsamic vinegar, and seasoning. Roast seasoned vegetables on a cookie sheet for 30 minutes, turning occasionally and mounding to keep them from drying out. Steam spinach until just wilted. Bake tortilla or pita directly on an oven rack for 5 to 7 minutes or just until crisp. Spread a thin layer of pasta sauce on a tortilla or on top of the pita bread, and distribute roasted vegetables and spinach. Sprinkle with Nutritarian Parmesan or nondairy mozzarella. Bake for an additional 3 to 5 minutes or until toppings are warm and cheese is melted, checking occasionally to avoid browning the vegetables.

Note: To make Nutritarian Parmesan, place ¼ cup walnuts and ¼ cup nutritional yeast in a food processor and pulse until it resembles the texture of grated Parmesan cheese.

PER SERVING: CALORIES 416; PROTEIN 24g; CARBOHYDRATE 53g; TOTAL FAT 13.5g; SATURATED FAT 2.2g; CHOLESTEROL 1.3mg; SODIUM 251mg; FIBER 13.9g; BETA-CAROTENE 5570mcg; VITAMIN C 193mg; CALCIUM 192mg; IRON 7.6mg; FOLATE 252mcg; MAGNESIUM 170mg; ZINC 5.4mg; SELENIUM 12.8mcg

Salad-Stuffed Pita

Serves: 4

For the Dressing (see Note):
    1 cup unsweetened soy, hemp, or almond milk
    1 cup raw almonds or ½ cup raw almond butter
    ¼ cup balsamic vinegar
    2 tablespoons fresh lemon juice
    ¼ cup raisins
    2 teaspoons Dijon mustard

For the Sandwich:
    2 cups shredded lettuce
    2 cups shredded spinach
    1 tomato, chopped
    1 avocado, chopped
    ½ cup thinly sliced red onion, if desired
    4 (100% whole grain) pitas (or wraps)

Combine dressing ingredients in a high-powered blender until smooth and creamy. Combine lettuce, spinach, tomato, avocado, and onion. Toss with desired amount of dressing. Reserve leftover dressing for another use. Stuff into whole grain pitas. If making wraps, place on wrap, roll up tightly, and cut in half.

Note: You can substitute any of my healthful nut- and seed-based dressings for the dressing in this recipe.

PER SERVING: CALORIES 390; PROTEIN 12g; CARBOHYDRATE 37g; TOTAL FAT 24.3g; SATURATED FAT 2.2g; SODIUM 141mg; FIBER 9.2g; BETA-CAROTENE 2859mcg; VITA-MIN C 17mg; CALCIUM 168mg; IRON 3.3mg; FOLATE 128mcg; MAGNESIUM 139mg; ZINC 1.6mg; SELENIUM 5.1mcg

Seasoned Kale Chips and Popcorn

Serves: 4

6 to 7 leaves kale, tough stems and center ribs removed
6 cups air-popped popcorn
Olive oil
Water
1 tablespoon nutritional yeast
1 to 2 teaspoons chili powder or other no-salt seasoning

Preheat the oven to 200°F. Tear kale into uniform, chip-size pieces and spread evenly on a baking sheet without overlapping the pieces. Bake for 50 minutes or until kale is crispy and dry, stirring occasionally to prevent burning. Remove the kale from the oven and, when cool, combine with the popcorn. Mix one part olive oil and two parts water in a spray bottle, shake very well, then lightly spray the popcorn and kale and sprinkle with a mixture of nutritional yeast and chili powder.

PER SERVING: CALORIES 116; PROTEIN 6g; CARBOHYDRATE 20g; TOTAL FAT 2.6g; SATURATED FAT 0.3g; SODIUM 46mg; FIBER 4.2g; BETA-CAROTENE 9287mcg; VITAMIN C 121mg; CALCIUM 143mg; IRON 2.5mg; FOLATE 33mcg; MAGNESIUM 56mg; ZINC 1.2mg; SELENIUM 0.9mcg

Seasoned Sweet Potato Fries

Serves: 4

> 2 tablespoons water
> ½ teaspoon Bragg Liquid Aminos
> ½ teaspoon dried thyme
> ½ teaspoon dried oregano
> ½ teaspoon dried basil
> ½ teaspoon paprika
> 2 tablespoons nutritional yeast
> Freshly ground black pepper, to taste
> 2 large sweet potatoes, peeled and cut into fries or long wedges

Preheat the oven to 375°F. In a large mixing bowl, whisk together the water, Bragg Liquid Aminos, dried herbs, paprika, nutritional yeast, and pepper. Add the sweet potatoes and toss until thoroughly coated. Place the sweet potatoes in a single layer on a nonstick baking sheet (or one that is lined with a nonstick baking mat) and bake for 45 minutes or until baked through and lightly browned, giving them a stir every 15 minutes.

PER SERVING: CALORIES 73; PROTEIN 3g; CARBOHYDRATE 15g; TOTAL FAT 0.3g; SATURATED FAT 0.1g; SODIUM 65mg; FIBER 3.1g; BETA-CAROTENE 5613mcg; VITAMIN C 2mg; CALCIUM 34mg; IRON 1.1mg; FOLATE 9mcg; MAGNESIUM 24mg; ZINC 1mg; SELENIUM 0.4mcg

Seeded Crackers with Dried Tomatoes

Serves: 15

1 cup sunflower seeds, soaked for 4 to 6 hours, then drained
1 large onion, chopped
1 clove garlic, minced
1 tablespoon dried basil
1 tablespoon dried thyme
1 tablespoon dried oregano
1 teaspoon Bragg Liquid Aminos
1 cup flaxseeds, soaked 4 to 6 hours, then drained
2 cups buckwheat or oat groats
½ cup unhulled sesame seeds, toasted
¾ cup chopped unsulfured, no-salt-added dried tomatoes

Preheat the oven to the lowest setting (such as 175°F). Place sunflower seeds, onion, and garlic in a food processor and process until well blended. Add a little water if necessary. Place sunflower mixture in a bowl, add remaining ingredients, and mix well. If mixture is too dry, add a little more water. Spread onto a parchment-lined baking sheet to about ⅛ inch thickness. It is easier to spread if you keep your hands wet. Bake for about 4½ hours or until desired crispness, stirring occasionally. If using a dehydrator, dry at 105°F for 6 hours, turn, and continue drying for an additional 3 to 4 hours or until desired crispness. Break into pieces.

PER SERVING: CALORIES 227; PROTEIN 7g; CARBOHYDRATE 25g; TOTAL FAT 12.9g; SATURATED FAT 1.4g; SODIUM 24mg; FIBER 7.4g; BETA-CAROTENE 19mcg; VITAMIN C 2mg; CALCIUM 98mg; IRON 3.1mg; FOLATE 49mcg; MAGNESIUM 126mg; ZINC 1.9mg; SELENIUM 6.4mcg

Taco Salad Wraps

Serves: 4

For the Dressing:
>   2 ripe avocados
>   2 tablespoons nutritional yeast
>   ¼ cup unsweetened soy, hemp, or almond milk
>   2 tablespoons lime juice
>   ½ teaspoon cumin
>   ½ teaspoon chili powder, regular or chipotle

For the Wraps:
>   1 cup cooked red kidney or black beans or low-sodium canned
>   beans, drained
>   4 (100% whole grain) flour tortillas
>   1 cup frozen corn kernels, thawed
>   4 plum tomatoes, chopped
>   2 cups shredded romaine lettuce

Blend dressing ingredients in a blender until smooth and creamy. With a fork or potato masher, mash beans, leaving slightly chunky. Spread desired amount of dressing on each tortilla and then top with bean mixture, corn, chopped tomato, and lettuce. Fold up the bottom edge of the tortilla until it partially covers the filling, then fold in the left and right sides of the tortilla and roll up. Slice in half diagonally.

Note: You can refrigerate leftover dressing for another use in the next three days.

PER SERVING: CALORIES 335; PROTEIN 15g; CARBOHYDRATE 50g; TOTAL FAT 9.9g; SATURATED FAT 1.4g; SODIUM 165mg; FIBER 13.6g; BETA-CAROTENE 1600mcg; VITAMIN C 17mg; CALCIUM 83mg; IRON 4.6mg; FOLATE 145mcg; MAGNESIUM 57mg; ZINC 1.8mg; SELENIUM 1.8mcg

Three-Seed Burgers
Serves: 4

½ cup raw pumpkin seeds
⅓ cup raw sunflower seeds
¼ cup unhulled sesame seeds
¾ cup cooked lentils
2 tablespoons rolled oats
3 tablespoons tomato paste, in BPA-free packaging
¼ cup chopped scallions
2 tablespoons tahini
1 tablespoon chopped flat-leaf parsley
Pinch of cayenne pepper

Preheat the oven to 350°F. In a food processor, combine pumpkin seeds, sunflower seeds, and sesame seeds and process until coarsely chopped. Add lentils, rolled oats, tomato paste, scallions, tahini, parsley, and cayenne. Process until mixture is blended. Shape mixture into four patties. Lightly oil a baking sheet with a little olive oil. Place patties on the sheet and bake for 10 minutes; turn and bake another 8 minutes.

PER SERVING: CALORIES 318; PROTEIN 14g; CARBOHYDRATE 20g; TOTAL FAT 22.7g; SATURATED FAT 3.3g; SODIUM 17mg; FIBER 6.5g; BETA-CAROTENE 209mcg; VITAMIN C 6mg; CALCIUM 150mg; IRON 6.1mg; FOLATE 126mcg; MAGNESIUM 169mg; ZINC 3.5mg; SELENIUM 6.3mcg

DESSERTS

Almond Chocolate Dip

Serves: 10

1⅓ cups raw almonds or ⅔ cup raw almond butter
1 cup unsweetened soy, hemp, or almond milk
1 teaspoon alcohol-free vanilla flavoring
1 tablespoon natural cocoa powder
⅔ cup dates, pitted
Strawberries or other fresh fruit for dipping

Blend all ingredients except fruit for dipping in a high-powered blender until smooth and creamy, adding more nondairy milk if needed to adjust consistency. Serve with fresh fruit.

PER SERVING: CALORIES 163; PROTEIN 5g; CARBOHYDRATE 17g; TOTAL FAT 10g; SATURATED FAT 0.8g; SODIUM 11mg; FIBER 4.2g; BETA-CAROTENE 6mcg; VITAMIN C 42mg; CALCIUM 104mg; IRON 1.2mg; FOLATE 28mcg; MAGNESIUM 67mg; ZINC 0.8mg; SELENIUM 1.1mcg

Almond Coconut Macaroons
Serves: 18

2 cups finely shredded unsweetened coconut
2 cups finely ground blanched almonds (see Note)
¼ cup unsweetened soy, hemp, or almond milk
1 tablespoon orange zest
1 teaspoon almond extract
2½ tablespoons ground flaxseed simmered with 3 tablespoons
    water for 2 minutes
½ cup pitted dates
¼ cup hot water

Preheat the oven to 325°F. In a large bowl, combine shredded coconut, ground blanched almonds, nondairy milk, orange zest, and almond extract. Cut in flaxseed mixture. Place dates and hot water in a food processor and process until mixture forms a ball. Add to bowl and mix well. The dough should be firm and slightly moist. If it is dry, add a little nondairy milk. Form round balls of dough and flatten into small patties. Line a baking sheet with parchment paper. Bake for 15 minutes. Makes about 36 macaroons.

Note: Use a food processor to grind almonds to a fine powder. You can substitute almond pulp from making homemade almond milk for the ground almonds and nondairy milk.

PER SERVING: CALORIES 182; PROTEIN 5g; CARBOHYDRATE 9g; TOTAL FAT 15.5g; SATURATED FAT 6.5g; SODIUM 9mg; FIBER 3.9g; BETA-CAROTENE 1mcg; VITAMIN C 1mg; CALCIUM 46mg; IRON 1mg; FOLATE 11mcg; MAGNESIUM 59mg; ZINC 0.7mg; SELENIUM 2.9mcg

Apple Oat Flaxseed Bars

Serves: 9

4 Medjool or 8 regular dates, pitted and chopped
3 tablespoons raw cashew butter
1 apple, peeled, cored, and chopped
1 cup old-fashioned rolled oats
½ cup raisins
½ cup chopped almonds, walnuts, or cashews
¼ cup unsweetened soy, hemp, or almond milk
2 tablespoons ground flaxseeds

Preheat the oven to 300°F. In a food processor, process dates and cashew butter until a paste forms. Add apple and pulse until mixture is well combined. Place in a bowl and mix in remaining ingredients. Press into a 9 × 9-inch baking dish. Bake for 30 minutes. Remove from oven and press once again. Allow to cool before slicing.

PER SERVING: CALORIES 201; PROTEIN 5g; CARBOHYDRATE 29g; TOTAL FAT 9.3g; SATURATED FAT 1.2g; SODIUM 5mg; FIBER 3.2g; BETA-CAROTENE 15mcg; VITAMIN C 1mg; CALCIUM 37mg; IRON 3.5mg; FOLATE 16mcg; MAGNESIUM 44mg; ZINC 0.7mg; SELENIUM 4.4mcg

Apple Strudy

Serves: 4

½ cup unsweetened vanilla soy, hemp, or almond milk
¾ teaspoon alcohol-free vanilla flavoring
1 teaspoon cinnamon
3 apples, peeled, cored, and chopped
¼ cup raisins, chopped
½ cup old-fashioned rolled oats
¼ cup ground raw walnuts
2 tablespoons ground flaxseeds

Preheat the oven to 350°F. In a bowl, mix the nondairy milk, vanilla, and cinnamon until combined. Stir in the chopped apples, raisins, oats, ground walnuts, and flaxseeds.

Pour into an 8 × 8-inch baking dish. Bake, covered, for 1 hour.

PER SERVING: CALORIES 176; PROTEIN 4g; CARBOHYDRATE 29g; TOTAL FAT 6.2g; SATURATED FAT 0.7g; SODIUM 14mg; FIBER 4.3g; BETA-CAROTENE 22mcg; VITAMIN C 5mg; CALCIUM 69mg; IRON 3.3mg; FOLATE 8mcg; MAGNESIUM 35mg; ZINC 0.5mg; SELENIUM 1.2mcg

Banana Pineapple Sorbet

Serves: 2

1 ripe banana, frozen (see Note)
1 cup fresh pineapple chunks

Blend the banana and pineapple and serve immediately.

Note: Freeze the banana at least 4 hours in advance. Peel and seal in a plastic bag before freezing.

PER SERVING: CALORIES 94; PROTEIN 1g; CARBOHYDRATE 24g; TOTAL FAT 0.3g; SATURATED FAT 0.1g; SODIUM 1mg; FIBER 2.7g; BETA-CAROTENE 44mcg; VITAMIN C 45mg; CALCIUM 14mg; IRON 0.4mg; FOLATE 27mcg; MAGNESIUM 26mg; ZINC 0.2mg; SELENIUM 0.7mcg

Chia Pudding
Serves: 4

  1 cup unsweetened soy, hemp, or almond milk
  ½ cup unsweetened, shredded coconut
  1 cup water
  4 Medjool dates or 8 regular dates, pitted
  ½ teaspoon alcohol-free vanilla flavoring
  ½ to ¾ teaspoon ground cardamom
  ½ cup chia seeds, divided

Blend milk, coconut, water, dates, vanilla, cardamom, and ¼ cup
of the chia seeds in a high-powered blender. Add additional milk if
needed to adjust consistency. Stir in remaining ¼ cup chia seeds.
Refrigerate for 15 minutes and stir again to distribute seeds evenly. If
desired, top with fresh berries and/or toasted unsweetened coconut.

For a parfait, alternate layers of berries with pudding in a wine glass.
For a chocolate chia pudding, blend in 2 tablespoons natural cocoa
powder.

PER SERVING: CALORIES 280; PROTEIN 7g; CARBOHYDRATE 34g; TOTAL FAT 15g;
SATURATED FAT 7.3g; SODIUM 42mg; FIBER 11.1g; BETA-CAROTENE 23mcg; VITA-
MIN C 1mg; CALCIUM 171mg; IRON 2.7mg; FOLATE 16mcg; MAGNESIUM 111mg;
ZINC 1.4mg; SELENIUM 16.8mcg

Chocolaty Brownies

Serves: 9

For the Brownie:
    ½ cup natural cocoa powder
    ½ cup chestnut flour or almond flour
    1¾ cups mashed cooked sweet potato
    ½ teaspoon cinnamon
    1 teaspoon alcohol-free vanilla flavoring
    ½ teaspoon baking soda
    ½ teaspoon baking powder
    ⅔ cup roughly chopped walnuts
    1 tablespoon ground flaxseeds, hemp seeds, or chia seeds
    3 tablespoons unsweetened soy, hemp, or almond milk

For the Icing:
    6 regular or 3 Medjool dates, pitted
    2 tablespoons tahini
    2 tablespoons natural cocoa powder
    4 to 5 tablespoons water to thin icing

For the brownie, preheat the oven to 350°F. Mix together the cocoa powder and flour and then mix into the mashed sweet potato. Stir in cinnamon, vanilla, baking soda, baking powder, walnuts, seeds, and nondairy milk. Press dough into a lightly oiled 9 × 9-inch baking dish and bake for 30 minutes. The brownies will firm up after they have cooled.

For the icing, process dates with a food processor until they form a paste, then add remaining ingredients. Spread on brownies after they have cooled. Cut into squares.

PER SERVING: CALORIES 199; PROTEIN 6g; CARBOHYDRATE 25g; TOTAL FAT 11.2g; SATURATED FAT 1.5g; SODIUM 95mg; FIBER 6g; BETA-CAROTENE 6032mcg; VITAMIN C 8mg; CALCIUM 84mg; IRON 2mg; FOLATE 23mcg; MAGNESIUM 81mg; ZINC 1.2mg; SELENIUM 2mcg

Pinoli Cookies

Serves: 13

> 1½ cups cooked chickpeas or 1 (15-ounce) can low-sodium
> or no-salt-added chickpeas, drained
> 1 cup raw almonds
> 4 Medjool dates or 8 regular dates, pitted
> 1 apple, cored
> 1½ teaspoons almond extract
> ¼ cup water
> ¾ cup old-fashioned rolled oats
> ⅓ cup pine nuts, or pinoli (see Note)

Preheat the oven to 350°F. Blend chickpeas, almonds, dates, apple, almond extract, and water in a high-powered blender until smooth. Place in a bowl and mix in oats. Drop on a lightly oiled or parchment-lined baking sheet in 2-tablespoon scoopfuls. Flatten a little with a fork and top with pine nuts, pressing nuts into the dough to secure. Bake for 12 minutes. Makes 26 cookies.

Note: Mediterranean Stone Pine Nuts have a higher protein content and better flavor than other varieties of pine nuts. They are available at www.DrFuhrman.com.

PER SERVING: CALORIES 160; PROTEIN 6g; CARBOHYDRATE 19g; TOTAL FAT 7.7g; SATURATED FAT 0.7g; SODIUM 2mg; FIBER 4.3g; BETA-CAROTENE 15mcg; VITAMIN C 1mg; CALCIUM 45mg; IRON 2.4mg; FOLATE 41mcg; MAGNESIUM 51mg; ZINC 0.9mg; SELENIUM 1mcg

Strawberry Banana Ice Cream

Serves: 4

3 ripe bananas, frozen (see Note)
⅓ cup unsweetened soy, hemp, or almond milk
2 cups frozen strawberries (or blueberries, for Blueberry Banana
   Ice Cream)
2 tablespoons chopped walnuts
1 tablespoon ground flaxseed
½ teaspoon alcohol-free vanilla flavoring

Blend all ingredients in a high-powered blender until smooth and creamy. Add additional nondairy milk if needed to adjust consistency.

Note: Freeze ripe bananas at least 4 hours in advance. Peel bananas and seal in a plastic bag before freezing.

PER SERVING: CALORIES 146; PROTEIN 3g; CARBOHYDRATE 29g; TOTAL FAT 3.4g; SATURATED FAT 0.4g; SODIUM 13mg; FIBER 4.6g; BETA-CAROTENE 44mcg; VITAMIN C 38mg; CALCIUM 29mg; IRON 1.1mg; FOLATE 39mcg; MAGNESIUM 49mg; ZINC 0.4mg; SELENIUM 3mcg

Vanilla or Chocolate Nice Cream

Serves: 4

¼ cup raw walnuts

2 ripe bananas, frozen (see Note)

⅓ cup unsweetened soy, hemp, or almond milk (frozen ahead
of time)

2 Medjool or 4 regular dates, pitted

1 teaspoon alcohol-free vanilla flavoring or 2 tablespoons natural
nonalkalized cocoa powder

Using a high-powered blender, blend walnuts to a fine powder.
Add remaining ingredients and blend on high speed until smooth
and creamy. Serve immediately or store in the freezer for later use.
If desired, substitute raw almonds, cashews, or hazelnuts for the
walnuts.

Note: Freeze ripe bananas at least 4 hours in advance. Peel bananas
and seal in a plastic bag before freezing.

PER SERVING: CALORIES 141; PROTEIN 2g; CARBOHYDRATE 25g; TOTAL FAT 4.6g;
SATURATED FAT 0.5g; SODIUM 11mg; FIBER 2.9g; BETA-CAROTENE 27mcg; VITAMIN
C 5mg; CALCIUM 22mg; IRON 0.6mg; FOLATE 23mcg; MAGNESIUM 38mg; ZINC
0.4mg; SELENIUM 1.9mcg (analysis for Vanilla Nice Cream)

Vanilla Zabaglione with Fresh Fruit
Serves: 8

1¾ cups raw cashews
½ to ¾ cup coconut water, or as needed
8 Medjool dates or 16 regular dates, pitted
1 vanilla pod, pulp scraped out, pod discarded
1 teaspoon alcohol-free vanilla flavoring
1 teaspoon ground chia seeds
12 cups your choice of fruit

Soak cashews overnight in coconut water. Drain and reserve the coconut water. In a high-powered blender, combine cashews, dates, vanilla pulp, vanilla flavoring, and chia seeds. Blend until very smooth, adding the reserved coconut water as needed to achieve a thick but pourable mixture. Refrigerate. For a nice presentation, alternate layers of fruit and zabaglione in a clear glass parfait dish. Or just spoon over your choice of fresh fruit in a bowl.

PER SERVING: CALORIES 179; PROTEIN 4g; CARBOHYDRATE 26g; TOTAL FAT 8.2g; SATURATED FAT 1.1g; SODIUM 5mg; FIBER 2.9g; BETA-CAROTENE 14mcg; VITAMIN C 1mg; CALCIUM 33mg; IRON 3.1mg; FOLATE 14mcg; MAGNESIUM 39mg; ZINC 0.7mg; SELENIUM 3.9mcg

Wild Blueberry Rice Pudding

Serves: 3

¼ cup raisins
1 banana
2 cups frozen wild blueberries
2 tablespoons chia seeds
½ teaspoon alcohol-free vanilla flavoring
1 cup cooked wild rice
¼ teaspoon cinnamon

In a high-powered blender, blend raisins and banana until raisins are completely ground. Add blueberries, chia seeds, and vanilla and blend until smooth. Place in a bowl and fold in wild rice. Sprinkle with cinnamon before serving.

PER SERVING: CALORIES 209; PROTEIN 4g; CARBOHYDRATE 46g; TOTAL FAT 2.6g; SATURATED FAT 0.3g; SODIUM 7mg; FIBER 9g; BETA-CAROTENE 44mcg; VITAMIN C 5mg; CALCIUM 70mg; IRON 1.7mg; FOLATE 23mcg; MAGNESIUM 61mg; ZINC 1.8mg; SELENIUM 4.7mcg

CHAPTER TEN

Your Questions Answered

Now that you have read this book and understand the role that nutritional excellence plays in preventing and reversing heart disease, you may have some questions about specific conditions and therapies. In this Q&A chapter, I give in-depth answers to common questions about issues related to cardiovascular health: How much should I exercise? Should I be worried about the mercury levels in fish? Does wine really have heart-healthy benefits? Do cruciferous vegetables harm the thyroid? What kind of supplements should I take, and how much? Read on for answers to these and other important questions.

How much exercise, and what type, is best for my heart or for my heart condition?

The answer is much like the answer of how much vitamin D or DHA is appropriate—that is, not too much, and not too little. If you have heart disease, you should exercise regularly, and you should not spend most of the day sitting. You should try to structure your day so that you spend at least fifteen minutes standing for each hour that you sit.

Plenty of competitive runners, including marathoners, develop heart disease. Running so much may actually give these "over-exercisers" free rein to eat more heart disease–causing foods without becoming overweight, promoting food-caused atherosclerosis and premature death.

For example, James Fixx, the author of the 1977 bestseller *The Complete Book of Running,* ran ten miles a day in addition to other vigorous exercise. Friends described him as being in top physical condition, yet Fixx had a fatal heart attack at the age of 52 while jogging near his home in Vermont. Although he had no symptoms, autopsy results revealed that his left circumflex coronary artery was almost totally blocked. About 80 percent of the blood flow in his right coronary artery was blocked, and half of the left anterior descending artery was blocked in places. All of his exercise did not protect him. Even though a fatal heart attack at age 52 is unusual, this example is a reminder that many individuals with superior fitness still develop heart disease. Being fit is not the same thing as being healthy. An important take-home point is that exercise is almost worthless if you don't eat right.

Though vigorous exercise over a limited time is associated with longer life span, extremely vigorous exercise for long periods of time, such as training for and racing in marathons regularly, is not. Iron Man triathlons and twenty-six-mile marathon races are pushing the value of exercise too far, resulting in more stress than the body can compensate for. Accumulating evidence from multiple studies indicates that developing peak performance for success in high-intensity, prolonged endurance competitions may increase a person's risk of developing atrial fibrillation in later life and is not life span–favorable.[1] Cardiorespiratory fitness for heart health and longevity does not require such intensity and draconian effort.

According to a 2015 analysis, even jogging at a very moderate pace goes a long way to enhancing longevity.[2] The results also suggest that strenuous running—done more frequently, for longer periods, or at a greater intensity—was not associated with any additional mortality benefits. The study demonstrated that joggers who ran 1 to 2.4 hours per week had the lowest risk of mortality, with a significant 71 percent lower risk of death compared with sedentary nonjoggers. Individuals who ran less than one hour per week still had a significantly (53 percent) lower risk of all-cause mortality, so less jogging is still good, too. However, running (or jogging) more than 2.5 hours a week did not result in any life span benefits. Running too fast (more than seven miles per hour) surprisingly obliterated the benefits. Jogging two to three times per week gave the most favorable life span–enhancing results.[3] The bottom line here is that running too much, too often, or too fast was not favorable.

Accumulating Evidence Against Doing Too Much

This is not the first study to show that more exercise isn't necessarily better in terms of health and longevity. In 2012, a study including more than fifty-two thousand men and women showed that the benefits of running are best accumulated in shorter distances—specifically, at fewer than twenty miles per week.[4]

At longer distances, the researchers observed a U-shaped relationship between all-cause mortality and running, with longer weekly distances trending in the wrong direction toward less mortality benefit. A later study, which followed more than fifty-five thousand people for fifteen years showed that just five to ten minutes of daily running, performed even at very slow speeds, significantly lowered an individual's risk of premature death and added about three years of life expectancy.[5]

Interval Training Is Beneficial

Interval training means that you exercise in bursts of energy for short periods of time, such as one to three minutes, but you exercise at an increased intensity to elevate your heart rate more than you would be capable of doing if you had to sustain the effort much longer. I recommend playing a song with a good, fast beat and either jumping or jogging in place, picking up your knees higher and at a faster rate as your exercise tolerance improves. Be sure to increase the intensity of the exertion further over the last minute so that you are out of breath at the end. That's it: After one song, you are done with the interval and can now walk or do some calisthenics or abdominal exercises. Incorporating intervals into your exercise program has large benefits.

- Doing intervals regularly encourages fat loss and you lose body fat more easily.[6]

- Interval training is effective at increasing exercise tolerance and heart function.[7]

- Intervals are effective at lowering blood pressure and/or preventing high blood pressure from developing, thus preventing strokes and heart attacks.[8]

It is also advantageous to do one interval, recover your heart rate, and then do other exercises in your repertoire, such as push-ups, leg raises, and abdominal crunches; then toward the end of your workout do another two- to four-minute interval and exert yourself.

The studies referenced above suggest that the ability of exercise to lower blood pressure and keep it low is proportional to the exertion expended (for a short period of time). In other words, if you are in good health without significant heart disease, then it is healthful and life-extending to exert yourself and elevate your heart rate doing high-intensity intervals.

To summarize my exercise recommendations:

1. Work part of the day standing up. Stay active and out of a chair as much as possible.

2. Twice a week, walk fast and eventually jog (at a comfortable pace for you) for fifteen to twenty minutes.

3. Twice a week, increase the intensity and do a few intervals of three to four minutes. This can be jumping and/or jogging in place, while picking your knees up to increase the exertion; or using equipment in a gym that requires exertion, such as a stair climber or a bicycle set at high resistance.

4. Exercise multiple body parts a few times a week, too. Don't forget your hamstrings, lower back, and abdominal muscles.

If you have heart disease, always err by doing too little, not too much. If you have heart failure, decreased ejection fraction, cardiomyopathy, or other indications of serious heart disease, check with your doctor so she or he can guide you to the extent and level at which you can safely exercise.

If I am still overweight, should I limit my intake of nuts and seeds to only 1 ounce a day? What about snacking?

I advise overweight individuals to limit their intake of nuts and seeds in order to limit their calorie intake. Nuts and seeds have about 180 calories in an ounce. I suggest that overweight women limit their intake to 1 ounce a day and men to 1½ ounces a day. However, this is not a rigid rule. If you are eating less of other foods, some extra nuts or seeds are still permissible. I don't have a limit for people who are slim and don't need to lose weight.

Just to clarify this topic: The calories from nuts and seeds are not more fattening than equal amounts of calories from grains, root vegetables, or fruit. So if an overweight individual chooses to eat 2–3 ounces of nuts or seeds a day, this amount can still be acceptable as long as that person correspondingly removes an equal amount of calories from other foods.

So let's say you choose to eat 3 ounces of seeds/nuts for 540 calories, and then you eat 560 other calories in the day from a healthy diet of greens, beans, onions, mushrooms, berries, beets, carrots, and tomatoes. That would still be a total of 1,100 calories for the day, which may be appropriate if you are a woman who is eating only when hungry. Likewise, you could eat half that amount of seeds and nuts (1½ ounces), for 270 calories, and then have more calories that day from boiled beets, carrots, winter squash, or steel cut oats for the same 1,100 calories. The point is, either dietary pattern can work. But it is important to eat only when you are hungry and not to eat haphazardly. You don't want to take in more calories than your body needs or use nuts and seeds to enable overeating.

Since fat loss from the body is enhanced when glycogen stores are lower, it is always best to eat only when you are hungry and not to snack or eat recreationally between meals when you are not hungry. It is also best to finish dinner at least three hours before bedtime.

Remember, the micronutrient and phytochemical benefits of nutrient-rich foods are enhanced when you eat nuts and seeds with the same meal, because the fat aids absorption of many beneficial anticancer nutrients. This means that most of your nut and seed intake should occur during lunch and dinner, or during the meal when you are eating the nutrient-rich vegetables. The enhanced absorption of antioxidants and phytochemicals from food in the same meal is an important reason why fat-containing foods have life span–enhancing benefits.

Never snack on nuts and seeds. If you are unable to make it to a meal and you must have a snack, choose something like carrots, tomatoes, or an apple. I recommend that you mostly eat nuts and seeds as an ingredient in a salad dressing. Measure out how many ounces you add to the blender, and from that, you can calculate how many ounces of nuts and seeds are in each serving of salad dressing. There's no perfect method that meets everyone's needs, so understand the principles and modify your eating style so it works for you.

Remember, despite false claims to the contrary, there is zero evidence to date that more fat in your diet from seeds and nuts has any detrimental health effects or increases the risk of any disease, especially heart disease. In fact, the opposite is true—more seeds and nuts in your diet is cardioprotective.

Fish is generally regarded as heart disease–favorable food. Why do you limit its consumption to only 6 ounces or less per week?

Today, almost all current nutritional advisors include fish as a cornerstone of a healthful diet. But my recommendations are slightly different from those of other respected health authorities. Although the differences may seem minor, they are significant, and I contend that they will make it possible for you to achieve both extraordinarily good health and an extraordinarily long life span.

Fish and shellfish have high concentrations of protein and other essential nutrients, are low in saturated fat, and contain the valuable omega-3 fatty acids EPA and DHA. These food factors are thought to contribute to heart health and to children's proper brain growth and development. Overwhelming evidence confirms the health benefits of omega-3 fatty acids, which is why fish and shellfish are considered to be an important part of a well-balanced diet.

Unfortunately, fish also supplies us with industrial contaminants; nearly all fish and shellfish contain mercury and other pollutants. All the seas in the world are polluted, and not a single fish is spared. Even in the North and South Poles, the marine life is more heavily polluted than humans are (yes, we are polluted too by the chemical toxins we have consumed). It is even affecting the animals eating the marine life, as studies have shown, for instance, that polar bears' ability to reproduce is negatively affected by industrial pollutants in the seals and fish that they eat. And the polar bears are not buying fish that have been raised in fish farms, where the dioxins and chemicals in the fish are *significantly* increased.

Nearly all fish and shellfish contain methylmercury. Mercury accumulates in fish when polluted water is filtered through their gills. The longer a fish lives, the more the mercury accumulates. Large fish eat small fish and accumulate all of the mercury that was in the small fish. Over a lifetime, this increases exponentially. Likewise, our tissues accumulate mercury from the fish we eat throughout our lifetimes.

Governmental health authorities do not advise what diet is ideal for maintaining excellent health for one hundred years. Instead, their advice is based on the relative risk of one food versus another, and they recommend avoiding only the most dangerous foods. Regardless, most governments warn us that pregnant women should not eat species of fish that contain high amounts of mercury. For everyone else (including women who are not pregnant), they advise that these higher-mercury-contaminated fish not be eaten too often. This weak admonition is based on the misguided notion that the benefits of eating fish outweigh the potential harm from mercury exposure.

Mercury is not the only toxic pollutant in fish—they can also contain polychlorinated biphenyls (PCBs) and dioxin. The simplest way of consuming less PCBs, dioxin, and mercury is to rarely eat fish—and when you do eat it, eat only the smaller, lower-mercury-containing species. Also, don't take unpurified fish oil supplements.

The advice given by governmental authorities for pregnant women includes:

1. *Never* eat shark, swordfish, king mackerel, or tilefish because they contain high levels of mercury.

2. Check advisories about the safety of eating local fish caught by family and friends in local rivers and coastal waterways. If unsure, don't eat more than 6 ounces at a meal, and don't eat any other fish during that week.

The U.S. Environmental Protection Agency (EPA) makes recommendations for what it considers an acceptable level of mercury in a pregnant woman's body. In the past twenty years, awareness has increased that mercury causes brain damage, so the EPA has lowered the "acceptable" level more than once.

I have been telling patients for years that if something can damage a fetus and result in childhood learning abnormalities, it can't be good for long-term brain health and longevity in adults. You can't have it both ways. The developing fetus should be viewed as a sensitive indicator of the potential of toxins to cause cellular damage in the short run. But this potential damage is a risk to adult cells, as well. We may not see the damage in adults in as short a period of time, but subtle cellular damage from mercury can be a contributory factor, in combination with other negative influences, that leads to the development of brain diseases seen later in life. It is not just youngsters who are at risk of brain damage from mercury.

No fish is completely free of mercury and other pollutants. If you eat generous portions of fish regularly, your body is undoubtedly high in mercury. You cannot remove the mercury from the fish by trimming the fat or by cooking, because it is deposited throughout the fish's tissues. I've observed that a person's mercury level correlates exceptionally well with the amount of fish they consume, and medical studies back up this observation.[9]

Individuals eating fish a few times a week have been found to have blood mercury levels exceeding the maximum level recommended by the National Academy of Sciences (blood level less than 5 micrograms).

Women eating seafood more than twice a week have been found to have seven times the blood mercury levels compared with women who rarely eat fish, and children eating fish regularly have been found to have mercury levels forty times higher than the national mean.[10] Even people eating only wild fish from the isolated waters of French Polynesia were found to have these higher mercury levels.[11]

Mercury poisons the brain. The Food and Drug Administration (FDA) wants us to think that eating a variety of fish with different amounts of mercury means we will not be harmed by mercury poisoning. But it does not guarantee that after eating fish for many years, we won't suffer from dementia or other diseases of brain aging associated with the continual accumulation of mercury and other pollutants in fish. High body stores of mercury cause brain damage and memory impairment, leading to dementia in later life.

The risk of brain damage from mercury increases with age. Besides the risk of neurological disease, other risks associated with mercury include hypertension, heart disease, mental disorders, and endocrine diseases.[12] Mercury accumulates in the bloodstream over time. It can be removed from the body naturally (the kidneys continually excrete mercury into our urine), but even after we eliminate mercury-containing fish from our diets, it may take years for the levels in our bodies to drop significantly.

Like mercury, other pollutants, including PCBs, accumulate in fish and in the body tissues of people who eat fish regularly. PCBs are neurotoxic, hormone-disrupting carcinogens that were banned in the 1970s, but they are resistant to degradation and are still in our environment. They are found at levels seven times higher in farmed salmon than in wild ones, according to a 2005 study.[13]

PCBs are persistent organic pollutants (POPs), which accumulate in animal fat. Because most farmed salmon are raised on feed that includes ground-up fish—and sometimes other animals, such as cattle—their bodies collect POPs. Farmed salmon are also less active and are fed to grow at an accelerated rate, so they contain more fat, which is filled with these fat-adhering chemicals. Other POPs found in fish include the organochlorine pesticide dieldrin and dioxins, which result from chlorine paper bleaching and the manufacturing and incineration of polyvinyl chloride (PVC).

Clearly, you should avoid commercially raised salmon unless it is raised and fed more naturally and is tested and documented to be lower in pollutants. As concerns have been raised about the high levels of pollution in fish, as well as the artificial colors used to make farm-raised salmon pink, the demand for wild salmon (and therefore, its price) has skyrocketed in recent years.

Wild salmon may have been suddenly appearing in restaurants and food stores everywhere, but where was it all coming from?

An article in the *New York Times* confirmed that most so-called "wild Pacific" or "Alaskan" salmon is just farm-raised salmon with a misleading label. In March 2005, the *Times* tested salmon sold in eight New York City stores, where it was sold for as much as $29 a pound. The reporters found that most of the fish was farm-raised, not wild. Only one sample tested wild.[14]

Investigators for the *Times* article were able to tell the farm-raised salmon from the wild salmon because of the presence in the farm-raised fish of the artificial pink food dye canthaxanthin, manufactured by Hoffmann-La Roche. This pharmaceutical company developed the SalmoFan (which is a color chart, similar to paint store swatches) so fish farmers could choose among various shades used to make the salmon have that "natural" pink-orange color. Salmon in the wild are colored naturally from eating pink crustaceans, but those raised commercially have gray flesh from eating fish meal. Europeans are suspicious of canthaxanthin, which has been linked to retinal discoloration in people who ingested it as a sunless tanning pill.[15] Try to avoid these polluted fish:

Farmed trout and salmon—polluted with PCBs and dioxin from the fish meal they are fed

Tuna, tilefish, swordfish, and shark—large predatory fish, polluted with mercury

Shrimp—can contain antibiotics, mostly illegal drug residues

So eating fish may be an advantage for people who are eating meat (and eating poorly in general) because it has anticlotting effects. But its benefits may be apparent only when compared with people who eat more meat and dairy products. There would be no cardiovascular advantage to eating fish when the diet is already excellent or near-ideal and basic omega-3 needs are met with another source, such as DHA from algae.

If you have heart disease and you still want to eat fish, limit it to a small amount per week. Both the type of fish you eat and where it is caught matter. Avoid eating fish in restaurants, which use the least expensive, farmed fish. Instead, buy frozen fish from a reputable market that can prove the source. Most fresh-looking fish in markets is typically just defrosted frozen fish. It is best not to thaw and refreeze fish, so purchasing frozen fish is the most sensible and economical way to go, since you can use small amounts while the remainder stays frozen.

Only eat the fish on the lowest-mercury list, because even fish with moderate mercury levels, eaten regularly, can contribute to the development of dementia. Lower-mercury seafoods include Arctic char, butterfish, catfish, clams, crawfish, flounder, herring, king crab, mackerel, mullet, mussels, oysters, pollock, porgy, salmon, sand dabs, sardines, scallops, shad, shrimp, smelt, sole, squid, striped bass, sturgeon, tilapia, river trout, and whiting.[16]

I have always heard that drinking wine is good for the heart. Should I have one glass daily?

The brief answer is, *no, drinking alcohol will not protect your heart.* For some time, observational studies have suggested that only heavy drinking was detrimental to cardiovascular health and that light consumption may actually be beneficial. This has led some people to drink moderately, believing that it will lower their risk of heart disease.

Contrary to what earlier studies have shown, however, it now appears, with better studies and more complete analysis, that any exposure to alcohol likely has an overall negative effect on the heart. In a 2014 study researchers analyzed evidence from more than fifty studies and data from 261,991 individuals to find out whether there is a link between drinking habits and cardiovascular health. They concluded that a *reduction* in alcohol consumption "may be beneficial for cardiovascular health. Our results therefore challenge the concept of a cardioprotective effect associated with light to moderate alcohol consumption reported in observational studies and suggest that this effect may have been due to residual confounding or selection bias."[17] Plus, they demonstrated that individuals who consume less alcohol can lower their weight.

Other important recent studies corroborated these findings. A 2014 meta-analysis was particularly valuable because it tried to create a closer approximation of theorized lifetime cumulative exposure to alcohol than studies using only baseline consumption. It demonstrated that the J-shaped curve used to claim that light drinking was life span–promoting was not seen, and that even 40 grams, or a fifth of a cup a day, was found to be life span–shortening.[18]

Alcohol is the fifth-leading risk factor for death and disability, accounting for 4 percent of life years lost because of disease.[19] Alcohol consumption is believed to be associated with adverse effects on the heart, including detrimental effects on blood pressure and contributing to cardiac arrhythmias. However, the major adverse effect of alcoholic beverages is their carcinogenicity. The harmful effects of alcohol on conditions such as liver cirrhosis, injuries, and cancers of the liver, bowel, breast, and esophagus have been firmly established.[20]

There is strong scientific consensus regarding even limited amounts of alcohol and increased risk of various cancers. For example, a pooled analysis of fifty-three studies indicated that for each daily alcoholic drink, the risk of breast cancer increased 7 percent, with two to three drinks increasing breast cancer risk 20 percent over nondrinkers.[21]

Even if the blood-thinning effects of alcohol were a cardiovascular advantage for people eating a very poor diet, drinking alcohol still would be helpful only for those continuing to eat badly, while further promoting their likelihood of getting a serious cancer. The bottom line is this: Do not drink expecting heart-health benefits— there are none.

*What if I have to take Coumadin (the blood thinner warfarin)
for atrial fibrillation or valve replacement and have been advised
not to eat green vegetables?*

Multiple individuals have asked me to give them a complete answer
with guidelines for people taking Coumadin (warfarin is the generic
name) who have been told by their health professionals to avoid green
vegetables because of the interaction between warfarin and vitamin K.
As a proponent of a diet rich in leafy greens, broccoli, and other foods
rich in vitamin K, my dietary recommendations often contradict the
advice of dietitians, nurses, and doctors who advise their patients
taking this medication to avoid foods that contain this vitamin.

The reason that health professionals recommend their patients on
warfarin avoid vitamin K–containing foods is that warfarin produces
its blood-thinning effects by interfering with the activation of a vitamin K–dependent enzyme that is needed to build clotting factors.
When you ingest more vitamin K from green vegetables, you can decrease the effectiveness of this medication. A higher dose of the drug
will then be required to maintain the recommended degree of blood
thinning. (The term "blood thinning" is a lay term that means a reduction in the natural ability of the body to form a blood clot.)

These definitions are important to know in order to understand
this issue:

> *Coagulation*—The formation of blood clots made by clot-
> ting factors and platelets, a normal body reaction when, for
> example, you cut yourself. Coumadin (warfarin) is called
> an *anticoagulant* because it works against the formation of
> blood clots.
>
> *Thrombus (singular) / thrombi (plural)*—Clots formed inside
> blood vessels, typically to seal a defect in the vessel wall.
> These clots, when formed in the blood vessels that supply
> the heart with oxygen, cause heart attacks.
>
> *Embolus (singular) / emboli (plural)*—A traveling clot, usually
> caused by a thrombus that breaks off and travels to a dis-

tal portion of the artery where it is narrower—occluding it, leading to a stroke, pulmonary infarction (death of lung tissue), or heart attack.

In many cases, warfarin is used as a preventive treatment to reduce the chance of emboli forming that could cause a stroke. Warfarin is most often prescribed for patients with atrial fibrillation, a common irregularity in the heart rate. When you have this irregular heartbeat, the turbulent flow of blood makes the formation of an embolus—which can travel to the brain and cause a stroke—more likely. This treatment is also used by people who have experienced a serious blood clot.

Since warfarin is given to prevent clots, the major side effect is bleeding. When you are taking it, you will not stop bleeding easily if you are cut. So, for instance, you could more easily bleed to death if you were in a car accident or if other bleeding occurs inside the body for a variety of reasons. The main problem with this medication is its very narrow therapeutic range: If you take too much, you can suffer from a major bleeding episode; if you take too little, it could be ineffective at preventing embolic events. People taking this drug have to be closely monitored with blood tests and their dose adjusted accordingly to make sure they are taking the correct amount.

According to current estimates, 70 percent of people on warfarin tend to stop taking the medicine because of frustration with blood tests, dosage changes, and side effects. Although monitoring is a medical necessity, often the demands of heavy patient loads can make it very challenging for busy physicians to follow patients as closely as they need to be followed. Besides the risk of a major bleed, another serious but more infrequent complication of warfarin therapy is drug-induced limb gangrene and skin necrosis (death of skin tissue). Other adverse reactions that occur infrequently include white blood cell diseases, hair loss, allergic reactions, diarrhea, dizziness, hepatitis and abnormal liver function, skin rash, headache, nausea and/or vomiting, and itching.

Physicians treat patients with warfarin primarily to decrease the occurrence of thromboembolism. They perceive that this risk has a greater clinical effect than the risk of drug-induced bleeding. However, only recently has the extent of the risks of bleeding been thoroughly investigated. A recent meta-analysis that pooled data from thirty-three studies examined the bleeding rates of patients who received at least three months of anticoagulation therapy. Major bleeding occurred at a rate of 7.22 per 100 patient-years, and fatal bleeding occurred at the rate of 1.3 per 100 patient-years.[22] This means that if ten people were put on warfarin therapy for ten years each, seven of the ten would suffer a bleeding event and one would die from taking the drug.

Before 1990, warfarin therapy for the prevention of stroke for people with atrial fibrillation was limited to those who also had additional risk factors, such as rheumatic heart disease and prosthetic heart valves. In recent years, however, hundreds of thousands of people with atrial fibrillation, including those without significant accompanying risk factors, except for their age, have been placed on this medication to decrease the risk of embolic stroke.

Medical studies have shown that patients with atrial fibrillation who also had other risk factors for strokes did have a survival advantage and a reduced risk of strokes when warfarin was prescribed. The results were considerably better than aspirin in these high-risk patients but not considerably better than aspirin for patients with only atrial fibrillation and no other serious risk factors.

Younger patients with atrial fibrillation and those without cardiac risk factors have not been shown to live longer as a result of taking warfarin, mainly because strokes are more infrequent. Recently, there has been more concern that aspirin is not an adequate treatment option because the risk of hemorrhagic strokes is still associated with its use and it does not sufficiently protect against clots forming in the heart.

Today some new blood thinners—Pradaxa (dabigatran), Xarelto (rivaroxaban), and Eliquis (apixaban)—may be better options than both aspirin and warfarin; they do not interact with vitamin K and thus do not require the restriction of green vegetable intake. More and more physicians have begun using these newer, but more expensive, blood-thinning medications instead of warfarin. These drugs seem a bit safer regarding the chances of a hemorrhagic bleed in the brain developing, and they also do not require frequent blood testing to monitor their levels.

The drawback to these newer medications is that their effect cannot be reversed quickly, as warfarin can be in the case of a bleeding episode, accident, or fall that could result in internal or external bleeding. With warfarin, you can use vitamin K to counter its effects fairly quickly.

Of course, all the factors determining your risk must be considered, and that is the job of your physician. Whether your doctor advises treatment, and which treatment, is guided by your risk of developing thromboembolic events.

It is not beneficial to use any blood thinner, even if you have atrial fibrillation, if you are at a relatively low risk for thromboembolic events. This would not include people who have diabetes, suffer from advanced atherosclerosis, have poorly controlled blood pressure, have an enlarged heart, or are obese and those who smoke or have had a recent embolic event. Doctors also consider a person's age in making these decisions. However, I contend that those people eating an NDPR diet are at considerably lower risk, regardless of age. A produce-rich diet has already been demonstrated in medical studies to have a powerful effect on decreasing the risk of embolic stroke and heart attack. In fact, in the Nurses' Health Study, a measly five servings of vegetables and fruits a day reduced the risk of embolic stroke by 30 percent, and this is still a poor diet by my standards.[23] Another study looking at the daily consumption of greens, vegetables, and fruit found a radical decrease in stroke incidence approaching 50 percent with higher fruit and vegetable intake.[24]

When you change your diet to include more vegetation and fewer animal products and refined foods, your cholesterol drops, your blood pressure typically decreases, and your risk of a heart attack or embolic stroke plummets.

My dietary recommendations, which are extremely low in salt and offer the equivalent of more than ten servings a day of stroke-protective produce, have been demonstrated to dramatically lower cholesterol, and I believe they offer a greater resistance to both strokes and heart attacks than any type of blood-thinning therapy. For healthier people following my nutritional advice, after a few months, the use of medications for the prevention of emboli with atrial fibrillation may not have a favorable benefit-to-risk ratio. In other words, it may be safer for such people to use no drug therapy.

Significant evidence supports my assertion that many people taking warfarin today would be safer if they ate an ideal diet with lots of vitamin K–containing greens and stopped the warfarin. Eating right will not cause you to bleed to death, and you will also experience a portfolio of benefits that can save your life.

If you absolutely must take warfarin because of a recent thrombotic event or a mechanical heart valve, you should still eat very healthfully, even if the drug dose has to be increased slightly to accommodate some green vegetables included in a healthful diet. As long as the amount of greens you eat is consistent, your doctor can adjust the medication dose to accommodate it.

So if you must stay on warfarin, your diet must be consistent from day to day to avoid fluctuations in the effectiveness of the drug. To keep the vitamin K amount constant, it is sensible to eat one large, raw salad a day and one serving of dark green vegetables, such as asparagus or string beans. However, leave out the very dark green leafy vegetables, such as steamed kale, collard greens, and spinach. Adding some of these to a soup is okay, however.

The goal is to keep your vitamin K level stable so that the amount of blood thinning does not swing into a danger zone. A dangerous level of blood thinning can occur if the dose of warfarin is adjusted to a high vitamin K intake and then suddenly you do not eat much vitamin K–containing foods for a few days. *The main goal is to eat the same amount of vitamin K–containing foods every day.*

> Many people following my dietary and health
> guidelines find that their health and risk factors
> improve so much that they no longer need to
> take warfarin (Coumadin).

In summary, the evidence indicates that warfarin is more effective than aspirin in high-risk patients, but it is associated with a higher rate of serious bleeding. A diet high in processed foods and animal products, though it is low in vitamin K, will still increase your risk of a heart attack and stroke even if you are taking blood-thinning drugs. If you must remain on warfarin, eat a beneficial but not an excess amount of those high-vitamin-K-containing foods. And, if at all possible, get off the warfarin. Work with your doctor to decide whether one of the newer blood-thinning medications is appropriate for you, or even no blood thinners, if you are healthy enough, eating right, and are at low risk of developing a clot.

What about chelation therapy for heart disease?

Intravenous (IV) chelation therapy has been widely used as a standard medical treatment for heavy-metal poisoning for more than fifty years. Chelation consists of a series of IV infusions of ethylenediaminetetra-acetic acid (EDTA), often in combination with other substances, including vitamins and minerals.

Today, some health practitioners offer the option of chelation with oral agents. A minority of nonmainstream or alternative physicians promote chelation as an alternative treatment for arteriosclerosis, including CAD, peripheral vascular disease (blockage or narrowing of blood vessels in the legs), and the mental deterioration caused by small strokes. It has been claimed to be an effective adjunct to treating and improving blood flow, decreasing angina, and preventing cardiac events and death.

Over the years, suggesting chelation therapy for anything other than heavy-metal poisoning has been met with considerable resistance. The results of studies have been mixed and heavily criticized for bias and lack of scientific validity. Despite the disagreements, interest in chelation as an alternative treatment for heart and vascular problems has continued to grow, with thousands of people seeking out the therapy annually as an option to coronary bypass surgery and balloon angioplasty. While word of mouth has resulted in many "believers" in this therapy, many patients are still confused.

The Trial to Assess Chelation Therapy (TACT) was the first large-scale, randomized multicenter study designed to determine the safety and efficacy of EDTA chelation therapy for individuals with CAD and prior myocardial infarction.[25] This study was funded by the National Heart, Lung, and Blood Institute and the National Center for Complementary and Alternative Medicine at a cost of more than $30 million. The results were presented at the American Heart Association Scientific Sessions in November 2012.

The study was conducted at 134 research sites in the United States and Canada. The sites represented a mix of clinical settings: university or teaching hospitals, clinical practices or cardiology research centers, and chelation practices. A total of 1,708 patients were randomized—839 patients to chelation and 869 patients to placebo. Participants were at least 50 years old, had experienced a myocardial infarction at least six weeks before enrollment, and had not had coronary or carotid revascularization procedures within the previous six months or smoked cigarettes within the previous three months. The study population had a high rate of diabetes (31 percent), with 84 percent on aspirin and 73 percent on statin drugs. Sixty-five percent of patients completed all forty infusions.

The study found marginal benefits for the chelation group, including a minimal effect on standard measures of quality of life at six, twelve, and twenty-four months, with the exception of a slight improvement in self-reported angina symptoms at one year.

The marginal benefits for the chelation group have been discussed, dissected, and debated by both sides of this issue. Noted was the lower LDL cholesterol at baseline in the chelation group; this difference alone could account for most of the difference in outcome over five years. Additionally, the placebo group was infused with a solution that contained glucose, which may have led to an adverse outcome in the placebo group, especially in those diabetic or prediabetic subjects. Even after $30 million was spent, the study still had flaws and did not settle the debate.

The TACT study, according to the researchers presenting the results, is not conclusive and should not change clinical practice. They did state that the results warrant further study, especially in patients with diabetes or prior anterior heart attack because of a finding of some benefit in these subgroups. These results provide evidence to guide further research, but they are not sufficient to support the routine use of chelation therapy for treatment of people who have had a heart attack.

The bottom line is that if chelation therapy has benefits, then those benefits are primarily symptomatic and minor. It is expensive and not without risk, but it may have some anticlotting, antiplatelet effects, thereby lowering the risk of clots. It may also have some sustained vasodilation effects from binding calcium, which can lessen symptoms. However, it does not reverse obstructive lesions. I do not think it will add further benefits to aggressive dietary treatment and will add only minor benefit to any standard care.

If my LDL level is favorable, is low HDL a risk factor for heart disease?

HDL is considered the "good" cholesterol because HDL particles remove cholesterol, and some physicians are concerned when it is too low. When you are eating a most favorable diet and naturally lower your LDL, do not be concerned if your HDL lowers, too. Think of it this way: You don't need to keep lots of snow shovels in your garage if you live in Florida.

It is true that a higher HDL level offers some degree of protection for a person with an abnormally high cholesterol. However, for people who drop their LDL cholesterol below 100 mg/dl with nutritional excellence, the HDL will typically lower as well. This lower HDL is *not* a risk factor for heart disease. Populations from around the world who demonstrate complete freedom from heart disease as a consequence of their natural, plant-based diets have very low HDL levels. Populations with the highest HDL levels typically have the highest rates of heart disease because their LDL is high, too. So the high HDL is a marker for people with lots of harmful LDL that needs to be carried away.

Among people with relatively high cholesterol levels who are at risk because of their diet, those with a genetically favorable high HDL will have a mild advantage. This is a reflection of the body's efforts to lessen the risk of all that SAD-generated cholesterol. However, when you do not have an atherosclerotic burden and have no vulnerable plaque, you do not need a high HDL to remove stored lipids within the plaque because there aren't any. If there is no soft plaque, more HDL is not needed, and the body has no need to generate HDL.

Dietary improvements that significantly drop your total cholesterol are still favorable if your HDL drops as well. When your total cholesterol falls to the ranges seen in these heart attack–proof populations around the world (less than 140 mg/dl), the HDL level no longer matters. Genetically favorable HDL levels are also less beneficial than thought in the past. Some genetic mechanisms that raise plasma HDL cholesterol do not lower the risk of myocardial infarction.[26] The lack of significance of HDL for people with favorable LDL cholesterol is supported by recent studies showing that once statin drugs effectively lower LDL into favorable ranges, a higher or lower HDL is of no consequence.[27]

Can cruciferous vegetables harm the thyroid?

Cruciferous vegetables contain compounds called *glucosinolates,* which are metabolized into isothiocyanates (ITCs). These compounds have powerful protective effects against many cancers, including breast, prostate, colorectal, bladder, and lung cancers[28]—*and* thyroid cancer.[29] Concerns about the potential effects of cruciferous vegetables on thyroid function arose from animal studies, followed by findings suggesting that certain breakdown products of glucosinolates could interfere with thyroid hormone synthesis or compete with iodine for uptake by the thyroid. However, this is only a hypothetical issue. The scientific consensus is that even a very high intake of cruciferous vegetables could be detrimental to thyroid function only in cases of iodine deficiency.[30]

Iodine deficiency could be a concern for people who follow a healthful, plant-based diet since iodine is not naturally abundant in foods, except for seafood and seaweeds. Iodized salt is the chief source of iodine in the Western diet. Vegans and other people eating mostly plant-based diets may not get enough iodine unless they take supplements, especially if they avoid salt.[31] Also, pregnant women may require a greater amount of iodine than the general population because of the iodine needs of the fetus.[32]

Even though animal studies suggested the hypothetical thyroid issue from eating very large amounts of cruciferous vegetables, no human study has demonstrated a deficiency in thyroid function resulting from consuming cruciferous vegetables. Only one such study seems to have been conducted, with large amounts of cooked Brussels sprouts, and showed no effects on thyroid function.[33] Raw cruciferous vegetables have not been investigated. The only case report I could find relating cruciferous vegetables to thyroid harm suggests that it would be almost impossible to consume enough of these vegetables to cause damage. This case was that of an 88-year-old woman who developed hypothyroidism after eating four to five pounds of raw bok choy every day for several months—an excessive and unreasonable intake.[34]

Recent results from the Adventist Health Study revealed that vegan Adventists were less likely than omnivore Adventists to have hypothyroidism.[35] Similarly, a 2011 study of Boston-area vegetarians and vegans found that vegans had higher urinary thiocyanate (indicative of higher cruciferous intake) and lower iodine intake, but no abnormalities or differences in thyroid function.[36]

The fear of eating cruciferous vegetables, or the fear that people with hypothyroidism should reduce or avoid eating kale or other cruciferous vegetables (a rumor circulating on the Internet), is unfounded. Whether you have normal thyroid function or hypothyroidism, there is no reason for you to avoid or restrict your intake of cruciferous vegetables. Eating cruciferous vegetables is not optional. They have numerous anticancer benefits, a high micronutrient-to-calorie ratio, and are associated with reduced risk of premature death.[37] The effective functioning of your immune system depends on your consumption of cruciferous vegetables. Eat one or two servings of cruciferous vegetables daily (and make some of them raw), in the context of a healthful variety of vegetables, beans, fruit, nuts, and seeds. And be sure to get adequate iodine, too (see the answer to the next question for more on iodine supplementation).

What nutritional supplements do you recommend besides a low dose of DHA-EPA?

It is wise to be conservative and not take too much of any one nutrient. For most nutrients, there is a sweet spot in the middle between too much and too little that is best for maximizing health. Don't forget: Too much of a nutrient can be just as harmful as too little, so don't take high doses of supplements that could drive your intake too high. The exception to this rule is vitamin B12, a nutrient with no apparent ill effects if too much is taken. A diet low or lacking in animal products has the risk of being low in vitamin B12 and, for many people, also low in zinc.

An adequate zinc intake is especially important for normal immune function. Absorption of zinc, as well as resistance to infection, can decrease with aging.[38] This increased need for zinc with some individuals, and with aging, can be exacerbated if a person eats a low-calorie, vegan, or near-vegan diet. That's because phytic acid in beans, seeds, and nuts can bind zinc, reducing its absorption. Supplementing with about 15 milligrams daily is conservative and sensible.

Iodine is found extensively in seafood and seaweed and can be low in a person who doesn't consume iodinated salt or seaweed. Some people add a pinch of kelp to a salad each day, which is an effective way to meet their iodine requirements.

Vitamin D is another common deficiency found in people who don't get sufficient sun exposure. The proper blood test to assure optimal vitamin D levels is a 25-hydroxy vitamin D test. Optimal levels are between 30 and 50 mg/dl.

For most people who are eating healthfully with few animal products to supply sufficient vitamin B12, I recommend a supplement that contains adequate vitamin D, vitamin B12, vitamin K2, zinc, and iodine.

In addition, I recommend an algae-derived DHA and EPA supplement with at least 100 milligrams of DHA.

I generally suggest 150 micrograms of iodine daily, and 100 micrograms daily of vitamin B12 for vegans. I also recommend confirming with a blood test that vitamin B12 status is adequate when a person is older than 75, as absorption can decrease with aging. Methylmalonic acid and homocysteine could both be elevated in response to a vitamin B12 deficiency. These tests can be valuable in the elderly, whose needs are difficult to determine because the B12 blood test can still be in the normal range even with deficiency present.

I do *not* recommend that people supplement with folic acid, beta-carotene, vitamin A, and vitamin E. Most multivitamins contain these cancer-promoting, synthetic vitamins that have been demonstrated to increase the rate of death.[39] The increased risk of cancer shown in trials examining this issue is likely significantly underestimated because of the limited years of follow-up in most trials. The confusion and confounding effects are especially apparent when comparing folate that comes from real food to folic acid from supplements. Cancer evolution is a slow process, and outcomes twenty to thirty years later (or more) are more accurate in determining risk, in contrast to a five-year analysis, which is worthless for evaluating this risk.

Since a Nutritarian diet is exceedingly high in natural folate, and all people eating healthfully will expose themselves to an optimal intake of folate, there is no reason to incur the enhanced risk of taking synthetic folic acid when you are eating relatively healthfully. Multiple studies have indicated that folic acid supplements place users at higher risk of breast, prostate, and colorectal cancers.[40]

In summary, I recommend the following supplements and daily doses:

Vitamin B12: 100–500 mcg

Vitamin D: 1,000–3,000 IU (depending on blood work)

Zinc: 15–30 mg

Vitamin K2: 25–50 mcg

Iodine: 150–300 mcg

DHA and EPA: 200–300 mg

What is vitamin K2? Do I need both vitamins K1 and K2?

There are two forms of vitamin K. It is easy to get enough vitamin K1 (also called *phylloquinone*) when following a Nutritarian diet, since it is abundant in leafy green vegetables. Kale, collard greens, spinach, and mustard greens are some of the richest sources of K1. Vitamin K2 (a few different substances called *menaquinones*), on the other hand, is produced by microorganisms and is scarce in plant foods. High-K2 foods include dark-meat chicken, pork, and fermented foods like cheese, so K2 is more difficult to get from a Nutritarian diet. The human body can synthesize some K2 from K1, and intestinal bacteria can produce some K2, but these are very small amounts.[41]

Studies report that a causative factor of the low incidence of hip fracture in Japan was from *natto,* a fermented soy food that is rich in vitamin K2, in the diet. Following this observation, several studies found supplementation with vitamin K2 to be particularly effective at improving bone health. A review of randomized controlled trials found that vitamin K2 reduced both bone loss and the risk of fractures: vertebral fracture by 60 percent, hip fracture by 77 percent, and all nonvertebral fractures by 81 percent. In women who already had osteoporosis, K2 supplementation was shown to reduce the risk of fracture, reduce bone loss, and increase bone mineral density.[42]

A vitamin K–dependent protein binds up calcium to protect the soft tissues, including the arteries, from calcification. Vitamin K2 in particular helps to prevent the artery wall from stiffening and to maintain its elasticity. Higher K2 intake has been linked with a lower likelihood of coronary calcification; however, the same association was not found for K1.[43]

Coronary artery calcification is a predictor of cardiovascular events, as is arterial stiffness. In 2004, the Rotterdam Study revealed that increased dietary intake of vitamin K2 significantly reduced the risk of coronary heart disease by 50 percent as compared to low dietary K2 intake. Similar results were found in another study conducted in 2009.[44] Furthermore, a systematic review of several studies in 2010 found no association between K1 intake and coronary heart disease, but higher K2 intake was associated with lower risk.[45] Therefore, taking in supplemental vitamin K2, in addition to the vitamin K1 you get in eating vegetation, is likely beneficial to help protect against vascular calcification.

Should I take natural cholesterol-lowering supplements?

Plant sterols (also known as *phytosterols*) are another supplemental option for people who are eating ideally and whose cholesterol is still unfavorable. Plant sterols are the plant version of cholesterol. Plant cell membranes contain plant sterols, and animal cell membranes contain cholesterol. We produce cholesterol in the liver and consume some in animal-based foods. Plant sterols are naturally present in plant foods and are structurally similar to cholesterol. They serve functions in plant cell membranes that are similar to those of cholesterol in animal cell membranes.

Plant sterols naturally occur in a range of plant sources such as vegetables, beans, grains, seeds, and nuts. The richest whole-food sources of plant sterols are pistachio nuts, Mediterranean pine nuts and sunflower seeds. They are followed by cashews, split peas, kidney beans, almonds, and other nuts.

When we consume plant sterols, these substances appear similar to cholesterol to the cells lining the small intestine. This allows the plant sterols to bind to the sites on those small intestine cells that cholesterol would bind to in order to be absorbed. This is one way that plant sterols block the absorption of cholesterol from food and also block the reabsorption of cholesterol produced by the liver, which lowers cholesterol levels. More than forty human trials have collectively shown that plant sterol supplements can safely reduce LDL levels by up to 15 percent.[46] Plant sterols have long been recognized, and are FDA-approved, for their capacity to reduce LDL cholesterol. No negative health effects were reported in these studies.

Plant sterols are one of the many components of a healthful diet based on whole plant foods that keep cholesterol levels in check. For people who have difficulty getting their LDL cholesterol levels into a favorable range, plant sterol supplements are a safe and mildly effective additional choice. In addition to cholesterol-lowering effects, plant sterols have also been shown to have anticancer, anti-inflammatory, antiatherogenic, and antioxidant activities.[47]

Observational studies have shown that higher plant sterol intake is associated with a lower risk of cancers of the lung, esophagus, stomach, and breast.[48] Additionally, dietary plant sterols are reported to play a protective, therapeutic role in benign prostatic hypertrophy (enlarged prostate), a common medical condition in older men.[49] Clinical symptoms of this condition have been improved by plant sterol supplementation.

Most people, even those with a history of high cholesterol in the past, who are following the Nutritarian diet-style would not require additional plant sterols because the diet is already so effective at lowering cholesterol, and the sterol exposure from the beans and nuts is adequate.

Red yeast rice is also effective at lowering cholesterol, though I rarely recommend it because it has the same active ingredient, and same potential for side effects, as low-dose statin drugs. It is like a baby statin, and the active ingredient and strength can vary from brand to brand.

What do you say to someone who insists that the Nutritarian diet-style is too radical, despite its effectiveness? What do you say to someone who says they would rather die younger, if need be, to enjoy life more and eat without restrictions?

I say: I hope you live close to a good hospital—because you'll need it.

Seriously, those comments reflect a personal ignorance about the relationship between food preferences and pleasure. The first thing to keep in mind is that eating healthfully does *not* result in reduced pleasure in life or even reduced pleasure from eating. That is a complete myth, spoken by someone whose eating behavior is likely driven by food addiction.

Taste preferences are not fixed; they can, and do, change. The main issue here is that your taste gets more sensitive as you get healthier and as you stop eating concentrated sweets and highly salted foods. Starting at three weeks and generally within three to six months, you will likely enjoy the new foods and new recipes as much or more compared with your old diet. That was the overwhelming consensus of more than seven hundred people who were polled after they had eaten a Nutritarian diet for a minimum of six months.[50] It takes some time for this shift to occur and for the drive to consume unhealthy foods to lessen—*but the change will happen.*

Certainly, I respect the right of all individuals to run their lives the way they see fit, and to live within their own risk tolerance. However, since conventional food is so addictive and unhealthy, many people feel that the addiction controls them and that they can't live without those health-destroying foods. But that furtive love affair quickly dissipates after the lovers have been separated for a few months. In fact, with time, many food addicts are pleasantly surprised how good they feel and how easy it was to give up their previous comfort foods.

My experience is that most people are in denial about the true risks associated with their preferred eating style. As much as they resist altering their unhealthy diet, they often quickly change their minds once they have their first serious health incident, such as a heart attack or cancer diagnosis. At that point, they curse their former choices and wish they had made better ones. Think about that for a minute: How would the future you want you to eat?

My goal and expectation is not to change the diet of all Americans, or even the majority. Most people will not change their fixed beliefs about food, no matter how overwhelming the evidence—and there are too many commercial interests and naysayers to support their desire to eat the way they want.

I believe that I have a responsibility—and this is a responsibility that all good physicians share—to properly educate my patients and the public and to provide them with the information they need to make the right choices. Then it is up to them. The problem is that most people are not informed or educated enough about this issue.

Remember, when you are deciding to jump on board with either 60 percent of my advice or with 100 percent, be aware that if you continue to eat highly flavored, sweetened, calorically concentrated, unhealthy foods often, you will continue to crave them. You will not be able to get the full pleasure that is possible from eating a Nutritarian diet.

So many people have reported that it is much easier to embrace this diet-style 100 percent. This allows your addictions to fade away and gives your taste buds the ability to reach their full potential. It takes time to learn how to cook delicious food fitting these guidelines. But remember, when it comes to almost anything you enjoy eating that is destructive to your health, you'll find that a Nutritarian version of that same food tastes just as good, or better. And the bonus is that the Nutritarian version is healthful as well as delicious.

For example, if you're afraid of giving up ice cream, try a Vanilla or Chocolate Nice Cream (Chapter 9), made with walnuts, bananas, non-dairy milk, and dates. You will be amazed at the flavor. Are you afraid you'll miss a burger barbecue on July 4th? Try one of my Black Bean (a hint of turkey or meat added, optional) Burgers made with mush-rooms, rolled oats, and black beans. Then after barbecuing those, you can use a pita pocket (or slice both sides of a whole grain bun in half so you use half the bread) and pile on thinly sliced red onion, sliced tomato, and some low-sugar, low-salt ketchup. You'll be astonished to discover that this tastes better than a whole beef burger!

My books and website offer you thousands of creatively delicious recipes. Even a growing number of excellent restaurants specialize in Nutritarian food. There is no reason why healthy food has to take a backseat when it comes to taste. My experience is that this way of eating is the tastiest and most enjoyable way to eat. Many other people agree, once their palates adjust to enjoying the taste of delicious whole foods. I focus more on breaking food addictions and helping people who are struggling with obstacles to dietary change in my book *The End of Dieting*.

For decades I have seen and experienced that the Nutritarian diet is simply the healthiest and most delicious way to enjoy life. What you eat affects every part of your life, and good, natural food is the best way to thrive every single day. Those of us who eat this way don't wish we were eating other food. I promise you: If you follow this plan, you will soon enjoy and even crave greens, beans, berries, and seeds combined in creative dishes.

And the amazing bonus is that this diet-style will reverse disease and keep you living longer and stronger. Heart disease, diabetes, and CAD (and angina) are not the inevitable consequence of aging. They are the direct result of bad dietary choices.

The solution is not at the doctor's office, at the pharmacy, or in the operating room; it is in your hands, and I hope these pages have helped make this clear.

Now that you know the facts, let's get to it! You can stop this No. 1 killer—from affecting you and your loved ones.

A Letter of Promise

Dear Reader,

Thank you for reading this book. It does not merely represent years of research and writing, but also decades of working with people who have serious illnesses and are fighting to save their lives. At times, this fight was carried on despite their own internal conflicts and the opposition they may have faced in their surrounding sphere of influence—their friends, family, and co-workers.

The problem of the standard American diet (SAD) affects all of us. I am sure that heart attacks and strokes have happened needlessly in your family and have had a devastating effect on you and your loved ones. I have certainly experienced this pain within my own family. My hope is that once you read these pages, you will have the in-depth knowledge you need to protect yourself and those you care about. We can all work together to save millions of lives and bring health back to our suffering population.

I am grateful to have earned your trust and thereby have this opportunity to potentially have a positive influence on your life. I feel very strongly that this message needs to be widely known.

Do not underestimate the powerful economic forces and the many individuals in powerful positions working against this. The information in these pages smacks some people right across their pocketbooks and egos and can result in vicious responses. It also upsets many who have strong food preferences, food allegiances, and food addictions that are not shaken by any amount of facts or evidence. They believe only the information they wish to believe.

Many will attack the science, deny the consistent superior results, and risk their lives by making the very same food choices that led them to get sick in the first place. People who embrace the status quo will experience the typical health outcomes that befall other Americans; in plain terms, their lives become a crapshoot.

Some will claim that this approach is too severe and that seeking excellent health and being committed to living a life free of heart attack and stroke is "crazy" or "extreme." It's amazing that suffering from heart attacks, living in fear and with disability, taking multiple drugs, and having your chest opened for bypass surgery are not considered extreme, but eating healthfully is.

There are even those who promote the idea that people who choose a long life, instead of suffering a slow, premature death from SAD food, are "orthorexic" (that is, they are obsessive about eating healthy food). This is insane given the reality that the majority of people in this country are eating a diet that will certainly lead to an early death. The question of what is "normal" needs to be reconsidered. Being in the majority should not be the criterion for normalcy; the fact that the use of alcohol, cigarettes, and drugs is so pervasive in our society is a good example of this. Addiction to fast food, commercially baked goods, alcohol, and even drugs is the common practice; such addictions are glorified and are certainly more popular than healthy eating. These harmful behaviors might be popular, but that doesn't make them normal.

Undoubtedly, this is an uphill battle, but we are slowly winning. The most accurate and effective information does not die. It may be knocked down for a while, but it rises up and inevitably plods forward. You can expect those attacks to continue, but they will never win. Butter, bacon, meat, cheese, chips, candy, and cake will never be the secret to a long life free of heart disease.

This is a fight against disease that we should all embrace enthusiastically, together. Today, not only are more people adopting a Nutritarian lifestyle, but there is also more and more support for it, such as more health food stores, prepared food options, health-based restaurants, and even Nutritarian meal-delivery services. More information about social connections, events, meet-ups, supportive services, and products can be found at www.DrFuhrman.com. My mission is to help remove the obstacles to your implementing healthful living.

I applaud every doctor who has incorporated nutrition into his or her practice in a significant way. All doctors recognize that we enjoy our careers more if we are successful in helping people avoid discomfort, get well, and live longer. All people who add more whole plant material to their diet have moved in the right direction, and all people who have adopted a diet, even if it is not one that I consider ideal, still have done something positive. Something is better than nothing, and at the least they are demonstrating that they care about what they put in their mouths. With added guidance, encouragement, and information, most people will make more changes in the right direction and be enthused with the results they accomplish.

Every step in the right direction will reduce risk and bear health dividends. This need not be an all-or-nothing plan, but when doctors ask patients for compliance, they should be aware that the more they ask for, the more they get; moderate changes most often result in insignificant benefits. Moderation can lead to heart attacks and needless death. It is much more difficult to navigate these waters when a person has one foot in a stream moving north and the other in a stream moving south. And dabbling in dangerous eating often leads to more stress and bad decision-making—it makes following this program harder to do, not easier.

We should know about the potential of smart nutrition to free us from the merry-go-round of more treatments and more disease. Too often, I have observed doctors take a paternalistic view and decide that the Nutritarian program is too difficult or too radical for a particular person or population they serve. However, I have found this not to be true; people of all types—from different educational backgrounds, ethnicities, economic groups, and nationalities—have embraced this program when they understand all the facts. Every person deserves the opportunity to make the choice for himself or herself.

I know that when a knowledgeable friend, doctor, or health professional sees this book in their patient's hands, they will be excited to know that this person will be able to achieve spectacular results in improving his or her health. They will share a knowing and happy smile with that patient, reflecting a mutual desire to help and wish the best for each other.

Smiling has substantial physiological health benefits. I am wishing you all those smiles that radiate inward, to aid your health, and outward, to connect with others. It brings a smile to my face to think that the knowledge in this book will lead you to a healthy, fully rewarding, and most pleasurable life.

Yours in health,

Joel Fuhrman, M.D.

Acknowledgments

I would like to acknowledge my team at DrFuhrman.com that aided me in the development of this book, specifically Lisa Fuhrman and Eileen Murphy, for their editing prowess; Lauren Russell and Tim Shay, who developed the diagrams and graphs; Linda Pospescu, R.D.; who assisted with recipes/menus; and Deana Ferreri, Ph.D., our staff cardiovascular research scientist, who is invaluable with research collection and interpretation.

Then HarperOne has a wonderful team of talented professionals with whom I work, including executive editor Gideon Weil, production editor Lisa Zuniga, and director of publicity Melinda Mullin.

References

Introduction: The Heart of the Matter

1. Boden WE, O'Rourke RA, Teo KK, et al. Optimal medical therapy with or without PCI for stable coronary disease. *N Engl J Med.* 2007;356(15):1503–16.

2. Fuhrman J, Singer M. Cardiovascular case studies, and user survey with a nutrient-dense, plant-rich (NDPR) diet-style. Fuhrman J, Singer M. Improved cardiovascular parameter with a nutrient-dense, plant-rich diet-style: a patient survey with illustrative cases. *J Lifestyle Med.* 2015. doi: 10.1177/1559827615611024.

3. Musini VM, Nazer M, Bassett K, et al. Blood pressure–lowering efficacy of mono-therapy with thiazide diuretics for primary hypertension. *Cochrane Database Syst Rev.* 2014;29:5. Wong GW, Wright JM. Blood pressure lowering efficacy of nonselective beta-blockers for primary hypertension. *Cochrane Database Syst Rev.* 2014;28:2.

4. Mozaffarian D, Benjamin EJ, Go AS, et al. American Heart Association Statistics Committee and Stroke Statistics Subcommittee. Heart disease and stroke statistics—2015 update: a report from the American Heart Association. *Circulation.* 2015 Jan 27;131(4):e29–322.

5. Butt DA, Mamdani M, Austin PC, et al. The risk of hip fracture after initiating anti-hypertensive drugs in the elderly. *Arch Intern Med.* doi: 10.1001/2013.

Chapter 1: Food Can Either Kill or Heal, the Choice Is Yours

1. Oliva A, Flores J, Merigioli S, et al. Autopsy investigation and Bayesian approach to coronary artery disease in victims of motor-vehicle accidents. *Atherosclerosis.* 2011 Sep;218(1):28–32. Joseph A, Ackerman D, Talley JD, et al. Manifestations of coronary atherosclerosis in young trauma victims: an autopsy study. *J Am Coll Cardiol.* 1993 Aug;22(2):459–67.

2. Martínez-González MA, Sánchez-Tainta A, Corella D, et al. A provegetarian food pattern and reduction in total mortality in the Prevención con Dieta Mediterránea (PREDIMED) study. *Am J Clin Nutr.* 2014;100(suppl 1):320S–28S.

3. Lagiou P, Sandin S, Lof M, et al. Low carbohydrate–high protein diet and incidence of cardiovascular diseases in Swedish women: prospective cohort study. *BMJ.* 2012;344:e4026.

4. Kritchevsky D. Dietary protein, cholesterol and atherosclerosis: a review of the early history. *J Nutr.* 1995;125(suppl 3):589S–93S.

5. Carroll KK. Dietary protein in relation to plasma cholesterol levels and atherosclerosis. *Nutr Rev.* 1978;36:1–5.

6. Kelemen LE, Kushi LH, Jacobs DR Jr, et al. Associations of dietary protein with disease and mortality in a prospective study of postmenopausal women. *Am J Epidemiol.* 2005;161(3):239–49.

7. Fenech MF. Dietary reference values of individual micronutrients and nutriomes for genome damage prevention: current status and a road map to the future. *Am J Clin Nutr.* 2010 May;91(5):1438S–54S. Ames BN. Prevention of mutation, cancer, and other age-associated diseases by optimizing micronutrient intake. *J Nucleic Acids.* 2010 Sep 22;2010:1–11. Ames BN, Atamna H, Killilea DW. Mineral and vitamin deficiencies can accelerate the mitochondrial decay of aging. *Mol Aspects Med.* 2005;26(4–5):363–78. Paul L. Diet, nutrition and telomere length. *J Nutr Biochem.* 2011;22(10):895–901. Troesch B, Hoeft B, McBurney M, et al. Dietary surveys indicate vitamin intakes below recommendations are common in representative Western countries. *Br J Nutr.* 2012;108(4):692–98. Cogsell ME, Zang Z, Carriquiry AL, et al. Sodium and potassium intakes among US adults: NHANES 2003–2008. *Am J Clin Nutr.* 2012;96(3):647–57. Bailey RL, Fulgoni VL, Keast DR, et al. Examination of vitamin intakes among US adults by dietary supplement use. *J Acad Nutr Diet.* 2012;112(5):657–63.e4. Yang Q, Cogswell ME, Hamner HC, et al. Folic acid source, usual intake, and folate and vitamin B-12 status in US adults: National Health and Nutrition Examination Survey (NHANES) 2003–2006. *Am J Clin Nutr.* 2010;91(1):64–72. Burnett-Hartman AN, Fitzpatrick AL, Gao K, et al. Supplement use contributes to meeting recommended dietary intakes for calcium, magnesium, and vitamin C in four ethnicities of middle-aged and older Americans: the Multi-Ethnic Study of Atherosclerosis. *J Am Diet Assoc.* 2009;109(3):422–29. Ford ES, Mokdad AH. Dietary magnesium intake in a national sample of US adults. *J Nutr.* 2003;133(9):2879–82.

8. Fuhrman J, Sarter B, Glaser D, et al. Changing perceptions of hunger on a high nutrient density diet. *Nutr J.* 2010;9:51.

9. Jenkins DJ, Kendall CW, Banach M, et al. Nuts as a replacement for carbohydrates in the diabetic diet. *Diabetes Care.* 2011;34:861–66.

10. Hu FB. Globalization of diabetes: the role of diet, lifestyle, and genes. *Diabetes Care.* 2011;34(6):1249–57.

11. Mirrahimi A, de Souza RJ, Chiavaroli L, et al. Associations of glycemic index and load with coronary heart disease events: a systematic review and meta-analysis of prospective cohorts. *J Am Heart Assoc.* 2012;1:e000752. Yu D, Shu X, Honglan LI, et al. Dietary carbohydrates, refined grains, glycemic load, and risk of coronary heart disease in Chinese adults. *Am J Epidemiol.* 2013;178(10):1542–49. Roberts CK, Liu S. Effects of glycemic load on metabolic health and type 2 diabetes mellitus. *J Diabetes Sci Technol.* 2009;3(4):697–704.

12. Rebello SA, Koh H, Chen C, et al. Amount, type, and sources of carbohydrates in relation to ischemic heart disease mortality in a Chinese population: a prospective cohort study. *Am J Clin Nutr.* 2014;100:53–64.

13. Jacobs DR Jr, Marquart L, Slavin J, et al. Whole-grain intake and cancer: an expanded review and meta-analysis. *Nutr Cancer.* 1998;30(2):85–90. Chatenoud L, Tavani A, La Vecchia C, et al. Whole grain intake and cancer risk. *Int J Cancer.* 1998;77(1):24–28.

14. Nordestgaard BG, Benn M, Schnohr P, et al. Nonfasting triglycerides and risk of myocardial infarction, ischemic heart disease, and death in men and women. *JAMA.* 2007;298:299–308. Bansal S, Buring JE, Rifai N, et al. Fasting compared with nonfasting triglycerides and risk of cardiovascular events in women. *JAMA.* 2007;298:309–16.

15. Teff KL, Grudziak J, Townsend RR, et al. Endocrine and metabolic effects of consuming fructose- and glucose-sweetened beverages with meals in obese men and women: influence of insulin resistance on plasma triglyceride responses. *J Clin Endocrinol Metab.* 2009;94:1562–69.

16. Jenkins DJ, Kendall CW, Popovich DG, et al. Effect of a very-high-fiber vegetable, fruit, and nut diet on serum lipids and colonic function. *Metabolism.* 2001;50(4):494–503.

17. Naruszewicz M, Zapolska-Downar D, Kośmider A, et al. Chronic intake of potato chips in humans increases the production of reactive oxygen radicals by leukocytes and increases plasma C-reactive protein: a pilot study. *Am J Clin Nutr.* 2009 Mar;89(3):773–77.

18. Sluijs I, van der Schouw YT, van der A DL, et al. Carbohydrate quantity and quality and risk of type 2 diabetes in the European Prospective Investigation into Cancer and Nutrition-Netherlands (EPIC-NL) study. *Am J Clin Nutr.* 2010;92(4):905–11. Barclay AW, Petocz P, McMillan-Price J, et al. Glycemic index, glycemic load, and chronic disease risk: a meta-analysis of observational studies. *Am J Clin Nutr.* 2008 Mar;87(3):627–37. Gnagnarella P, Gandini S, La Vecchia C, et al. Glycemic index, glycemic load, and cancer risk: a meta-analysis. *Am J Clin Nutr.* 2008;87:1793–1801. Sieri S, Krogh V, Berrino F, et al. Dietary glycemic load and index and risk of coronary heart disease in a large Italian cohort: the EPICOR study. *Arch Intern Med.* 2010;170:640–47. Kaushik S, Wang JJ, Flood V, et al. Dietary glycemic index and the risk of age-related macular degeneration. *Am J Clin Nutr.* 2008 Oct;88(4):1104–10.

19. Gnagnarella P, Gandini S, La Vecchia C, et al. Glycemic index, glycemic load, and cancer risk: a meta-analysis. *Am J Clin Nutr.* 2008 Jun;87(6):1793–801.

20. Dong JY, Qin LQ. Dietary glycemic index, glycemic load, and risk of breast cancer: meta-analysis of prospective cohort studies. *Breast Cancer Res Treat.* 2011 Apr;126(2):287–94. Sieri S, Pala V, Brighenti F, et al. Dietary glycemic index, glycemic load, and the risk of breast cancer in an Italian prospective cohort study. *Am J Clin Nutr.* 2007 Oct;86(4):1160–66.

21. Yun SH, Kim K, Nam SJ, et al. The association of carbohydrate intake, glycemic load, glycemic index, and selected rice foods with breast cancer risk: a case-control study in South Korea. *Asia Pac J Clin Nutr.* 2010;19(3):383–92.

22. Jakobson MU, Dethlefsen C, Joensen AM, et al. Intake of carbohydrates compared with intake of saturated fatty acids and risk of myocardial infarction: importance of the glycemic index. *Am J Clin Nutr.* 2010;91:1764–68. Liu S, Willett WC, Stampfer MJ, et al. A prospective study of dietary glycemic load, carbohydrate intake, and risk of coronary heart disease in US women. *Am J Clin Nutr.* 2000;71:1455–61. Hu FB. Are refined carbohydrates worse than saturated fat? *Am J Clin Nutr.* 2010;91:1541–42.

23. Atkinson FS, Foster-Powell K, Brand-Miller JC. International tables of glycemic index and glycemic load values: 2008. *Diabetes Care.* 2008 Dec;31(12):2281–83. Foster-Powell K, Holt SH, Brand-Miller JC. International table of glycemic index and glycemic load values: 2002. *Am J Clin Nutr.* 2002 Jul;76(1):5–56.

24. Halton TL, Willett WC, Liu S, et al. Potato and French fry consumption and risk of type 2 diabetes in women. *Am J Clin Nutr.* 2006;83(2):284–90.

25. Williams CD, Satia JA, Adair LS, et al. Dietary patterns, food groups, and rectal cancer risk in whites and African-Americans. *Cancer Epidemiol Biomarkers Prev.* 2009 May;18(5):1552–61.

26. Mozaffarian D, Hao T, Rimm EB, et al. Changes in diet and lifestyle and long-term weight gain in women and men. *N Engl J Med.* 2011 Jun 23;364(25):2392–2404.

27. Carbohydrates in human nutrition. Report of a joint FAO/WHO expert consultation, Rome, Italy, 14–18 April 1997. FAO food and nutrition paper 66. World Health Organization. 1998. ISBN 9251041148.

28. Bednar GE, Patil AR, Murray SM, et al. Starch and fiber fractions in selected food and feed ingredients affect their small intestinal digestibility and fermentability and their large bowel fermentability in vitro in a canine model. *J Nutr.* 2001;131(2):276–86.

29. Jenkins DJ, Kendall CW, Augustin LS, et al. Effect of legumes as part of a low glycemic index diet on glycemic control and cardiovascular risk factors in type 2 diabetes mellitus: a randomized controlled trial. *Arch Intern Med.* 2012;172(21):1653–60.

30. Mollard RC, Wong CL, Luhovyy BL, et al. First and second meal effect of pulses on blood glucose appetite and food intake at a later meal. *Appl Physiol Nutr Metab.* 2011;36(5):634–42. Wolever TM, Jenkins DJ, Ocana AM, et al. Second-meal effect: low-glycemic-index foods eaten at dinner improve subsequent breakfast glycemic response. *Am J Clin Nutr.* 1988;48(4):1041–47. Brighenti F, Benini L, Del Rio D, et al. Colonic fermentation of indigestible carbohydrates contributes to the second-meal effect. *Am J Clin Nutr.* 2006;83(4):817–22.

31. Darmadi-Blackberry I, Wahlqvist ML, Kouris-Blazos A, et al. Legumes: the most important dietary predictor of survival in older people of different ethnicities *Asia Pac J Clin Nutr.* 2004;13(2):217–20.

32. Maffucci T, Piccolo E, Cumashi A, et al. Inhibition of the phosphatidylinositol 3-kinase/Akt pathway by inositol pentakisphosphate results in antiangiogenic and antitumor effects. *Cancer Res.* 2005;65(18):8339–49. Singh J, Basu PS. Non-nutritive bioactive compounds in pulses and their impact on human health: an overview. *Food Nutr Sci.* 2012;3(12):1664–72. Zhang Z, Song Y, Wang XL. Inositol hexaphosphate-induced enhancement of natural killer cell activity correlates with suppression of colon carcinogenesis in rats. *World J Gastroenterol.* 2005;11(32):5044–46.

33. Mollard RC, Luhovyy BL, Panahi S, et al. Regular consumption of pulses for 8 weeks reduces metabolic syndrome risk factors in overweight and obese adults. *Br J Nutr.* 2012;108(suppl 1):S111–S22.

34. Chitnis MM, Yuen JS, Protheroe AS, et al. The type 1 insulin-like growth factor receptor pathway. *Clin Cancer Res.* 2008;14:6364–70. Werner H, Bruchim I. The insulin-like growth factor-I receptor as an oncogene. *Arch Physiol Biochem.* 2009;115:58–71. Davies M, Gupta S, Goldspink G, et al. The insulin-like growth factor system and colorectal cancer: clinical and experimental evidence. *Int J Colorectal Dis.* 2006;21:201–8. Sandhu MS, Dunger DB, Giovannucci EL. Insulin, insulin-like growth factor-I (IGF-I), IGF binding proteins, their biologic interactions, and colorectal cancer. *J Natl Cancer Inst.* 2002;94:972–80. Rowlands MA, Gunnell D, Harris R, et al. Circulating insulin-like growth factor peptides and prostate cancer risk: a systematic review and meta-analysis. *Int J Cancer.* 2009;124(10):2416–29.

35. Werner H, Bruchim I. The insulin-like growth factor–1 receptor as an oncogene. *Arch Physiol Biochem.* 2009;115(2):58–71. Chitnis MM, Yuen JS, Protheroe AS, et al. The type 1 insulin-like growth factor receptor pathway. *Clin Cancer Res.* 2008;14(20):6364–70.

36. Bartke A. Minireview: role of the growth hormone/insulin-like growth factor system in mammalian aging. *Endocrinology.* 2005;146:3718–23.

37. Rinaldi S, Peeters PH, Berrino F, et al. IGF-I, IGFBP-3 and breast cancer risk in women: the European Prospective Investigation into Cancer and Nutrition (EPIC). *Endocr Relat Cancer.* 2006;13:593–605.

38. Hankinson SE, Willett WC, Colditz GA, et al. Circulating concentrations of insulin-like growth factor-I and risk of breast cancer. *Lancet.* 1998;351:1393–96.

39. Lann D, LeRoith D. The role of endocrine insulin-like growth factor-I and insulin in breast cancer. *J Mammary Gland Biol Neoplasia.* 2008;13:371–79. Allen NE, Roddam AW, Allen DS, et al. A prospective study of serum insulin-like growth factor-I (IGF-I), IGF-II, IGF-binding protein–3 and breast cancer risk. *Br J Cancer.* 2005;92:1283–87. Fletcher O, Gibson L, Johnson N, et al. Polymorphisms and circulating levels in the insulin-like growth factor system and risk of breast cancer: a systematic review. *Cancer Epidemiol Biomarkers Prev.* 2005;14:2–19. Renehan AG, Zwahlen M, Minder C, et al. Insulin-like growth factor (IGF)-I, IGF binding protein–3, and cancer risk: systematic review and meta-regression analysis. *Lancet.* 2004;363(9418):1346–53. Shi R, Yu H, McLarty J, et al. IGF-I and breast cancer: a meta-analysis. *Int J Cancer.* 2004;111(3):418–23. Sugumar A, Liu YC, Xia Q, et al. Insulin-like growth factor (IGF)-I and IGF-binding protein 3 and the risk of premenopausal breast cancer: a meta-analysis of literature. *Int J Cancer.* 2004;111(2):293–97. Endogenous Hormones and Breast Cancer Collaborative Group, Key TJ, Appleby PN, et al. Insulin-like growth factor 1 (IGF1), IGF binding protein 3 (IGFBP3), and breast cancer risk: pooled individual data analysis of 17 prospective studies. *Lancet Oncol.* 2010;11(6):530–42.

40. Thissen JP, Ketelslegers JM, Underwood LE. Nutritional regulation of the insulin-like growth factors. *Endocr Rev.* 1994;15:80–101. Tsilidis KK, Travis RC, Appleby PN, et al. Insulin-like growth factor pathway genes and blood concentrations, dietary protein and risk of prostate cancer in the NCI Breast and Prostate Cancer Cohort Consortium (BPC3). *Int J Cancer.* 2013;133(2):495–504.

41. Qun LQ, He K, Xu JY. Milk consumption and circulating insulin-like growth factor–1 levels: a systematic literature review. *Int J Food Sci Nutr.* 2009;60(suppl 7):330–40. Heaney RP, McCarron DA, Dawson-Hughes B, et al. Dietary changes favorably affect bone remodeling in older adults. *J Am Diet Assoc.* 1999;99:1228–33.

42. Roddam AW, Allen NE, Appleby P, et al. Insulin-like growth factors, their binding proteins, and prostate cancer risk: analysis of individual patient data from 12 prospective studies. *Ann Intern Med.* 2008;149(7):461–71. Sim HG, Cheng CW. Changing demography of prostate cancer in Asia. *Eur J Cancer.* 2005;41(6):834–45.

43. Song Y, Chavarro JE, Cao Y, et al. Whole milk intake is associated with prostate cancer-specific mortality among U.S. male physicians *J Nutr.* 2013;143(2):189–96.

44. Giovannucci E, Pollak M, Liu Y, et al. Nutritional predictors of insulin-like growth factor I and their relationships to cancer in men. *Cancer Epidemiol Biomarkers Prev.* 2003;12:84–89. Holmes MD, Pollak MN, Willett WC, et al. Dietary correlates of plasma insulin-like growth factor I and insulin-like growth factor binding protein

3 concentrations. *Cancer Epidemiol Biomarkers Prev.* 2002;11:852–61. Allen NE, Appleby PN, Davey GK, et al. The associations of diet with serum insulin-like growth factor I and its main binding proteins in 292 women meat-eaters, vegetarians, and vegans. *Cancer Epidemiol Biomarkers Prev.* 2002;11:1441–48. Kaklamani VG, Linos A, Kaklamani E, et al. Dietary fat and carbohydrates are independently associated with circulating insulin-like growth factor 1 and insulin-like growth factor-binding protein 3 concentrations in healthy adults. *J Clin Oncol.* 1999;17:3291–98. Larsson SC, Wolk K, Brismar K, et al. Association of diet with serum insulin-like growth factor I in middle-aged and elderly men. *Am J Clin Nutr.* 2005;81:1163–67.

45. Andreassen M, Raymond I, Kistorp C, et al. IGF-1 as predictor of all cause mortality and cardiovascular disease in an elderly population. *Eur J Endocrinol.* 2009;160:25–31.

46. Van Bunderen CC, van Nieuwpoort IC, van Schoor NM, et al. The association of serum insulin-like growth factor-I with mortality, cardiovascular disease, and cancer in the elderly: a population-based study. *J Clin Endocrinol Metab.* 2010;95(10):4616–24.

47. Levine ME, Suarez JA, Brandhorst S, et al. Low protein intake is associated with a major reduction in IGF-1, cancer, and overall mortality in the 65 and younger but not older population. *Cell Metab.* 2014:19(3);407–17.

48. Andreassen M, Raymond I, Kistorp C, et al. IGF-1 as predictor of all cause mortality and cardiovascular disease in an elderly population. *Eur J Endocrinol.* 2009;160:25–31. Chisalita SI, Dahlström U, Arnqvist HJ, et al. Increased IGF1 levels in relation to heart failure and cardiovascular mortality in an elderly population: impact of ACE inhibitors. *Eur J Endocrinol.* 2011;165(6):891–98.

49. Salvioli S, Capri M, Bucci L, et al. Why do centenarians escape or postpone cancer? The role of IGF-1, inflammation and p53. *Cancer Immunol Immunother.* 2009;58(12):1909–17.

50. Crowe FL, Key TJ, Allen NE, et al. The association between diet and serum concentrations of IGF-I, IGFBP-1, IGFBP-2, and IGFBP-3 in the European Prospective Investigation into Cancer and Nutrition. *Cancer Epidemiol.* 2009;18(5):1333–40. Tsilidis KK, Travis RC, Appleby PN, et al. Insulin-like growth factor pathway genes and blood concentrations, dietary protein and risk of prostate cancer in the NCI Breast and Prostate Cancer Cohort Consortium (BPC3). *Int J Cancer.* 2013;133(2):495–504.

51. Tonding SF, Silva FM, Antonio JP, et al. Adiposity markers and risk of coronary heart disease in patients with type 2 diabetes mellitus. *Nutr J.* 2014;13:124.

52. Chiba Y, Saitoh S, Takagi S, et al. Relationship between visceral fat and cardiovascular disease risk factors: the Tanno and Sobetsu Study. *Hypertens Res.* 2007;30:229–36.

53. Logue J, Murray HM, Welsh P, et al. Obesity is associated with fatal coronary heart disease independently of traditional risk factors and deprivation. *Heart.* 2011;97:564–68.

Chapter 2: Bypassing Angioplasty

1. Ettinger PO, Wu CF, De La Cruz C Jr, et al. Arrhythmias and the "Holiday Heart": alcohol-associated cardiac rhythm disorders. *Am Heart J.* 1978; 95(5):555–62.

2. Phillips DP, Jarvinen JR, Abramson IS, et al. Cardiac mortality is higher around Christmas and New Year's than at any other time: the holidays as a risk factor for death. *Circulation.* 2004;110:3781–88. Kloner RA. The "Merry Christmas Coronary" and "Happy New Year Heart Attack" phenomenon. *Circulation.* 2004;110:3744–45.

3. Movahed MR, Hashemzadeh M, Jamal M, et al. Decreasing in-hospital mortality of patients undergoing percutaneous coronary intervention with persistent higher mortality rates in women and minorities in the United States. *J Invasive Cardiol.* 2010;22(2):58–60.

4. Forrester JS, Shah PK. Lipid lowering versus revascularization: an idea whose time (for testing) has come. *Circulation.* 1997;96:1360–62.

5. Danenberg HD, Welt FG, Walker, M, et al. Systemic inflammation induced by lipopolysaccharide increases neointimal formation after balloon and stent injury in rabbits. *Circulation.* 2002;105(24):2917–22. Hoshida S, Nishino M, Takeda T, et al. A persistent increase in C-reactive protein is a risk factor for restenosis in patients with stable angina who are not receiving statins. *Atherosclerosis.* 2004;173(2):285–90.

6. Peters S. Can angiotensin receptor antagonists prevent restenosis after stent placement? *Am J Cardiovasc Drugs.* 2002;2(3):143–48.

7. Naghavi M, Libby P, Falk E, et al. From vulnerable plaque to vulnerable patient: a call for new definitions and risk assessment strategies: part II. *Circulation.* 2003;108(15):1772–78. Naghavi M, Libby P, Falk E, et al. From vulnerable plaque to vulnerable patient: a call for new definitions and risk assessment strategies: part I. *Circulation.* 2003;108(14):1664–72. Wexberg P, Gyongyosi M, Sperker W, et al. Pre-existing arterial remodeling is associated with in-hospital and late adverse cardiac events after coronary interventions in patients with stable angina pectoris. *J Am Coll Cardiol.* 2000 Nov 15;36(6):1860–69.

8. Ornish D, Scherwitz IW, Billings JH, et al. Intensive lifestyle changes for reversal of coronary heart disease. *JAMA.* 1998;280:2001–7. Stefanick M, Mackey S, Sheehan M, et al. Effects of diet and exercise in men and postmenopausal women with low levels of HDL and high levels of LDL cholesterol. *N Engl J Med.* 1998;339(1):12–20.

9. Ambrose JA, Fuster V. Can we predict future coronary events in patients with stable coronary artery disease? *JAMA.* 1997;277:343–44. Forrester JS, Shah PK. Lipid lowering versus revascularization: an idea whose time (for testing) has come. *Circulation.* 1997;96:1360–62.

10. Finn SD, Blankenship JC, Alexander KP, et al. 2014 ACC/AHA/AATS/PCNA/SCAI/STS focused update of the guideline for the diagnosis and management of patient with stable ischemic heart disease. *JACC.* 2014;130:1749–67.

11. Boden WE, O'Rourke RA, Teo KK, et al. Optimal medical therapy with or without PCI for stable coronary disease. *N Engl J Med.* 2007;356(15):1503–16.

Chapter 3: Nutritional Excellence, Not Drugs

1. Shikany JM, Safford MM, Newby PK, et al. Southern dietary pattern is associated with hazard of acute coronary heart disease in the Reasons for Geographic and Racial Differences in Stroke (REGARDS) study. *Circulation.* 2015;132(9):804–14.

2. Yang Q, Zhong Y, Ritchy M, et al. Vital signs: predicted heart age and racial disparities in heart age amount US adults at the state level. *MMWR*. 2015 Sept;64(34): 950–58.

3. Shaw LJ, Merz CN, Pepine CJ, et al. Women's Ischemia Syndrome Evaluation (WISE) Investigators. The economic burden of angina in women with suspected ischemic heart disease: results from the National Institutes of Health–National Heart, Lung, and Blood Institute–sponsored Women's Ischemia Syndrome Evaluation. *Circulation*. 2006;114:894–904.

4. Yusaf S, Hawken S, Ounpuu S, et al. INTERHEART Study Investigators. Effect of potentially modifiable risk factors associated with myocardial infarction in 52 countries (the INTERHEART study): case-control study. *Lancet*. 2004;364(9438):937–52.

5. Chomistek AK, Chiuve SE, Eliassen AH, et al. Healthy lifestyle in the primordial prevention of cardiovascular disease among young women. *J Am Coll Cardiol*. 2015;65:43–51.

6. Chive SE, Rexrode KM, Speigelman D, et al. Primary prevention of stroke by healthy lifestyle. *Circulation*. 2008;18(9):947–54. Gorelick PB. Primary prevention of stroke: impact of healthy lifestyle. *Circulation*. 2008;118:904–6. Akesson A, Weismayer C, Newby PK, et al. Combined effect of low-risk dietary and lifestyle behaviors in primary prevention of myocardial infarction in women. *Arch Intern Med*. 2007;167(19):2122–27. Hu FB, Manson JE, Stampfer MJ, et al. Diet, lifestyle, and the risk of type 2 diabetes mellitus in women. *N Engl J Med*. 2001;345(11):790–97.

7. Go AS, Mozaffarian D, Roger VL, et al. Heart disease and stroke statistics—2013 update: a report from the American Heart Association. *Circulation*. 2013;127(1):e6–e245. National Center for Health Statistics (U.S.). *Health, United States, 2012: With Special Feature on Emergency Care*. Hyattsville, MD: National Center for Health Statistics, 2013 May. Report No.: 2013-1232; Table 92: Selected prescription drug classes used in the past 30 days, by sex and age.

8. Fuhrman J, Singer M. Improved cardiovascular parameter with a nutrient-dense, plant-rich diet-style: a patient survey with illustrative cases. *J Lifestyle Med*. 2015. doi: 10.1177/1559827615611024.

9. Li CI, Daling JR, Tang MT, et al. Use of antihypertensive medications and breast cancer risk among women aged 55 to 74 years. *JAMA Intern Med*. 2013;173(17):1629–37.

10. McDougall JA, Malone DE, Daling JR, et al. Long-term statin use and risk of ductal and lobular breast cancer among women 55 to 74 years of age. *Cancer Epidemiol Biomarkers Prev*. 2013;22(9):1529–37.

11. POISE Study Group. Effects of extended-release metoprolol succinate in patients undergoing non-cardiac surgery (POISE trial): a randomised controlled trial. *Lancet*. 2008;371(9627):1839–47.

12. Bangalore S, Messerli FH, Kostis JB, et al. Cardiovascular protection using beta-blockers. *J Am Coll Cardiol*. 2007;50(7):563–72.

13. Wiysonge CS, Bradley H, Mayosi BM, et al. Beta-blockers for hypertension. *Cochrane Database Syst Rev*. 2012;11:CD002003.

14. Shen L, Shah BR, Reyes EM, et al. Role of diuretics, ß blockers, and statins in increasing the risk of diabetes in patients with impaired glucose tolerance: reanalysis of data from the NAVIGATOR study. *BMJ*. 2013;347:f6745.

15. Tinetti ME, Han L, Lee DSH, et al. Antihypertensive medications and serious fall injuries in a nationally representative sample of older adults. *JAMA Intern Med*. 2014;174(4):588–95.

16. Mitchell GF, Vasan RS, Keyes MJ, et al. Pulse pressure and risk of new-onset atrial fibrillation. *JAMA*. 2007;297(7):709–15. Swaminathan RV, Alexander KP. Pulse pressure and vascular risk in the elderly: associations and clinical implications. *Am J Geriatr Cardiol*. 2006;15(4):226–32;quiz133–34.

17. Messerli FH, Mancia G, Conti CR, et al. Dogma disputed: can aggressively lowering blood pressure in hypertensive patients with coronary artery disease be dangerous? *Ann Intern Med*. 2006 Jun 20;144(12):884–93.

18. Tringali S, Oberer CW, Huang J. Low diastolic blood pressure as a risk for all-cause mortality in VA patients. *Int J Hypertens*. 2013;2013:178780.

19. Boschert S. A low systolic window in HT may be of limited benefit. *Family Practice News*. 2013;46(6):1,14.

20. University of Alabama at Birmingham. Blood pressure medications can lead to increased risk of stroke. *ScienceDaily*. 29 May 2015. Available at www.sciencedaily.com/releases/2015/05/150529193554.htm.

21. James PA, Oparil S, Carter BL, et al. 2014 Evidence-based guideline for the management of high blood pressure in adults. Report from the panel members appointed to the Eighth Joint National Committee (JNC 8). *JAMA*. 2014;311(5):507–20.

22. Loyola University Health System. More aggressive blood pressure treatment found to reduce heart disease, save lives. *ScienceDaily*. 18 September 2015. Available at www.sciencedaily.com/releases/2015/09/150918111448.htm.

23. The Accord Study Group. Effects of intensive blood-pressure control in type 2 diabetes mellitus. *N Eng J Med*. 2010;362:1575–85.

24. Lamarche B, Desroches S, Jenkins DJ, et al. Combined effects of a dietary portfolio of plant sterols, vegetable protein, viscous fibre and almonds on LDL particle size. *Br J Nutr*. 2004;92(4):657–63. Damasceno NR, Sala-Vila A, Cofán M, et al. Mediterranean diet supplemented with nuts reduces waist circumference and shifts lipoprotein subfractions to a less atherogenic pattern in subjects at high cardiovascular risk. *Atherosclerosis*. 2013;230(2):347–53. Kaliora AC, Dedoussis GV, Schmidt H. Dietary antioxidants in preventing atherogenesis. *Atherosclerosis*. 2006;187(1):1–17.

25. Superko HR, Gadesam RR. Is it LDL particle size or number that correlates with risk of cardiovascular disease? *Curr Atheroscler Rep*. 2008:10(5):377–85.

26. Papanikolaou Y, Fulgoni VL III. Bean consumption is associated with greater nutrient intake, reduced systolic blood pressure, lower body weight, and a smaller waist circumference in adults: results from the National Health and Nutrition Examination Survey 1999–2002. *J Am Coll Nutr*. 2008;27(5):569–76. Streppel MT, Arends LR, van 't Veer P, et al. Dietary fiber and blood pressure: a meta-analysis of randomized

placebo-controlled trials. *Arch Intern Med.* 2005;165(2):150–56. Frisoli TM, Schmieder RE, Grodzicki T, et al. Beyond salt: lifestyle modifications and blood pressure. *Eur Heart J.* 2011;32(24):3081–87. Alonso A, de la Fuente C, Martín-Arnau AM, et al. Fruit and vegetable consumption is inversely associated with blood pressure in a Mediterranean population with a high vegetable-fat intake: the Seguimiento Universidad de Navarra (SUN) Study. *Br J Nutr.* 2004;92(2):311–19. Pettersen BJ, Anousheh R, Fan J, et al. Vegetarian diets and blood pressure among white subjects: results from the Adventist Health Study–2 (AHS-2). *Public Health Nutr.* 2012;15(10):1909–16. Utsugi MT, Ohkubo T, Kikuya M, et al. Fruit and vegetable consumption and the risk of hypertension determined by self measurement of blood pressure at home: the Ohasama study. *Hypertens Res.* 2008;31(7):1435–43. Cassidy A, O'Reilly ÉJ, Kay C, et al. Habitual intake of flavonoid subclasses and incident hypertension in adults. *Am J Clin Nutr.* 2011;93(2):338–47. O'Neil CE, Keast DR, Nicklas TA, et al. Nut consumption is associated with decreased health risk factors for cardiovascular disease and metabolic syndrome in U.S. adults: NHANES 1999–2004. *J Am Coll Nutr.* 2011;30(6):502–10. Lidder S, Webb AJ. Vascular effects of dietary nitrate (as found in green leafy vegetables and beetroot) via the nitrate–nitrite–nitric oxide pathway. *Br J Clin Pharmacol.* 2013;75(3):677–96.

27. Macready AL, George TW, Chong MF, et al. FLAVURS Study Group. Flavonoid-rich fruit and vegetables improve microvascular reactivity and inflammatory status in men at risk of cardiovascular disease—FLAVURS: a randomized controlled trial. *Am J Clin Nutr.* 2014;99(3):479–89. Martin KR. Both common and specialty mushrooms inhibit adhesion molecule expression and in vitro binding of monocytes to human aortic endothelial cells in a pro-inflammatory environment. *Nutr J.* 2010;9:29. Zakkar M, van der Heiden K, Luong le A, et al. Activation of Nrf2 in endothelial cells protects arteries from exhibiting a proinflammatory state. *Arterioscler Thromb Vasc Biol.* 2009;29(11):1851–57. Lee WJ, Ou HC, Hsu WC, et al. Ellagic acid inhibits oxidized LDL–mediated LOX-1 expression, ROS generation, and inflammation in human endothelial cells. *J Vasc Surg.* 2010;52(5):1290–300. Chen XL, Dodd G, Kunsch C. Sulforaphane inhibits TNF-alpha-induced activation of p38 MAP kinase and VCAM–1 and MCP–1 expression in endothelial cells. *Inflamm Res.* 2009;58(8):513–21.

28. Dunaief DM, Fuhrman J, Dunaief JL, et al. Glycemic and cardiovascular parameters improved in type 2 diabetes with the high nutrient density (HND) diet. *Open J Prev Med.* 2012;3:364–71.

29. Floegel A, Chung SJ, von Ruesten A, et al. Antioxidant intake from diet and supplements and elevated serum C-reactive protein and plasma homocysteine concentrations in US adults: a cross-sectional study. *Public Health Nutr.* 2011;14(11):2055–64. Brighenti F, Valtueña S, Pellegrini N, et al. Total antioxidant capacity of the diet is inversely and independently related to plasma concentration of high-sensitivity C-reactive protein in adult Italian subjects. *Br J Nutr.* 2005;93(5):619–25. Esmaillzadeh A, Kimiagar M, Mehrabi Y, et al. Fruit and vegetable intakes, C-reactive protein, and the metabolic syndrome. *Am J Clin Nutr.* 2006;84(6):1489–97. Zhu Y, Zhang Y, Ling W, et al. Fruit consumption is associated with lower carotid intima-media thickness and C-reactive protein levels in patients with type 2 diabetes mellitus. *J Am Diet Assoc.* 2011;111(10):1536–42. Salas-Salvadó J, Casas-Agustench P, Murphy MM, et al. The effect of nuts on

inflammation. *Asia Pac J Clin Nutr.* 2008;17(suppl 1):333–36. González R, Ballester I, López-Posadas R, et al. Effects of flavonoids and other polyphenols on inflammation. *Crit Rev Food Sci Nutr.* 2011;51(4):331–62. Margolis KL, Manson, JE, Greenland P, et al. Leukocyte count as a predictor of cardiovascular events and mortality in postmenopausal women: the Women's Health Initiative Observational Study. *Arch Intern Med.* 2005;165(5):500–8. Bloomer RJ, Kabir MM, Canale RE, et al. Effect of a 21 day Daniel Fast on metabolic and cardiovascular disease risk factors in men and women. *Lipids Health Dis.* 2010;9:94.

30. Mayne ST, Cartmel B, Scarmo S, et al. Noninvasive assessment of dermal carotenoids as a biomarker of fruit and vegetable intake. *Am J Clin Nutr.* 2010;92(4):794–800.

31. Lidder S, Webb AJ. Vascular effects of dietary nitrate (as found in green leafy vegetables and beetroot) via the nitrate-nitrite-nitric oxide pathway. *Br J Clin Pharmacol.* 2013;75:677–96.

32. Lamarche B, Desroches S, Jenkins DJ, et al. Combined effects of a dietary portfolio of plant sterols, vegetable protein, viscous fibre and almonds on LDL particle size. *Br J Nutr.* 2004;92(4):657–63. Damasceno NR, Sala-Vila A, Cofán M, et al. Mediterranean diet supplemented with nuts reduces waist circumference and shifts lipoprotein subfractions to a less atherogenic pattern in subjects at high cardiovascular risk. *Atherosclerosis.* 2013;230(2):347–53. Kaliora AC, Dedoussis GV, Schmidt H. Dietary antioxidants in preventing atherogenesis. *Atherosclerosis.* 2006;187(1):1–17.

33. Jenkins DJ, Kendall CW, Popovich DG, et al. Effect of a very-high-fiber vegetable, fruit, and nut diet on serum lipids and colonic function. *Metabolism.* 2001;50(4):494–503.

34. Candore G, Colonna-Romano G, Balistreri CR, et al. Biology of longevity: role of the innate immune system. *Rejuvenation Res.* 2006;9(1):143–48.

35. DeFilippis AP, Young R, Carrubba CJ, et al. An analysis of calibration and discrimination among multiple cardiovascular risk scores in a modern multiethnic cohort. *Ann Intern Med.* 2015;162(4):266–75.

36. Ray KK, Seshasai SR, Erqou S, et al. Statins and all-cause mortality in high-risk primary prevention: a meta-analysis of 11 randomized controlled trials involving 65,229 participants. *Arch Intern Med.* 2010;170(12):1024–31.

37. Okuyama H, Langsjoen PH, Hamazaki T, et al. Statins stimulate atherosclerosis and heart failure: pharmacological mechanisms. *Expert Rev Clin Pharmacol.* 2015;8:189–99.

38. Naci H, Brugts JJ, Fleurence R, et al. Comparative benefits of statins in the primary and secondary prevention of major coronary events and all-cause mortality: a network meta-analysis of placebo-controlled and active-comparator trials. *Eur J Prev Cardiol.* 2013;20(4):641–57.

39. Naci H, Ioannidis JPA. Comparative effectiveness of exercise and drug interventions on mortality outcomes: metaepidemiological study. *BMJ.* 2013;347:f5577.

40. Qu Q, Paulose-Rom R, Burt VL, et al. Prescription cholesterol-lowering medication use in adults aged 40 and over: United States, 2003–2012. NCHS Data Brief #177 Dec 2014.

41. Sugiyama T, Tsugawa Y, Tseng C, et al. Different time trends of caloric and fat intake between statin users and nonusers among us adults: gluttony in the time of statins? *JAMA Intern Med.* 2014;174(7):1038–45.

42. Hippisley-Cox J, Coupland C. Unintended effects of statins in men and women in England and Wales: population based cohort study using the QResearch database. *BMJ.* 2010;340:c2197.

43. Mikus CR, Boyle LJ, Borengasser SJ, et al. Simvastatin impairs exercise training adaptations. *J Am Coll Cardiol.* 2013;62:709–14.

44. Golomb BA, Evans MA. Statin adverse effects: a review of the literature and evidence for a mitochondrial mechanism. *Am J Cardiovasc Drugs.* 2008;8:373–418.

45. Kelley BJ, Glasser S. Cognitive effects of statin medications. *CNS Drugs.* 2014;28:411–19.

46. Zhang H, Plutzky J, Turchin A. Discontinuation of statins in routine care settings. *Ann Intern Med.* 2013;159:75–76.

47. Sattar N, Preiss D, Murray H, et al. Statins and risk of incident diabetes: a collaborative meta-analysis of randomised statin trials. *Lancet.* 2010;375:735–42. Preiss D, Seshasai SR, Welsh P, et al. Risk of incident diabetes with intensive-dose compared with moderate-dose statin therapy: a meta-analysis. *JAMA.* 2011;305(24):2556–64.

48. McDougall JA, Malone KE, Daling JR, et al. Long-term statin use and risk of ductal and lobular breast cancer among women 55 to 74 years of age. *Cancer Epidemiol Biomarkers Prev.* 2013;22(9):1529–37.

49. Culver AL, Ockene IS, Balasubramanian R, et al. Statin use and risk of diabetes mellitus in postmenopausal women in the Women's Health Initiative. *Arch Intern Med.* 2012;172:144–52.

50. Dormuth CR, Filion KB, Paterson JM, et al. Higher potency statins and the risk of new diabetes: multicentre, observational study of administrative databases. *BMJ.* 2014;348:g3244.

51. Corrao G, Ibrahim B, Nicotra F, et al. Statins and the risk of diabetes: evidence from a large population-based cohort study. *Diabetes Care.* 2014;37(8):2225–32.

52. Abramson JD, Redberg RF. Don't give more patients statins. *New York Times.* Opinion Pages. 13 Nov 2013. Available at http://www.nytimes.com/2013/11/14/opinion /dont-give-more-patients-statins.html?_r=1&).

53. Abramson JD, Rosenberg HG, Jewell N, et al. Should people at low risk of cardiovascular disease take a statin? *BMJ.* 2013;347:f6123.

54. Zhang H, Plutzky J, Skentzos S, et al. Discontinuation of statins in routine care settings: a cohort study. *Ann Intern Med.* 2013;158:526–34.

55. Okuyama H, Langsjoen PH, Hamazaki T, et al. Statins stimulate atherosclerosis and heart failure: pharmacological mechanisms. *Expert Rev Clin Pharmacol.* 2015;8:189–99.

56. Welin L, Wilhelmsen L, Björnberg A, et al. Aspirin increases mortality in diabetic patients without cardiovascular disease: a Swedish record linkage study. *Pharmacoepidemiol Drug Saf.* 2009;18(12):1143–49.

57. Fowkes FG, Price JF, Stewart MC, et al. Aspirin for prevention of cardiovascular events in a general population screened for a low ankle brachial index: a randomized controlled trial. *JAMA*. 2010 Mar 3;303(9):841–48.

58. Ikeda Y, Shimada K, Teramoto T, et al. Low-dose aspirin for primary prevention of cardiovascular events in Japanese patients 60 years or older with atherosclerotic risk factors: a randomized clinical trial. *JAMA*. 2014;312(23):2510–12.

59. Gaziano JM, Greenland P. When should aspirin be used for prevention of cardiovascular events? Editorial. *JAMA*. 2014;312(23):2503–4.

Chapter 4: The Nutritional Path to Reversing Disease

1. Hung HC, Joshipura KJ, Jiang R, et al. Fruit and vegetable intake and risk of major chronic disease. *J Natl Cancer Inst*. 2004;96:1577–84. Joshipura KJ, Hu FB, Manson JE, et al. The effect of fruit and vegetable intake on risk for coronary heart disease. *Ann Intern Med*. 2001;134:1106–14.

2. Zhang X, Shu XO, Xiang YB, et al. Cruciferous vegetable consumption is associated with a reduced risk of total and cardiovascular disease mortality. *Am J Clin Nutr*. 2011;94:240–46.

3. Donovan EL, McCord JM, Reuland DJ, et al. Phytochemical activation of Nrf2 protects human coronary artery endothelial cells against an oxidative challenge. *Oxid Med Cell Longev*. 2012;2012:132931. Han SG, Han SS, Toborek M, et al. EGCG protects endothelial cells against PCB 126-induced inflammation through inhibition of AhR and induction of Nrf2-regulated genes. *Toxicol Appl Pharmacol*. 2012;261:181–88.

4. Zakkar M, van der Heiden K, Luong le A, et al. Activation of Nrf2 in endothelial cells protects arteries from exhibiting a proinflammatory state. *Arterioscler Thromb Vasc Biol*. 2009;29:1851–57.

5. Huang CS, Lin AH, Liu CT, et al. Isothiocyanates protect against oxidized LDL–induced endothelial dysfunction by upregulating Nrf2-dependent antioxidation and suppressing NFkappaB activation. *Mol Nutr Food Res*. 2013;57:1918–30.

6. Zhao J, Moore AN, Redell JB, et al. Enhancing expression of Nrf2-driven genes protects the blood brain barrier after brain injury. *J Neurosci*. 2007;27:10240–48.

7. Han SG, Han SS, Toborek M, et al. EGCG protects endothelial cells against PCB 126–induced inflammation through inhibition of AhR and induction of Nrf2-regulated genes. *Toxicol Appl Pharmacol*. 2012;261:181–88. Cimino F, Speciale A, Anwar S, et al. Anthocyanins protect human endothelial cells from mild hyperoxia damage through modulation of Nrf2 pathway. *Genes Nutr*. 2013;8:391–99. Ungvari Z, Bagi Z, Feher A, et al. Resveratrol confers endothelial protection via activation of the antioxidant transcription factor Nrf2. *Am J Physiol Heart Circ Physiol*. 2010;299:H18–24.

8. Muthusamy VR, Kannan S, Sadhaasivam K, et al. Acute exercise stress activates Nrf2/ARE signaling and promotes antioxidant mechanisms in the myocardium. *Free Radic Biol Med*. 2012;52:366–76.

9. Fratta Pasini A, Albiero A, Stranieri C, et al. Serum oxidative stress-induced repression of Nrf2 and GSH depletion: a mechanism potentially involved in endothelial dysfunction of young smokers. *PLoS One.* 2012;7(1):e30291.

10. Galeone C, Pelucchi C, Levi F, et al. Onion and garlic use and human cancer. *Am J Clin Nutr.* 2006;84:1027–32.

11. Powolny A, Singh S. Multitargeted prevention and therapy of cancer by diallyl trisulfide and related Allium vegetable-derived organosulfur compounds. *Cancer Lett.* 2008;269:305–14.

12. Modem S, Dicarlo SE, Reddy TR. Fresh garlic extract induces growth arrest and morphological differentiation of MCF7 breast cancer cells. *Genes Cancer.* 2012;3:177–86. Na HK, Kim EH, Choi MA, et al. Diallyl trisulfide induces apoptosis in human breast cancer cells through ROS-mediated activation of JNK and AP-1. *Biochem Pharmacol.* 2012;84(10):1241–50. Malki A, El-Saadani M, Sultan AS. Garlic constituent diallyl trisulfide induced apoptosis in MCF7 human breast cancer cells. *Cancer Biol Ther.* 2009;8:2175–85.

13. Rahman K, Lowe GM. Garlic and cardiovascular disease: a critical review. *J Nutr.* 2006;136(30):736S–40S.

14. Slimestad R, Fossen T, Vagen IM. Onions: a source of unique dietary flavonoids. *J Agric Food Chem.* 2007;55:10067–80.

15. Kim DO, Heo HJ, Kim YJ, et al. Sweet and sour cherry phenolics and their protective effects on neuronal cells. *J Agric Food Chem.* 2005;53:9921–27. Gebhardt SE, Harnly JM, Bhagwat SA, et al. USDA's flavonoid database: flavonoids in fruit. 2003: http://www.ars.usda.gov/SP2UserFiles/Place/80400525/Articles/ADA2003_FruitFlav.pdf.

16. Erdman JW Jr, Balentine D, Arab L, et al. Flavonoids and heart health: proceedings of the ILSI North America Flavonoids Workshop, May 31–June 1, 2005, Washington, DC. *J Nutr.* 2007;137:718S–37S.

17. Higdon J, Drake VJ. Flavonoids. In: Higdon J, Drake VJ. *Evidence-Based Approach to Dietary Phytochemicals and Other Dietary Factors.* New York: Thieme; 2012:83–108.

18. Huxley RR, Neil HA. The relation between dietary flavonol intake and coronary heart disease mortality: a meta-analysis of prospective cohort studies. *Eur J Clin Nutr.* 2003;57:904–8. Knekt P, Kumpulainen J, Jarvinen R, et al. Flavonoid intake and risk of chronic diseases. *Am J Clin Nutr.* 2002;76:560–68. Mursu J, Voutilainen S, Nurmi T, et al. Flavonoid intake and the risk of ischaemic stroke and CVD mortality in middle-aged Finnish men: the Kuopio Ischaemic Heart Disease Risk Factor Study. *Br J Nutr.* 2008;100:890–95. Mink PJ, Scrafford CG, Barraj LM, et al. Flavonoid intake and cardiovascular disease mortality: a prospective study in postmenopausal women. *Am J Clin Nutr.* 2007;85:895–909.

19. Erdman JW Jr, Balentine D, Arab L, et al. Flavonoids and heart health: proceedings of the ILSI North America Flavonoids Workshop, May 31–June 1, 2005, Washington, DC. *J Nutr.* 2007;137:718S–37S. Martin KR, Bopp J, Burrell L, et al. The effect of 100% tart cherry juice on serum uric acid levels, biomarkers of inflammation and cardiovascular disease risk factors. *FASEB J.* 2011;25(meeting abstract suppl):339.2. Kelley DS, Rasooly R, Jacob RA, et al. Consumption of Bing sweet cherries lowers

circulating concentrations of inflammation markers in healthy men and women. *J Nutr.* 2006;136:981–86. Aviram M, Dornfeld L. Pomegranate juice consumption inhibits serum angiotensin converting enzyme activity and reduces systolic blood pressure. *Atherosclerosis.* 2001;158:195–98. Aviram M, Dornfeld L, Rosenblat M, et al. Pomegranate juice consumption reduces oxidative stress, atherogenic modifications to LDL, and platelet aggregation: studies in humans and in atherosclerotic apolipoprotein E–deficient mice. *Am J Clin Nutr.* 2000;71:1062–76. Aviram M, Rosenblat M, Gaitini D, et al. Pomegranate juice consumption for 3 years by patients with carotid artery stenosis reduces common carotid intima-media thickness, blood pressure and LDL oxidation. *Clin Nutr.* 2004;23:423–33. Aviram M, Volkova N, Coleman R, et al. Pomegranate phenolics from the peels, arils, and flowers are antiatherogenic: studies in vivo in atherosclerotic apolipoprotein E–deficient (E 0) mice and in vitro in cultured macrophages and lipoproteins. *J Agric Food Chem.* 2008;56:1148–57.

20. Johnson SA, Figueroa A, Navaei N, et al. Daily blueberry consumption improves blood pressure and arterial stiffness in postmenopausal women with pre- and stage 1-hypertension: a randomized, double-blind, placebo-controlled clinical trial. *J Acad Nutr Diet.* 2015;115:369.

21. Shukitt-Hale B. Blueberries and neuronal aging. *Gerontology.* 2012;58:518–23.

22. Krikorian R, Shidler MD, Nash TA, et al. Blueberry supplementation improves memory in older adults. *J Agric Food Chem.* 2010;58:3996–4000.

23. Kim DO, Heo HJ, Kim YJ, et al. Sweet and sour cherry phenolics and their protective effects on neuronal cells. *J Agric Food Chem.* 2005;53:9921–27. Traustadottir T, Davies SS, Stock AA, et al. Tart cherry juice decreases oxidative stress in healthy older men and women. *J Nutr.* 2009;139:1896–1900.

24. Bookheimer SY, Renner BA, Ekström A, et al. Pomegranate juice augments memory and FMRI activity in middle-aged and older adults with mild memory complaints. *Evid Based Complement Alternat Med.* 2013;2013:946298.

25. Burkhardt S, Tan DX, Manchester LC, et al. Detection and quantification of the antioxidant melatonin in Montmorency and Balaton tart cherries (Prunus cerasus). *J Agric Food Chem.* 2001;49:4898–902. Kolar J, Malbeck J. Levels of the antioxidant melatonin in fruits of edible berry species. *Planta Med.* 2009;75:PJ42.

26. Pigeon WR, Carr M, Gorman C, et al. Effects of a tart cherry juice beverage on the sleep of older adults with insomnia: a pilot study. *J Med Food.* 2010;13:579–83.

27. Martin KR, Bopp J, Burrell L, et al. The effect of 100% tart cherry juice on serum uric acid levels, biomarkers of inflammation and cardiovascular disease risk factors. *FASEB J.* 2011;25(meeting abstract suppl):339.2.

28. Krinsky NI, Johnson EJ. Carotenoid actions and their relation to health and disease. *Mol Aspects Med.* 2005;26:459–516.

29. Shardell MD, Alley DE, Hicks GE, et al. Low-serum carotenoid concentrations and carotenoid interactions predict mortality in US adults: the Third National Health and Nutrition Examination Survey. *Nutr Res.* 2011;31:178–89.

30. Canene-Adams K, Campbell JK, Zaripheh S, et al. The tomato as a functional food. *J Nutr.* 2005;135:1226–30.

31. Van Breemen RB, Pajkovic N. Multitargeted therapy of cancer by lycopene. *Cancer Lett.* 2008;269:339–51.

32. Rizwan M, Rodriguez-Blanco I, Harbottle A, et al. Tomato paste rich in lycopene protects against cutaneous photodamage in humans in vivo: a randomized controlled trial. *Br J Dermatol.* 2011;164(1):154–62.

33. Rissanen TH, Voutilainen S, Nyyssonen K, et al. Low serum lycopene concentration is associated with an excess incidence of acute coronary events and stroke: the Kuopio Ischaemic Heart Disease Risk Factor Study. *Br J Nutr.* 2001;85:749–54. Rissanen T, Voutilainen S, Nyyssonen K, et al. Lycopene, atherosclerosis, and coronary heart disease. *Exp Biol Med (Maywood).* 2002;227:900–7. Rissanen TH, Voutilainen S, Nyyssonen K, et al. Serum lycopene concentrations and carotid atherosclerosis: the Kuopio Ischaemic Heart Disease Risk Factor Study. *Am J Clin Nutr.* 2003;77:133–38.

34. Sesso HD, Buring JE, Norkus EP, et al. Plasma lycopene, other carotenoids, and retinol and the risk of cardiovascular disease in women. *Am J Clin Nutr.* 2004;79:47–53.

35. Hak AE, Ma J, Powell CB, et al. Prospective study of plasma carotenoids and tocopherols in relation to risk of ischemic stroke. *Stroke.* 2004;35:1584–88.

36. Karppi J, Laukkanen JA, Sivenius J, et al. Serum lycopene decreases the risk of stroke in men: a population-based follow-up study. *Neurology.* 2012;79:1540–47.

37. Karppi J, Laukkanen JA, Mäkikallio TH, et al. Low serum lycopene and ß-carotene increase risk of acute myocardial infarction in men. *Eur J Public Health.* 2012 Dec;22(6):835–40.

38. Gajendragadkar PR, Hubsch A, Maki-Petaja KM, et al. Effects of oral lycopene supplementation on vascular function in patients with cardiovascular disease and healthy volunteers: a randomised controlled trial. *PLoS One.* 2014;9:e99070.

39. Silaste ML, Alfthan G, Aro A, et al. Tomato juice decreases LDL cholesterol levels and increases LDL resistance to oxidation. *Br J Nutr.* 2007;98:1251–58. Burton-Freeman B, Talbot J, Park E, et al. Protective activity of processed tomato products on postprandial oxidation and inflammation: a clinical trial in healthy weight men and women. *Mol Nutr Food Res.* 2012;56(4):622–31. Hadley CW, Clinton SK, Schwartz SJ. The consumption of processed tomato products enhances plasma lycopene concentrations in association with a reduced lipoprotein sensitivity to oxidative damage. *J Nutr.* 2003;133:727–32.

40. Xaplanteris P, Vlachopoulos C, Pietri P, et al. Tomato paste supplementation improves endothelial dynamics and reduces plasma total oxidative status in healthy subjects. *Nutr Res.* 2012;32:390–94.

41. Gajendragadkar PR, Hubsch A, Maki-Petaja KM, et al. Effects of oral lycopene supplementation on vascular function in patients with cardiovascular disease and healthy volunteers: a randomised controlled trial. *PLoS One.* 2014;9:e99070.

42. Lycopene. Monograph. *Altern Med Rev.* 2003;8:336–42. Available at http://www.alt medrev.com/publications/8/3/336.pdf.

43. Ried K, Fakler P. Protective effect of lycopene on serum cholesterol and blood pressure: meta-analyses of intervention trials. *Maturitas.* 2011;68:299–310.

44. Palozza P, Parrone N, Catalano A, et al. Tomato lycopene and inflammatory cascade: basic interactions and clinical implications. *Curr Med Chem.* 2010;17:2547–63. Palozza P, Parrone N, Simone RE, et al. Lycopene in atherosclerosis prevention: an integrated scheme of the potential mechanisms of action from cell culture studies. *Arch Biochem Biophys.* 2010;504:26–33.

45. Canene-Adams K, Campbell JK, Zaripheh S, et al. The tomato as a functional food. *J Nutr.* 2005;135:1226–30.

46. Kris-Etherton PM, Lichtenstein AH, Howard BV, et al. Antioxidant vitamin supplements and cardiovascular disease. *Circulation.* 2004;110:637–41.

47. Heber D, Lu QY. Overview of mechanisms of action of lycopene. *Exp Biol Med (Maywood).* 2002;227:920–23.

48. USDA. United States Department of Agriculture Economic Research Service. Food availability (per capita) data system. Available at http://www.ers.usda.gov/data -products/food-availability-(per-capita)-data-system.aspx.

49. Brown MJ, Ferruzzi MG, Nguyen ML, et al. Carotenoid bioavailability is higher from salads ingested with full-fat than with fat-reduced salad dressings as measured with electrochemical detection. *Am J Clin Nutr.* 2004;80:396–403. Goltz SR, Campbell WW, Chitchumroonchokchai C, et al. Meal triacylglycerol profile modulates postprandial absorption of carotenoids in humans. *Mol Nutr Food Res.* 2012;56:866–77.

50. Van het Hof KH, de Boer BC, Tijburg LB, et al. Carotenoid bioavailability in humans from tomatoes processed in different ways determined from the carotenoid response in the triglyceride-rich lipoprotein fraction of plasma after a single consumption and in plasma after four days of consumption. *J Nutr.* 2000;130:1189–96.

51. Fuhrman J, Sarter B, Acocella S. et al. Changing perceptions of hunger on a high nutrient density diet. *Nutr J.* 2010;9:51.

52. Chobotova K. Aging and cancer: converging routes to disease prevention. *Integr Cancer Ther.* 2009;8:115–22. Devaraj S, Wang-Polagruto J, Polagruto J, et al. High-fat, energy-dense, fast-food-style breakfast results in an increase in oxidative stress in metabolic syndrome. *Metabolism.* 2008;57(6):867–70. Egger G, Dixon J. Inflammatory effects of nutritional stimuli: further support for the need for a big picture approach to tackling obesity and chronic disease. *Obesity Rev.* 2010;11(2):137–49. Esmaillzadeh A, Azadbakht L. Major dietary patterns in relation to general obesity and central adiposity among Iranian women. *J Nutr.* 2008;138(2):358–63.

53. Thompson HJ, Heimendinger J, Gillette C, et al. In vivo investigation of changes in biomarkers of oxidative stress induced by plant food rich diets. *J Agric Food Chem.* 2005;53:6126–32.

54. Peairs AT, Rankin JW. Inflammatory response to a high-fat, low-carbohydrate weight loss diet: effect of antioxidants. *Obesity.* 2008;16:1573–78. Patel C, Ghanim

H, Ravishankar S, et al. Prolonged reactive oxygen species generation and nuclear factor-kappaB activation after a high-fat, high-carbohydrate meal in the obese. *J Clin Endocrinol Metab.* 2007;92:4476–79.

55. Devaraj S, Mathur S, Basu A, et al. A dose-response study on the effects of purified lycopene supplementation on biomarkers of oxidative stress. *J Am Coll Nutr.* 2008;27:267–73. Esmaillzadeh A, Azadbakht L. Dietary flavonoid intake and cardiovascular mortality. *Br J Nutr.* 2008;100:695–97. Esmaillzadeh A, Kimiagar M, Mehrabi Y, et al. Fruit and vegetable intakes, C-reactive protein, and the metabolic syndrome. *Am J Clin Nutr.* 2006;84:1489–97. O'Keefe JH, Gheewala NM, O'Keefe JO, et al. Dietary strategies for improving post-prandial glucose, lipids, inflammation, and cardiovascular health. *J Am Coll Cardiol.* 2008;51:249–55. Bose KS, Agrawal BK, Bose KSC. Effect of lycopene from tomatoes (cooked) on plasma antioxidant enzymes, lipid peroxidation rate and lipid profile in grade-I hypertension. *Ann Nutr Metab.* 2007;51:477–81. Thompson HJ, Heimendinger J, Haegele A, et al. Effect of increased vegetable and fruit consumption on markers of oxidative cellular damage. *Carcinogenesis.* 1999;20:2261–66.

56. Khansari N, Shakiba Y, Mahmoudi M. Chronic inflammation and oxidative stress as a major cause of age-related diseases and cancer. *Recent Pat Inflamm Allergy Drug Discov.* 2009;3:73–80. Federico A, Morgillo F, Tuccillo C, et al. Chronic inflammation and oxidative stress in human carcinogenesis. *Int J Cancer.* 2007;121:2381–86. Willcox JK, Ash SL, Catignani GL, et al. Antioxidants and prevention of chronic disease. *Crit Rev Food Sci Nutr.* 2004;44:275–95. Guo W, Kong E, Meydani M, et al. Dietary polyphenols, inflammation, and cancer. *Nutr Cancer.* 2009;61:807–10.

57. Vives-Bauza C, Anand M, Shirazi AK, et al. The age lipid A2E and mitochondrial dysfunction synergistically impair phagocytosis by retinal pigment epithelial cells. *J Biol Chem.* 2008;283:24770–80. Bockowski L, Sobaniec W, Kulak W, et al. Serum and intraerythrocyte antioxidant enzymes and lipid peroxides in children with migraine. *Pharmacol Rep.* 2008;60:542–48.

58. Peairs AT, Rankin JW. Inflammatory response to a high-fat, low-carbohydrate weight loss diet: effect of antioxidants. *Obesity* 2008;16:1573–78. Patel C, Ghanim H, Ravishankar S, et al. Prolonged reactive oxygen species generation and nuclear factor-kappaB activation after a high-fat, high-carbohydrate meal in the obese. *J Clin Endocrinol Metab.* 2007:92:4476–79. Khansari N, Shakiba Y, Mahmoudi M. Chronic inflammation and oxidative stress as a major cause of age-related diseases and cancer. *Recent Pat Inflamm Allergy Drug Discov* 2009;3:73–80.

59. Olusi SO. Obesity is an independent risk factor for plasma lipid peroxidation and depletion of erythrocyte cytoprotective enzymes in humans. *Int J Obes Relat Metab Disord.* 2002;26:1159–64.

60. Rizos EC, Ntzani EE, Bika E, et al. Association between omega-3 fatty acid supplementation and risk of major cardiovascular disease events: a systematic review and meta-analysis. *JAMA.* 2012;308(10):1024–33.

61. Burr ML, Ashfield-Watt PA, Dunstan FD, et al. Lack of benefit of dietary advice to men with angina: results of a controlled trial. *Eur J Clin Nutr.* 2003;57(2):193–200.

62. Mozaffarian D, Lemaitre RN, King IB, et al. Plasma phospholipid long-chain omega-3 fatty acids and total and cause-specific mortality in older adults: the Cardiovascular Health Study. *Ann Intern Med.* 2013;158(7):515–25.

63. De Oliveira Otto MC, Wu JH, Baylin A, et al. Circulating and dietary omega-3 and omega-6 polyunsaturated fatty acids and incidence of CVD in the Multi-Ethnic Study of Atherosclerosis. *J Am Heart Assoc.* 2013;2(6):e000506. doi: 10.1161/JAHA .113.000506.

64. Wu JH, Lemaitre RN, King IB, et al. Association of plasma phospholipid long-chain omega-3 fatty acids with incident atrial fibrillation in older adults: the cardiovascular health study. *Circulation.* 2012;125:1084–93. Virtanen JK, Mursu J, Voutilainen S, et al. Serum long-chain n-3 polyunsaturated fatty acids and risk of hospital diagnosis of atrial fibrillation in men. *Circulation.* 2009;120:2315–21.

65. He Z, Yang L, Tian J, et al. Efficacy and safety of omega-3 fatty acids for the prevention of atrial fibrillation: a meta-analysis. *Can J Cardiol.* 2013;29:196–203. Metcalf RG, Skuladottir GV, Indridason OS, et al. U-shaped relationship between tissue docosahexaenoic acid and atrial fibrillation following cardiac surgery. *Eur J Clin Nutr.* 2014;68:114–18. Wu JH, Marchioli R, Silletta MG, et al. Plasma phospholipid omega-3 fatty acids and incidence of postoperative atrial fibrillation in the OPERA trial. *J Am Heart Assoc.* 2013;2:e000397.

66. Brasky TM, Darke AK, Song X, et al. Plasma phospholipid fatty acids and prostate cancer risk in the SELECT trial. *J Natl Cancer Inst.* 105:15:1132–41.

67. Crowe FL, Paul N, Appleby PN, et al. Circulating fatty acids and prostate cancer risk: individual participant meta-analysis of prospective studies. *J Natl Cancer Inst.* 2014;106(9):dju240.

68. Baydoun MA, Kaufman JS, Satia JA, et al. Plasma n-3 fatty acids and the risk of cognitive decline in older adults: the Atherosclerosis Risk in Communities Study. *Am J Clin Nutr.* 2007;85(4):1103–11. Connor WE, Connor SL. The importance of fish and docosahexaenoic acid in Alzheimer disease. *Am J Clin Nutr.* 2007;85(4):929–30. Cole GM, Ma QL, Frautschy SA, et al. Omega-3 fatty acids and dementia. *Prostaglandins Leukot Essent Fatty Acids.* 2009;81(2–3): 213–21. Van Gelder BM, Tijhuis M, Kalmijn S, et al. Fish consumption, n-3 fatty acids, and subsequent 5-y cognitive decline in elderly men: the Zutphen Elderly Study. *Am J Clin Nutr.* 2007;85(4):1142–47.

69. Pottala JV, Yaff K, Robinson JG, et al. Higher RBC EPA + DHA corresponds with larger total brain and hippocampal volumes. *Neurology.* 2014;82(5):435–42.

70. Sarter B, Kelsey KS, Schwartz TA, et al. Blood docosahexaenoic acid and eicosapentaenoic acid in vegans: associations with age and gender and effects of an algal-derived omega-3 fatty acid supplement. *Clin Nutr.* 2015;34(2):212–18.

71. McNamara RK, Strawn JR. Role of long-chain omega-3 fatty acids in psychiatric practice. *PharmaNutrition.* 2013;1(2):41–49. Grosso G, Galvano F, Marventano S, et al. Omega-3 fatty acids and depression: scientific evidence and biological mechanisms. *Oxid Med Cell Longev.* 2014;2014:313570. Grosso G, Pajak A, Marventano S, et al. Role of omega-3 fatty acids in the treatment of depressive disorders: a comprehensive meta-analysis of randomized clinical trials. *PLoS One.* 2014;9(5):e96905. doi: 10.1371/journal.pone.0096905.

72. Kiecolt-Glaser JK, Belury MA, Porter K, et al. Depressive symptoms, omega-6:omega-3 fatty acids, and inflammation in older adults. *Psychosom Med.* 2007;69(3):217–24. Mazza M, Pomponi M, Janiri L, et al. Omega-3 fatty acids and antioxidants in neurological and psychiatric diseases: an overview. *Prog Neuropsychopharmacol Biol Psychiatry.* 2007;31(1):12–26.

73. McNamara RK, Strimpfel J, Jandacek R, et al. Detection and treatment of long-chain omega-3 fatty acid deficiency in adolescents with SSRI-resistant major depressive disorder. *PharmaNutrition.* 2014;2(2):38–46. Kraguljac NV, Montori VM, Pavuluri M, et al. Efficacy of omega-3 fatty acids in mood disorders: a systematic review and meta analysis. *Psychopharmacol Bull.* 2009;42(3):39–54. Lin PY, Su KP. A meta-analytic review of double-blind, placebo-controlled trials of antidepressant efficacy of omega-3 fatty acids. *J Clin Psychiatry.* 2007;68(7):1056–61. Frangou S, Lewis M, McCrone P. Efficacy of ethyl-eicosapentaenoic acid in bipolar depression: randomised double-blind placebo-controlled study. *Br J Psychiatry.* 2006;188:46–50.

74. Wilson VK, Houston DK, Kilpatrick L, et al. Relationship between 25-hydroxyvitamin D and cognitive function in older adults: the Health, Aging and Body Composition Study. *J Am Geriatr Soc.* 2014;62(4):636–41.

75. Toffanello ED, Coin A, Egle Perissinotto E, et al. Vitamin D deficiency predicts cognitive decline in older men and women: the Pro.V.A. Study. *Neurology.* 2014;83(24):2292–98.

76. Swardfager W, Herrmann N, Mazereeuw G, et al. Zinc in depression: a meta-analysis. *Biol Psychiatry.* 2013;74(12):872–78.

77. Maserejian NN, Hall SA, McKinlay JB. Low dietary or supplemental zinc is associated with depression symptoms among women, but not men, in a population-based epidemiological survey. *J Affect Disord.* 2012;136(3):781–88.

78. Nowak G, Siwek M, Dudek D, et al. Effect of zinc supplementation on antidepressant therapy in unipolar depression: a preliminary placebo-controlled study. *Pol J Pharmacol.* 2003;55(6):1143–47. Ranjbar E, Kasaei MS, Mohammad-Shirazi M, et al. Effects of zinc supplementation in patients with major depression: a randomized clinical trial. *Iran J Psychiatry.* 2013;8(2):73–79.

Chapter 5: Fat-Food Nation: The Science of Fat

1. Chowdhury R, Warnakula S, Kunutsor S, et al. Association of dietary, circulating, and supplement fatty acids with coronary risk: a systematic review and meta-analysis. *Ann Intern Med.* 2014;160:398–406.

2. Pan A, Sun Q, Bernstein AM, et al. Red meat consumption and mortality: results from 2 prospective cohort studies. *Arch Intern Med.* 2012;172(7):555–63. Sinha R, Cross AJ, Graubard BI, et al. Meat intake and mortality: a prospective study of over half a million people. *Arch Intern Med.* 2009;169:562–71. Major JM, Cross AJ, Doubeni CA, et al. Socioeconomic deprivation impact on meat intake and mortality: NIH-AARP Diet and Health Study. *Cancer Causes Control.* 2011;22:1699–1707. Key TJ, Fraser GE, Thorogood M, et al. Mortality in vegetarians and nonvegetarians: detailed findings from a collaborative analysis of 5 prospective studies. *Am J Clin Nutr.* 1999;70:516S–24S. Fraser GE. Associations between diet and cancer, ischemic

heart disease, and all-cause mortality in non-Hispanic white California Seventh-day Adventists. *Am J Clin Nutr.* 1999;70:532S–38S. Vogel RA, Corretti MC, Plotnick GD. Effect of a single high-fat meal on endothelial function in healthy subjects. *Am J Cardiol.* 1997;79:350–54. Hall WL. Dietary saturated and unsaturated fats as determinants of blood pressure and vascular function. *Nutr Res Rev.* 2009;22:18–38.

3. U.S. Department of Agriculture and U.S. Department of Health and Human Services. *Dietary Guidelines for Americans, 2010.* 7th ed. Washington, DC: U.S. Government Printing Office, December 2010. Available at health.gov/dietaryguidelines /dga2010/dietaryguidelines2010.pdf.

4. Lawrence GD. Dietary fats and health: dietary recommendations in the context of scientific evidence. *Adv Nutr.* 2013;4:294–302. Hegsted DM, McGandy RB, Myers ML, et al. Quantitative effects of dietary fat on serum cholesterol in man. *Am J Clin Nutr.* 1965;17:281–95.

5. Hegsted DM, Ausman LM, Johnson JA, et al. Dietary fat and serum lipids: an evaluation of the experimental data. *Am J Clin Nutr.* 1993;57:875–83. Hodson L, Skeaff CM, Chisholm WA. The effect of replacing dietary saturated fat with polyunsaturated or monounsaturated fat on plasma lipids in free-living young adults. *Eur J Clin Nutr.* 2001;55:908–15. Mensink RP, Zock PL, Kester AD, et al. Effects of dietary fatty acids and carbohydrates on the ratio of serum total to HDL cholesterol and on serum lipids and apolipoproteins: a meta-analysis of 60 controlled trials. *Am J Clin Nutr.* 2003;77:1146–55. Mensink RP, Katan MB. Effect of dietary fatty acids on serum lipids and lipoproteins: a meta-analysis of 27 trials. *Arterioscler Thromb.* 1992;12:911–19. Micha R, Mozaffarian D. Saturated fat and cardiometabolic risk factors, coronary heart disease, stroke, and diabetes: a fresh look at the evidence. *Lipids.* 2010;45:893–905.

6. Chowdhury R, Warnakula S, Kunutsor S, et al. Association of dietary, circulating, and supplement fatty acids with coronary risk: a systematic review and meta-analysis. *Ann Intern Med.* 2014;160(6):398–406.

7. Astrup A, Dyerberg J, Elwood P, et al. The role of reducing intakes of saturated fat in the prevention of cardiovascular disease: where does the evidence stand in 2010? *Am J Clin Nutr.* 2011;93(4):684–88. Siri-Tarino PW, Sun Q, Hu FB, et al. Saturated fatty acids and risk of coronary heart disease: modulation by replacement nutrients. *Curr Atheroscler Rep.* 2010;12:384–90.

8. Jakobsen MU, O'Reilly EJ, Heitmann BL, et al. Major types of dietary fat and risk of coronary heart disease: a pooled analysis of 11 cohort studies. *Am J Clin Nutr.* 2009;89:1425–32.

9. Mozaffarian D, Micha R, Wallace S. Effects on coronary heart disease of increasing polyunsaturated fat in place of saturated fat: a systematic review and meta-analysis of randomized controlled trials. *PLoS Med.* 2010;7(3):e1000252.

10. Jakobsen MU, Dethlefsen C, Joensen AM, et al. Intake of carbohydrates compared with intake of saturated fatty acids and risk of myocardial infarction: importance of the glycemic index. *Am J Clin Nutr.* 2010;91:1764–68.

11. Siri-Tarino PW, Sun Q, Hu FB, et al. Saturated fat, carbohydrate, and cardiovascular disease. *Am J Clin Nutr.* 2010;91:502–9. Siri PW, Krauss RM. Influence of dietary

carbohydrate and fat on LDL and HDL particle distributions. *Curr Atheroscler Rep.* 2005;7:455–59.

12. Halton TL, Willett WC, Liu S, et al. Low-carbohydrate-diet score and the risk of coronary heart disease in women. *N Engl J Med.* 2006;355:1991–2002. Barclay AW, Petocz P, McMillan-Price J, et al. Glycemic index, glycemic load, and chronic disease risk: a meta-analysis of observational studies. *Am J Clin Nutr.* 2008;87:627–37. Mirrahimi A, de Souza RJ, Chiavaroli L, et al. Associations of glycemic index and load with coronary heart disease events: a systematic review and meta-analysis of prospective cohorts. *J Am Heart Assoc.* 2012;1(5):e000752. Fan J, Song Y, Wang Y, et al. Dietary glycemic index, glycemic load, and risk of coronary heart disease, stroke, and stroke mortality: a systematic review with meta-analysis. *PLoS One.* 2012;7(12):e52182.

13. Hu FB. Are refined carbohydrates worse than saturated fat? *Am J Clin Nutr.* 2010;91:1541–42.

14. Hu FB, Stampfer MJ. Nut consumption and risk of coronary heart disease: a review of epidemiologic evidence. *Curr Atheroscler Rep.* 1999;1(3):204–9.

15. Jenkins DJ, Kendall CW, Popovich DG, et al. Effect of a very-high-fiber vegetable, fruit, and nut diet on serum lipids and colonic function. *Metabolism.* 2001;50:494–503.

16. Albert CM, Gaziano JM, Willett WC, et al. Nut consumption and decreased risk of sudden cardiac death in the Physicians' Health Study. *Arch Intern Med.* 2002;162(12):1382–87.

17. Kennedy A, Martinez K, Chuang CC, et al. Saturated fatty acid–mediated inflammation and insulin resistance in adipose tissue: mechanisms of action and implications. *J Nutr.* 2009;139:1–4. Jimenez-Gomez Y, Lopez-Miranda J, Blanco-Colio LM, et al. Olive oil and walnut breakfasts reduce the postprandial inflammatory response in mononuclear cells compared with a butter breakfast in healthy men. *Atherosclerosis.* 2009;204:e70–76. Perez-Martinez P, Lopez-Miranda J, Blanco-Colio L, et al. The chronic intake of a Mediterranean diet enriched in virgin olive oil decreases nuclear transcription factor kappaB activation in peripheral blood mononuclear cells from healthy men. *Atherosclerosis.* 2007;194:e141–46. Masson CJ, Mensink RP. Exchanging saturated fatty acids for (n-6) polyunsaturated fatty acids in a mixed meal may decrease postprandial lipemia and markers of inflammation and endothelial activity in overweight men. *J Nutr.* 2011;141(5):816–21.

18. Sieri S, Chiodini P, Agnoli C, et al. Dietary fat intake and development of specific breast cancer subtypes. *J Natl Cancer Inst.* 2014;106(5):dju068. doi: 10.1093/jnci/dju068 Farvid MS, Cho E, Chen WY, et al. Premenopausal dietary fat in relation to pre- and post-menopausal breast cancer. *Breast Cancer Res Treat.* 2014;145:255–65.

19. Boyd NF, Stone J, Vogt KN, et al. Dietary fat and breast cancer risk revisited: a meta-analysis of the published literature. *Br J Cancer.* 2003;89:1672–85.

20. Rosqvist F, Iggman D, Kullberg J, et al. Overfeeding polyunsaturated and saturated fat causes distinct effects on liver and visceral fat accumulation in humans. *Diabetes.* 2014;63:2356–68.

21. Bjermo H, Iggman D, Kullberg J, et al. Effects of n-6 PUFAs compared with SFAs on liver fat, lipoproteins, and inflammation in abdominal obesity: a randomized controlled trial. *Am J Clin Nutr*. 2012;95:1003–12.

22. Riccardi G, Giacco R, Rivellese AA. Dietary fat, insulin sensitivity and the metabolic syndrome. *Clin Nutr*. 2004;23:447–56.

23. National Cancer Institute. Applied Research: Cancer Control and Population Sciences. Table 4. Food Sources of Arachidonic Acid. Available at http://applied research.cancer.gov/diet/foodsources/fatty_acids/table4.html. Wynder EL, Rose DP, Cohen LA. Diet and breast cancer in causation and therapy. *Cancer*. 1986;58:1804–13. Makarem N, Chandran U, Bandera EV, et al. Dietary fat in breast cancer survival. *Ann Rev Nutr*. 2013;33:319–48. De Lorgeril M, Salen P. New insights into the health effects of dietary saturated and omega-6 and omega-3 polyunsaturated fatty acids. *BMC Med*. 2012;10:50.

24. Thissen JP, Ketelslegers JM, Underwood LE. Nutritional regulation of the insulin-like growth factors. *Endocr Rev*. 1994;15(1):80–101. Kaaks R. Nutrition, insulin, IGF-1 metabolism and cancer risk: a summary of epidemiological evidence. *Novartis Found Symp*. 2004;262:247–60, discussion 260–68.

25. Tang WH, Wang Z, Levison BS, et al. Intestinal microbial metabolism of phosphatidylcholine and cardiovascular risk. *N Engl J Med*. 2013;368:1575–84. Wang Z, Klipfell E, Bennett BJ, et al. Gut flora metabolism of phosphatidylcholine promotes cardiovascular disease. *Nature*. 2011;472:57–63. Richman EL, Kenfield SA, Stampfer MJ, et al. Choline intake and risk of lethal prostate cancer: incidence and survival. *Am J Clin Nutr*. 2012;96:855–63.

26. World Cancer Research Fund/American Institute for Cancer Research. *Food, Nutrition, Physical Activity, and the Prevention of Cancer: A Global Perspective*. Washington DC: AICR; 2007. Lunn JC, Kuhnle G, Mai V, et al. The effect of haem in red and processed meat on the endogenous formation of N-nitroso compounds in the upper gastrointestinal tract. *Carcinogenesis*. 2007;28:685–90. Kuhnle GG, Story GW, Reda T, et al. Diet-induced endogenous formation of nitroso compounds in the GI tract. *Free Radic Biol Med*. 2007;43:1040–47. Zheng W, Lee S-A. Well-done meat intake, heterocyclic amine exposure, and cancer risk. *Nutr Cancer*. 2009;61:437–46.

27. Brewer GJ. Iron and copper toxicity in diseases of aging, particularly atherosclerosis and Alzheimer's disease. *Exp Biol Med*. 2007;232:323–35. Brewer GJ. Risks of copper and iron toxicity during aging in humans. *Chem Res Toxicol*. 2010;23:319–26.

28. Hunnicutt J, He K, Xun P. Dietary iron intake and body stores are associated with risk of coronary artery disease in a meta-analysis of prospective cohort studies. *J Nutr*. 2014;144(3):359–66. doi: 10.3945/jn.113.185124.

29. Reaven PD, Grasse BJ, Tribble DL. Effects of linoleate-enriched and oleate-enriched diets in combination with alpha-tocopherol on the susceptibility of LDL and LDL subfractions to oxidative modification in humans. *Arterioscler Thromb*. 1994;14:557–66. Hargrove RL, Etherton TD, Pearson TA, et al. Low fat and high monounsaturated fat diets decrease human low density lipoprotein oxidative susceptibility in vitro. *J Nutr*. 2001;131:1758–63. Basu A, Rhone M, Lyons TJ. Berries: emerging impact on cardiovascular health. *Nutr Rev*. 2010;68:168–77. Kaliora AC, Dedoussis

GV, Schmidt H. Dietary antioxidants in preventing atherogenesis. *Atherosclerosis.* 2006;187:1–17.

30. Bernstein AM, Sun Q, Hu FB, et al. Major dietary protein sources and risk of coronary heart disease in women. *Circulation.* 2010;122:876–83.

31. Chen GC, Lv DB, Pang Z, et al. Red and processed meat consumption and risk of stroke: a meta-analysis of prospective cohort studies. *Eur J Clin Nutr.* 2013;67(1):91–95.

32. World Cancer Research Fund/American Institute for Cancer Research. Continuous Update Project Report. *Food, Nutrition, Physical Activity, and the Prevention of Colorectal Cancer.* 2011.

33. Mansson HL. Fatty acids in bovine milk fat. *Food Nutr Res.* 2008;52. doi: 10.3402 /fnr.v52i0.1821.

34. Huth PJ, Park KM. Influence of dairy product and milk fat consumption on cardiovascular disease risk: a review of the evidence. *Adv Nutr.* 2012;3:266–85.

35. Genkinger JM, Hunter DJ, Spiegelman D, et al. Dairy products and ovarian cancer: a pooled analysis of 12 cohort studies. *Cancer Epidemiol Biomarkers Prev.* 2006;15:364–72. Larsson SC, Orsini N, Wolk A. Milk, milk products and lactose intake and ovarian cancer risk: a meta-analysis of epidemiological studies. *Int J Cancer.* 2006;118:431–41. Ganmaa D, Cui X, Feskanich D, et al. Milk, dairy intake and risk of endometrial cancer: a 26-year follow-up. *Int J Cancer.* 2012;130(11):2664–71. Song Y, Chavarro JE, Cao Y, et al. Whole milk intake is associated with prostate cancer–specific mortality among U.S. male physicians. *J Nutr.* 2013;143:189–96. Raimondi S, Mabrouk JB, Shatenstein B, et al. Diet and prostate cancer risk with specific focus on dairy products and dietary calcium: a case-control study. *Prostate* 2010;70:1054–65. Qin LQ, Xu JY, Wang PY, et al. Milk consumption is a risk factor for prostate cancer in Western countries: evidence from cohort studies. *Asia Pac J Clin Nutr.* 2007;16:467–76.

36. Kris-Etherton PM, Hu FB, Ros E, et al. The role of tree nuts and peanuts in the prevention of coronary heart disease: multiple potential mechanisms. *J Nutr.* 2008;138:1746S–51S.

37. Fraser GE, Shavlik DJ. Ten years of life: is it a matter of choice? *Arch Intern Med.* 2001;161:1645–52. Baer HJ, Glynn RJ, Hu FB, et al. Risk factors for mortality in the Nurses' Health Study: a competing risks analysis. *Am J Epidemiol.* 2011;173:319–29. Guasch-Ferre M, Bullo M, Martinez-Gonzalez MA, et al. Frequency of nut consumption and mortality risk in the PREDIMED nutrition intervention trial. *BMC Med.* 2013;11:164. Salas-Salvado J, Casas-Agustench P, Murphy MM, et al. The effect of nuts on inflammation. *Asia Pac J Clin Nutr.* 2008;17(suppl 1):333–36. Ros E. Nuts and novel biomarkers of cardiovascular disease. *Am J Clin Nutr.* 2009;89:1649S–56S.

38. Sabate J, Oda K, Ros E. Nut consumption and blood lipid levels: a pooled analysis of 25 intervention trials. *Arch Intern Med* 2010;170:821–27.

39. Dreher ML, Davenport AJ. Hass avocado composition and potential health effects. *Crit Rev Food Sci Nutr.* 2013;53:738–50.

40. Luu HN, Blot WJ, Xiang Y, et al. Prospective evaluation of the association of nut/peanut consumption with total and cause-specific mortality. *JAMA Intern Med.* 2015;175(5):755–66. doi: 10.1001/jamainternmed.2014.8347.

41. Hu FB, Stampfer MJ, Manson JE, et al. Frequent nut consumption and risk of coronary heart disease in women: prospective cohort study. *BMJ.* 1998;317(7169):1341–45.

42. Albert CM, Gaziano JM, Willett WC, et al. Nut consumption and decreased risk of sudden cardiac death in the Physicians' Health Study. *Arch Intern Med.* 2002;162(12);1382–87.

43. Fraser GE. Nut consumption, lipids, and risk of a coronary event. *Clin Cardiol.* 1999;22(suppl 3):11–15. Fraser GE, Shavlik DJ. Risk factors for all-cause and coronary heart disease mortality in the oldest-old: the Adventist Health Study. *Arch Intern Med.* 1997;157(19):2249–58.

44. Jenkins DJ, Kendell CW, Banack MS, et al. Nuts as a replacement for carbohydrates in the diabetic diet. *Diabetes Care.* 2011;34(8):1706–11.

45. Mattes RD, Dreher ML. Nuts and healthy body weight maintenance mechanisms. *Asia Pac J Clin Nutr.* 2010;19(1):137–41. Bes-Rastrollo M, Sabaté J, Gomez-Gracia E, et al. Nut consumption and weight gain in a Mediterranean cohort: the SUN study. *Obesity (Silver Spring).* 2007;15:107–16. Bes-Rastrollo M, Wedick NM, Martinez-Gonzalez MA, et al. Prospective study of nut consumption, long-term weight change, and obesity risk in women. *Am J Clin Nutr.* 2009;89(6):1913–19.

46. Wien MA, Sabaté JM, Iklé DN, et al. Almonds vs. complex carbohydrates in a weight reduction program. *Int J Obes Relat Metab Disord.* 2003;27(11):1365–72. Mattes RD, Kris-Etherton PM, Foster GD. Impact of peanuts and tree nuts on body weight and healthy weight loss in adults. *J Nutr.* 2008;138(9):1741S–45S.

47. Mattes RD, Dreher ML. Nuts and healthy body weight maintenance mechanisms. *Asia Pac J Clin Nutr.* 2010;19(1):137–41. Bes-Rastrollo M, Sabaté J, Gomez-Gracia E, et al. Nut consumption and weight gain in a Mediterranean cohort: the SUN study. *Obesity (Silver Spring).* 2007;15:107–16. Bes-Rastrollo M, Wedick NM, Martinez-Gonzalez MA, et al. Prospective study of nut consumption, long-term weight change, and obesity risk in women. *Am J Clin Nutr.* 2009;89(6):1913–19.

48. Novotny JA, Gebauer SK, Baer DJ. Discrepancy between the Atwater factor predicted and empirically measured energy values of almonds in human diets. *Am J Clin Nutr.* 2012;96(2):296–301.

49. Sabate J et al. Nut consumption and blood lipid levels: a pooled analysis of 25 intervention trials. *Arch Intern Med.* 2010;170:821–27.

50. Sabate J, Oda K, Ros E. Nut consumption and blood lipid levels. *Arch Intern Med.* Salas-Salvado J, Guasch-Ferre M, Bullo M, et al. Nuts in the prevention and treatment of metabolic syndrome. *Am J Clin Nutr.* 2014;100(suppl 1):399S–407S.

51. Tsai CJ, Leitzmann MF, Hu FB, et al. A prospective cohort study of nut consumption and the risk of gallstone disease in men. *Am J Epidemiol.* 2004;160:961–68. Tsai CJ, Leitzmann MF, Hu FB, et al. Frequent nut consumption and decreased risk of cholecystectomy in women. *Am J Clin Nutr.* 2004;80:76–81.

52. Salas-Salvado J, Guasch-Ferre M, Bullo M, et al. Nuts in the prevention and treatment of metabolic syndrome. *Am J Clin Nutr.* 2014;100(suppl 1):399S–407S. Jenkins DJ, Ken-

dall CW, Banach MS, et al. Nuts as a replacement for carbohydrates in the diabetic diet. *Diabetes Care.* 2011;34:1706–11. Josse AR, Kendall CW, Augustin LS, et al. Almonds and postprandial glycemia: a dose-response study. *Metabolism.* 2007;56:400–4. Pan A, Sun Q, Manson JE, et al. Walnut consumption is associated with lower risk of type 2 diabetes in women. *J Nutr.* 2013;143:512–18. Kochar J, Gaziano JM, Djousse L. Nut consumption and risk of type II diabetes in the Physicians' Health Study. *Eur J Clin Nutr.* 2010;64:75–79. Salas-Salvado J, Bullo M, Babio N, et al. Reduction in the incidence of type 2 diabetes with the Mediterranean diet: results of the PREDIMED-Reus nutrition intervention randomized trial. *Diabetes Care.* 2011;34:14–19. Jenkins DJ, Kendall CW, Josse AR, et al. Almonds decrease postprandial glycemia, insulinemia, and oxidative damage in healthy individuals. *J Nutr.* 2006;136:2987–92. Wien MA, Sabate JM, Ikle DN, et al. Almonds vs. complex carbohydrates in a weight reduction program. *Int J Obes Relat Metab Disord.* 2003;27:1365–72. Jenkins DJ, Kendall CW, Marchie A, et al. Effect of almonds on insulin secretion and insulin resistance in non-diabetic hyperlipidemic subjects: a randomized controlled crossover trial. *Metabolism.* 2008;57:882–87. Wien M, Bleich D, Raghuwanshi M, et al. Almond consumption and cardiovascular risk factors in adults with prediabetes. *J Am Coll Nutr.* 2010;29:189–97. Jiang R, Manson JE, Stampfer MJ, et al. Nut and peanut butter consumption and risk of type 2 diabetes in women. *JAMA.* 2002;288:2554–60.

53. Wien MA, Sabate JM, Ikle DN, et al. Almonds vs. complex carbohydrates in a weight reduction program. *Int J Obes Relat Metab Disord.* 2003;27:1365–72. Mohammadi-fard N, Salehi-Abarghouei A, Salas-Salvado J, et al. The effect of tree nut, peanut, and soy nut consumption on blood pressure: a systematic review and meta-analysis of randomized controlled clinical trials. *Am J Clin Nutr.* 2015 May;101(5):966–82. Djousse L, Rudich T, Gaziano JM. Nut consumption and risk of hypertension in US male physicians. *Clin Nutr.* 2009;28:10–14. Estruch R, Martinez-Gonzalez MA, Corella D, et al. Effects of a Mediterranean-style diet on cardiovascular risk factors: a randomized trial. *Ann Intern Med.* 2006;145:1–11.

54. Jackson CL, Hu FB. Long-term associations of nut consumption with body weight and obesity. *Am J Clin Nutr.* 2014;100(suppl 1):408S–11S. Mattes RD, Dreher ML. Nuts and healthy body weight maintenance mechanisms. *Asia Pac J Clin Nutr.* 2010;19:137–41. Vadivel V, Kunyanga CN, Biesalski HK. Health benefits of nut consumption with special reference to body weight control. *Nutrition.* 2012;28:1089–97.

55. Zhang Z, Xu G, Wei Y, et al. Nut consumption and risk of stroke. *Eur J Epidemiol.* 2015;30:189–96.

56. Poulose SM, Miller MG, Shukitt-Hale B. Role of walnuts in maintaining brain health with age. *J Nutr.* 2014;144:561S–66S. O'Brien J, Okereke O, Devore E, et al. Long-term intake of nuts in relation to cognitive function in older women. *J Nutr Health Aging.* 2014;18:496–502. Pribis P, Shukitt-Hale B. Cognition: the new frontier for nuts and berries. *Am J Clin Nutr.* 2014;100(suppl 1):347S–52S. Martinez-Lapiscina EH, Clavero P, Toledo E, et al. Mediterranean diet improves cognition: the PREDIMED-NAVARRA randomised trial. *J Neurol Neurosurg Psychiatry.* 2013;84:1318–25. Barbour JA, Howe PR, Buckley JD, et al. Nut consumption for vascular health and cognitive function. *Nutr Res Rev.* 2014;27:131–58.

57. Falasca M, Casari I. Cancer chemoprevention by nuts: evidence and promises. *Front Biosci (Schol Ed)*. 2012;4:109–20. Gonzalez CA, Salas-Salvado J. The potential of nuts in the prevention of cancer. *Br J Nutr*. 2006;96(suppl 2):S87–94. Falasca M, Casari I, Maffucci T. Cancer chemoprevention with nuts. *J Natl Cancer Inst*. 2014;106(9). doi: 10.1093/jnci/dju238. Fillon M. Nuts may lower cancer risk. *J Natl Cancer Inst*. 2014;106(4):dju102. Sabate J, Ang Y. Nuts and health outcomes: new epidemiologic evidence. *Am J Clin Nutr*. 2009;89:1643S–48S. Buck K, Zaineddin AK, Vrieling A, et al. Meta-analyses of lignans and enterolignans in relation to breast cancer risk. *Am J Clin Nutr*. 2010;92:141–53. Velentzis LS, Cantwell MM, Cardwell C, et al. Lignans and breast cancer risk in pre- and post-menopausal women: meta-analyses of observational studies. *Br J Cancer*. 2009;100:1492–98. Saarinen NM, Tuominen J, Pylkkanen L, et al. Assessment of information to substantiate a health claim on the prevention of prostate cancer by lignans. *Nutrients*. 2010;2:99–115.

58. Guasch-Ferre M, Bullo M, Martinez-Gonzalez MA, et al. Frequency of nut consumption and mortality risk in the PREDIMED nutrition intervention trial. *BMC Med*. 2013;11:164. Van den Brandt PA, Schouten LJ. Relationship of tree nut, peanut and peanut butter intake with total and cause-specific mortality: a cohort study and meta-analysis. *Int J Epidemiol*. 2015. doi: 10.1093/ije/dyv039. Baer HJ, Glynn RJ, Hu FB, et al. Risk factors for mortality in the Nurses' Health Study: a competing risks analysis. *Am J Epidemiol*. 2011;173:319–29. Ellsworth JL, Kushi LH, Folsom AR. Frequent nut intake and risk of death from coronary heart disease and all causes in postmenopausal women: the Iowa Women's Health Study. *Nutr Metab Cardiovasc Dis*. 2001;11:372–77. Fraser GE, Shavlik DJ. Ten years of life: is it a matter of choice? *Arch Intern Med*. 2001;161:1645–52. Fraser GE, Shavlik DJ. Risk factors for all-cause and coronary heart disease mortality in the oldest-old: the Adventist Health Study. *Arch Intern Med*. 1997;157:2249–58. Luu HN, Blot WJ, Xiang YB, et al. Prospective evaluation of the association of nut/peanut consumption with total and cause-specific mortality. *JAMA Intern Med*. 2015;175(5):755–66. Sabate J. Nut consumption, vegetarian diets, ischemic heart disease risk, and all-cause mortality: evidence from epidemiologic studies. *Am J Clin Nutr*. 1999;70:500S–3S.

59. Fraser GE, Shavlik DJ. Ten years of life: is it a matter of choice? *Arch Intern Med*. 2001;161(13):1645–52.

60. Kris-Etherton PM, Hu FB, Ros E, et al. The role of tree nuts and peanuts in the prevention of coronary heart disease: multiple potential mechanisms. *J Nutr*. 2008;138: 1746S–51S.

61. Salas-Salvadó J, Casas-Agustench P, Murphy MM, et al. The effect of nuts on inflammation. *Asia Pac J Clin Nutr*. 2008;17(suppl 1):333–36. Casas-Agustench P, Bulló M, Salas-Salvadó J. Nuts, inflammation and insulin resistance. *Asia Pac J Clin Nutr*. 2010;19(1):124–30. Gopinath B, Buyken AE, Flood VM, et al. Consumption of polyunsaturated fatty acids, fish, and nuts and risk of inflammatory disease mortality. *Am J Clin Nutr*. 2011;93(5):1073–79. Ros E. Nuts and novel biomarkers of cardiovascular disease. *Am J Clin Nutr*. 2009 May;89(5):1649S–56S. Kris-Etherton PM, Hu FB, Ros E, et al. The role of tree nuts and peanuts in the prevention of coronary heart disease: multiple potential mechanisms. *J Nutr*. 2008;138(9):1746S–51S. O'Neil CE, Keast DR, Nicklas TA, et al. Nut consumption is associated with decreased health risk factors for cardiovascular disease and metabolic syndrome in U.S. adults: NHANES

1999–2004. *J Am Coll Nutr.* 2011;30(6):502–10. Falasca M, Casari I. Cancer chemoprevention by nuts: evidence and promises. *Front Biosci (Schol Ed).* 2012;1(4):109–20. González CA, Salas-Salvadó J. The potential of nuts in the prevention of cancer. *Br J Nutr.* 2006;96(suppl 2):S87–94.

62. Young VM, Toborek M, Yang F, et al. Effect of linoleic acid on endothelial cell inflammatory mediators. *Metabolism.* 1998;47(5):566–72. Simopoulos AP. The omega-6/omega-3 fatty acid ratio, genetic variation, and cardiovascular disease. *Asia Pac J Clin Nutr.* 2008;17(suppl 1):131–34. Herieka M, Erridge C. High-fat meal induced postprandial inflammation. *Mol Nutr Food Res.* 2014 Jan;58(1):136–46. Blankenhorn DH, Johnson R, Mack WI, et al. The influence of diet on the appearance of new lesions in human coronary arteries *JAMA.* 1990;263(12):1646–52.

63. Sala-Vila A, Romero-Mamani ES, Gilabert R, et al. Changes in ultrasound-assessed carotid intima-media thickness and plaque with a Mediterranean diet: a substudy of the PREDIMED trial. *Arterioscler Thromb Vasc Biol.* 2014;34(2):439-45.

64. Guasch-Ferré M, Bulló M, Martínez-González MA, et al. PREDIMED Study Group. Frequency of nut consumption and mortality risk in the PREDIMED nutrition intervention trial. *BMC Med.* 2013;11:164.

65. Poulose SM, Miller MG, Shukitt-Hale B. Role of walnuts in maintaining brain health with age. *J Nutr.* 2014;144(suppl 4):561S–66S.

66. Kris-Etherton PM. Walnuts decrease risk of cardiovascular disease: a summary of efficacy and biologic mechanisms. *J Nutr.* 2014;144(suppl 4):547S–54S.

67. Katz DL, Davidhi A, Ma Y, et al. Effects of walnuts on endothelial function in overweight adults with visceral obesity: a randomized, controlled, crossover trial. *J Am Coll Nutr.* 2012;31(6):415–23. West SG, Krick AL, Klein LC, et al. Effects of diets high in walnuts and flax oil on hemodynamic responses to stress and vascular endothelial function. *J Am Coll Nutr.* 2010;29(6):595–603.

68. Mozaffarian D, Wu JH. Omega-3 fatty acids and cardiovascular disease: effects on risk factors, molecular pathways, and clinical events. *J Am Coll Cardiol.* 2011;58:2047–67.

69. De Lorgeril M, Salen P. New insights into the health effects of dietary saturated and omega-6 and omega-3 polyunsaturated fatty acids. *BMC Med.* 2012;10:50. Berquin IM, Edwards IJ, Chen YQ. Multi-targeted therapy of cancer by omega-3 fatty acids. *Cancer Lett.* 2008;269:363–77.

70. Hu D, Huang J, Wang Y, et al. Fruits and vegetables consumption and risk of stroke: a meta-analysis of prospective cohort studies. *Stroke.* 2014;45:1613–19.

71. Cassidy A, O'Reilly EJ, Kay C, et al. Habitual intake of flavonoid subclasses and incident hypertension in adults. *Am J Clin Nutr.* 2011;93:338–47. Chong MF, Macdonald R, Lovegrove JA. Fruit polyphenols and CVD risk: a review of human intervention studies. *Br J Nutr.* 2010;104(suppl 3):S28–39.

72. Rodrigues-Leyva D, Weighell W, Edel AL, et al. Potent antihypertensive action of dietary flaxseed in hypertensive patients. *Hypertension.* 2013;62(6):1081–89.

73. Karppi J, Laukkanen JA, Sivenius J, et al. Serum lycopene decreases the risk of stroke in men: a population-based follow-up study. *Neurology.* 2012;79(15):1540–47. Li X,

Xu J. Dietary and circulating lycopene and stroke risk: a meta-analysis of prospective studies. *Sci Rep.* 2014 May 22;4:5031.

74. Li D, Mehta JL. Oxidized LDL, a critical factor in atherogenesis. *Cardiovasc Res.* 2005 Dec 1;68(3):353–54.

75. Yu-Poth S, Etherton TD, Reddy CC, et al. Lowering dietary saturated fat and total fat reduces the oxidative susceptibility of LDL in healthy men and women. *J Nutr.* 2000;130(9):2228–37.

76. Kris-Etherton PM, Hu FB, Ros E, et al. The role of tree nuts and peanuts in the prevention of coronary heart disease: multiple potential mechanisms. *J Nutr.* 2008;138(9):1746S–51S. Jenkins DJ, Kendall CW, Marchie A, et al. Almonds reduce biomarkers of lipid peroxidation in older hyperlipidemic subjects. *J Nutr.* 2008;138:908–13. Jenkins DJ, Kendall CW, Marchie A, et al. Dose response of almonds on coronary heart disease risk factors: blood lipids, oxidized low-density lipoproteins, lipoprotein(a), homocysteine, and pulmonary nitric oxide: a randomized, controlled, crossover trial. *Circulation.* 2002;106:1327–32.

77. Navar-Boggan AM, Peterson ED, D'Agostino RB, et al. Hyperlipidemia in early adulthood increases long-term risk of coronary heart disease. *Circulation.* 2015;131(5): 451–58.

78. Lloyd-Jones DM, Leip EP, Larson MG, et al. Prediction of lifetime risk for cardiovascular disease by risk factor burden at 50 years of age. *Circulation.* 2006;113(6):791–98.

79. Hyttinen L, Strandberg TE, Strandberg AY, et al. Effect of cholesterol on mortality and quality of life up to a 46-year follow-up. *Am J Cardiol.* 2011;108(5):677–81.

80. Li Y, Zhou C, Zhou X, et al. Egg consumption and risk of cardiovascular diseases and diabetes: a meta-analysis. *Atherosclerosis.* 2013;229(2):424–530.

81. Rong Y, Chen L, Zhu T, et al. Egg consumption and risk of coronary heart disease and stroke: dose-response meta-analysis of prospective cohort studies. *BMJ.* 2013;346:e8539.

82. Djousse L, Gaziano JM, Buring JE, et al. Egg consumption and risk of type 2 diabetes in men and women. *Diabetes Care.* 2009;32:295–300.

83. Shin JY, Xun P, Nakamura Y, et al. Egg consumption in relation to risk of cardiovascular disease and diabetes: a systematic review and meta-analysis. *Am J Clin Nutr.* 2013 Jul;98(1):146–59.

84. Virtanen JK, Mursu J, Tuomainen TP, et al. Egg consumption and risk of incident type 2 diabetes in men: the Kuopio Ischaemic Heart Disease Risk Factor Study. *Am J Clin Nutr.* 2015 May;101(5):1088–96.

85. Spence JD, Jenkins DJ, Davignon J. Dietary cholesterol and egg yolks: not for patients at risk of vascular disease. *Can J Cardiol.* 2010;26:e336–39.

86. Tang WH, Wang Z, Levison BS, et al. Intestinal microbial metabolism of phosphatidylcholine and cardiovascular risk. *N Engl J Med.* 2013;368:1575–84. Wang Z, Klipfell E, Bennett BJ, et al. Gut flora metabolism of phosphatidylcholine promotes cardiovascular disease. *Nature.* 2011;472:57–63.

87. Sharp SJ, Pocock SJ. Time trends in serum cholesterol before cancer death. *Epidemiology.* 1997 Mar;8:132–36. Zureik M, Courbon D, Ducimetiere P. Decline in

serum total cholesterol and the risk of death from cancer. *Epidemiology*. 1997 Mar;8(2):137–43.

88. Shirani J, Yousefi J, Roberts WC. Major cardiac findings at necropsy in 366 American octogenarians. *Am J Cardiol*. 1995;75(2):151–56.

89. Joseph A, Ackerman D, Talley JD, et al. Manifestations of coronary atherosclerosis in young trauma victims: an autopsy study. *J Am Coll Cardiol*. 1993;22(2):459–67.

90. Campbell TC, Parpia B, Chen J. Diet, lifestyle, and the etiology of coronary artery disease: the Cornel China Study. *Am J Cardiol*. 1998;82(10B):18–21T.

91. Micha R, Mozaffarian D. Saturated fat and cardiometabolic risk factors, coronary heart disease, stroke, and diabetes: a fresh look at the evidence. *Lipids*. 2010;45:893–905. Tholstrup T, Vessby B, Sandstrom B. Difference in effect of myristic and stearic acid on plasma HDL cholesterol within 24 h in young men. *Eur J Clin Nutr*. 2003;57:735–42.

92. Abbey M, Noakes M, Belling GB, et al. Partial replacement of saturated fatty acids with almonds or walnuts lowers total plasma cholesterol and low-density-lipoprotein cholesterol. *Am J Clin Nutr*. 1994;59:995–99. Spiller GA, Jenkins DA, Bosello O, et al. Nuts and plasma lipids: an almond-based diet lowers LDL-C while preserving HDL-C. *J Am Coll Nutr*. 1998;17:285–90. Sabate J, Oda K, Ros E. Nut consumption and blood lipid levels: a pooled analysis of 25 intervention trials. *Arch Intern Med*. 2010;170:821–27.

93. Micha R, Mozaffarian D. Saturated fat and cardiometabolic risk factors, coronary heart disease, stroke, and diabetes: a fresh look at the evidence. *Lipids*. 2010;45:893–905. Grundy SM. Influence of stearic acid on cholesterol metabolism relative to other long-chain fatty acids. *Am J Clin Nutr*. 1994;60:986S–90S. German JB, Dillard CJ. Saturated fats: what dietary intake? *Am J Clin Nutr*. 2004;80:550–59.

94. SELFNutritionData. Nutrient Search. Available at http://www.nutritiondata.com /tools/nutrient-search.

95. Rizzo M, Pernice V, Frasheri A, et al. Small, dense low-density lipoproteins (LDL) are predictors of cardio- and cerebro-vascular events in subjects with the metabolic syndrome. *Clin Endocrinol (Oxf)*. 2009;70:870–75. Austin MA, Breslow JL, Hennekens CH, et al. Low-density lipoprotein subclass patterns and risk of myocardial infarction. *JAMA*. 1988;260:1917–21.

96. Dreon DM, Fernstrom HA, Campos H, et al. Change in dietary saturated fat intake is correlated with change in mass of large low-density-lipoprotein particles in men. *Am J Clin Nutr*. 1998;67:828–36.

97. Kratz M, Gulbahce E, von Eckardstein A, et al. Dietary mono- and polyunsaturated fatty acids similarly affect LDL size in healthy men and women. *J Nutr*. 2002;132:715–18.

98. Siri PW, Krauss RM. Influence of dietary carbohydrate and fat on LDL and HDL particle distributions. *Curr Atheroscler Rep*. 2005;7:455–59.

99. Abbey M, Noakes M, Belling GB, et al. Partial replacement of saturated fatty acids with almonds or walnuts lowers total plasma cholesterol and low-density-lipoprotein cholesterol. *Am J Clin Nutr*. 1994;59:995–99.

100. Vega-Lopez S, Ausman LM, Jalbert SM, et al. Palm and partially hydrogenated soybean oils adversely alter lipoprotein profiles compared with soybean and canola oils in moderately hyperlipidemic subjects. *Am J Clin Nutr.* 2006;84:54–62.

Chapter 6: Salt Is a Four-Letter Word

1. Wang Y, Wang QJ. The prevalence of prehypertension and hypertension among adults according to the new joint National Committee guidelines. *Arch Intern Med.* 2004;164(19):2126–34.

2. Frohlich ED, Varagic J. The role of sodium in hypertension is more complex than simply elevating arterial pressure. *Nat Clin Pract Cardiovasc Med.* 2004;1(1):24–30.

3. Dickenson BD, Havas S. Reducing the population burden of cardiovascular disease by reducing sodium intake: a report of the Council on Science and Public Health. *Arch Intern Med.* 2007;167(14):1460–68.

4. Karppanen H, Mervaala E. Sodium intake and hypertension. *Prog Cardiovasc Dis.* 2006;49(2):59–75. Cutler JA, Roccell E. Salt reduction for preventing hypertension and cardiovascular disease. *Hypertension.* 2006;48(5):818–19.

5. Cook N, Cutler J, Obarzanek E, et al. Long term effects of dietary sodium reduction on cardiovascular disease outcomes: observational follow-up of the trails of hypertension prevention (TOHP). *BMJ.* 2007;334:885.

6. Havas S, Roccella EJ, Lenfant C. Reducing the public health from elevated blood pressure levels in the United States by lowering intake of dietary sodium. *Am J Public Health.* 2004;94(1):19–22.

7. Prospective Studies Collaboration. Age specific relevance of usual blood pressure to vascular mortality: a meta analysis of individual data for one million adults in 61 prospective studies. *Lancet.* 2002;360:1903–13.

8. Weinberger MH. Salt sensitivity is associated with an increased mortality in both normal and hypertensive humans. *J Clin Hypertens.* 2002;4(4):274–76.

9. Tuomilehto J, Jousilahti P, Rastenyte D, et al. Urinary sodium excretion and cardiovascular mortality in Finland: a prospective study. *Lancet.* 2001;357: 848–51.

10. Luke RG. President's address: salt—too much of a good thing? *Trans Am Clin Climatol Assoc.* 2007;118:1–22.

11. Freis E. The role of salt in hypertension. *Blood Pressure.* 1991;1:196–200.

12. National High Blood Pressure Education Program. The Seventh Report of the Joint National Committee on Prevention, Detection, Evaluation, and Treatment of High Blood Pressure. *Lifetime Risk of Hypertension.* Bethesda, MD: U.S. National Heart, Lung, and Blood Institute. 2004 Aug. Available at http://www.ncbi.nlm.nih.gov /books/NBK9636/.

13. National High Blood Pressure Education Program Working Group report on primary prevention of hypertension. *Arch Intern Med.* 1993 Jan 25;153(2):186–208. Henney JE, Taylor CL, Boon CS. *Strategies to Reduce Sodium Intake in the United States.* Institute of Medicine (U.S.) Committee on Strategies to Reduce Sodium Intake. Washington,

DC: National Academies Press, 2010. Available at http://iom.nationalacademies .org/Reports/2010/Strategies-to-Reduce-Sodium-Intake-in-the-United-states.aspx.

14. Centers for Disease Control and Prevention. Salt. 2015. Available at http://www .cdc.gov/salt/.

15. Oparil S. Low sodium intake: cardiovascular health benefit or risk? *N Engl J Med.* 2014; 371:677–79.

16. O'Donnell M, Mente A, Rangarajan S, et al. Urinary sodium and potassium excretion, mortality, and cardiovascular events. *N Engl J Med.* 2014;371:612–23.

17. O'Donnell M, et al. Urinary sodium and potassium excretion, mortality, and cardiovascular events. *N Engl J Med.* (referred to as Study A in the text). Mente A, O'Donnell MJ, Rangarajan S, et al. Association of urinary sodium and potassium excretion with blood pressure. *N Engl J Med.* 2014;371:601–11 (referred to as Study B).

18. Mozaffarian D, Fahimi S, Singh GM, et al. Global sodium consumption and death from cardiovascular causes. *N Engl J Med.* 2014;371:624–34.

19. Go AS, Mozaffarian D, Roger VL, et al. Heart disease and stroke statistics—2014 update: a report from the American Heart Association. *Circulation.* 2014;129:e28–e292.

20. Bibbins-Domingo K, Chertow GM, Coxson PG, et al. Projected effect of dietary salt reductions on future cardiovascular disease. *N Engl J Med.* 2010;362:590–99.

21. Van Rensbergen G, Nawrot T. Medical conditions of nursing home admissions. *BMC Geriatr.* 2010;10:46.

22. National Center for Health Statistics. *Health, United States, 2011: With Special Feature on Socioeconomic Status and Health.* Hyattsville, MD: 2012. Table 51. End-stage renal disease patients, by selected characteristics: United States, selected years 1980–2010, pp. 190–91. Available at http://www.cdc.gov/nchs/data/hus/hus11.pdf.

23. Cherubini A, Lowenthal DT, Paran E, et al. Hypertension and cognitive function in the elderly. *Am J Ther.* 2007;14(6):533–54.

24. Bui AL, Horwich TB, Fonarow GC. Epidemiology and risk profile of heart failure. *Nat Rev Cardiol.* 2011;8:30–41. Pfister R, Michels G, Sharp SJ, et al. Estimated urinary sodium excretion and risk of heart failure in men and women in the EPIC-Norfolk study. *Eur J Heart Fail.* 2014;16:394–402.

25. Hall MJ, Levant S, DeFrances CJ. Hospitalization for congestive heart failure: United States, 2000–2010. NCHS Data Brief. 2012;108:1–8. Available at http://www.cdc .gov/nchs/data/databriefs/db108.htm.

26. Zhao LQ, Liu SW. Atrial fibrillation in essential hypertension: an issue of concern. *J Cardiovasc Med (Hagerstown).* 2014;15:100–6. Gutierrez C, Blanchard DG. Atrial fibrillation: diagnosis and treatment. *Am Fam Physician.* 2011;83:61–68.

27. Sakhaee K, Maalouf NM, Sinnott B. Clinical review. Kidney stones 2012: pathogenesis, diagnosis, and management. *J Clin Endocrinol Metab.* 2012;97:1847–60.

28. Tsugane S, Sasazuki S. Diet and the risk of gastric cancer: review of epidemiological evidence. *Gastric Cancer.* 2007;10:75–83. D'Elia L, Rossi G, Ippolito R, et al. Habitual salt intake and risk of gastric cancer: a meta-analysis of prospective studies. *Clin Nutr.* 2012;31(4):489–98. Lu JB, Qin YM. Correlation between high salt intake and

mortality rates for oesophageal and gastric cancers in Henan Province, China. *Int J Epidemiol.* 1987;16(2):171–76. Deckers IAG, Van Den Brandt PA, van Engeland M, et al. Long-term dietary sodium, potassium and fluid intake: exploring potential novel risk factors for renal cell cancer in the Netherlands Cohort Study on diet and cancer. *Br J Cancer.* 2014;110:797–801.

29. Amer M, Woodward M, Appel LJ. Effects of dietary sodium and the DASH diet on the occurrence of headaches: results from randomised multicentre DASH-Sodium clinical trial. *BMJ Open.* 2014;4:e006671. Aanen MC, Bredenoord AJ, Smout A. Effect of dietary sodium chloride on gastro-oesophageal reflux: a randomized controlled trial. *Scand J Gastroenterol.* 2006;41(10):1141–46. Wu P, Zhao XH, Ai ZS, et al. Dietary intake and risk for reflux esophagitis: a case-control study. *Gastroenterol Res Pract.* 2013;2013:691026.

30. Himalayan Crystal Salt: http://www.himalayancrystalsalt.com.

31. Institute of Medicine Standing Committee on the Scientific Evaluation of Dietary Reference Intakes. *Dietary Reference Intakes for Calcium, Phosphorus, Magnesium, Vitamin D, and Fluoride.* Washington, DC: National Academies Press; 1997.

32. Havas S, Dickinson B, Wilson M. The urgent need to reduce sodium consumption. *JAMA.* 2007;298(12):1439–41.

33. Jacobson MF. Salt: the forgotten killer. Washington, DC: Center for Science in the Public Interest; 2005: 8. Available at https://cspinet.org/salt/saltreport.pdf.

34. Nestle M. *What to Eat.* New York: North Star; 2006: 365.

35. Goldstein LB. The complex relationship between cholesterol and brain hemorrhage. *Circulation.* 2009;119:2131–33.

36. Yano K, Reed D, MacLean C. Serum cholesterol and hemorrhagic stroke in the Honolulu Heart Program. *Stroke.* 1989;20(11):1460–65.

37. Heaney R. Role of dietary sodium in osteoporosis. *J Am Coll Nutr.* 2006;25(3): 271S–76S.

38. Tsugane S, Sasazuki S. Diet and the risk of gastric cancer: review of epidemiological evidence. *Gastric Cancer.* 2007;10(2):75–83. Joossens JV, Hill MJ, Elliot P, et al. European Cancer Prevention (ECP) and the INTERSALT Cooperative Research Group. Dietary salt, nitrate and stomach cancer mortality in 24 countries. *Int J Epidemiol.* 1996;25(3):494–504.

39. Burney P. A diet rich in sodium may potentiate asthma: epidemiologic evidence for a new hypothesis. *Chest.* 1987;91(suppl 2):143s–48s. Tribe RM, Barton JR, Poston L, et al. Dietary sodium intake, airway responsiveness, and cellular transport. *Am J Respir Crit Care Med.* 1994;149:1426–33.

40. Pistelli R, Forastiere F, Corbo GM, et al. Respiratory symptoms and bronchial responsiveness are related to dietary salt intake and urinary potassium excretion in male children. *Eur Respir J.* 1993;6:517–22. Demissie K, Ernst P, Gray DK, et al. Usual dietary salt intake and asthma in children: a case-control study. *Thorax.* 1996;51:59–63.

41. Sutter Health, Palo Alto Medical Foundation. Seasoning without salt. Available at http://www.pamf.org/heartfailure/lifestyle/diet/seasoning.html.

Chapter 7: Comparing Cardioprotective Diets

1. Nissen SE. Halting the progression of atherosclerosis with intensive lipid lowering: results from the Reversal of Atherosclerosis with Aggressive Lipid Lowering (REVERSAL) trial. *Am J Med.* 2005;118(S12A):22–27.

2. Tang WHW, Wang Z, Levison BS, et al. Intestinal microbial metabolism of phosphatidylcholine and cardiovascular risk. *N Engl J Med.* 2013; 368:1575–84. Keleman LE, Kushi LH, Jacobs DR Jr, et al. Association of dietary protein with disease and mortality in a prospective study of post-menopausal women. *Am J Epidemiol.* 2005;161(3):239–48. Lagiou P, Sandin S, Lof M, et al. Low-carbohydrate, high-protein diet and incidence of cardiovascular diseases in Swedish women: prospective cohort study. *BMJ.* 2012;344:e4026. American Heart Association. Vegetarian diets. 2015. Available at http://www.heart.org/HEARTORG/GettingHealthy/NutritionCenter/Vegetarian-Diets_UCM_306032_Article.jsp.

3. Grant WB. A multicounty ecological study of cancer incidence rates in 2008 with respect to various risk-modifying factors. *Nutrients.* 2014;6:163–89.

4. Public Radio International (PRI). Global cancer incidence. 2008. Available at http://globalcancermap.com.

5. Thompson RC, Allam AH, Lombardi GP, et al. Atherosclerosis across 4000 years of human history: the Horus study of four ancient populations. *Lancet.* 2013;381(9873):1211–22.

6. Bjerregaard P, Young TK, Hegele RA. Low incidence of cardiovascular disease among the Inuit: what is the evidence? *Atherosclerosis.* 2003;166(2):351–57.

7. Cheng TO. Changing prevalence of heart diseases in People's Republic of China. *Ann Intern Med.* 1974;80(1):108–9. Smith JM. Dietary decadence and dynastic decline in the Mongol Empire. *J Asian Hist.* 2000;34(1):35–52.

8. Ströhle A, Wolters M, Hahn A. Carbohydrates and the diet-atherosclerosis connection: more between earth and heaven. Comment on the article "The atherogenic potential of dietary carbohydrate." *Prev Med.* 2007 Jan;44(1):82–84; author reply 84–85. Shaper AG. Commentary: personal reflection on serum-cholesterol, diet and coronary heart-disease in Africans and Asians in Uganda. *Int J Epidemiol.* 2012;41(5):1225–28.

9. Levine ME, Suarez JA, Brandhorst S, et al. Low protein intake is associated with a major reduction in IGF-1, cancer, and overall mortality in the 65 and younger but not older population. *Cell Metab.* 2014;19(3):407–17.

10. For more, see the WCRF/AICR website at http://www.dietandcancerreport.org/cup.

11. Oyebode O, Gordon-Dseagu V, Walker A, et al. Fruit and vegetable consumption and all-cause, cancer and CVD mortality: analysis of Health Survey for England data. *J Epidemiol Community Health.* 2014;68(9):856–62. doi: 10.1136/jech-2013-203500.

12. Wang X, Ouyang Y, Liu J, et al. Fruit and vegetable consumption and mortality from all causes, cardiovascular disease, and cancer: systematic review and dose-response meta-analysis of prospective cohort studies. *BMJ.* 2014;349:g4490. Dauchet L, Amouyel P, Hercberg S, et al. Fruit and vegetable consumption and risk of coronary heart disease: a meta-analysis of cohort studies. *J Nutr.* 2006;136(10):2588–93. He

FJ, Nowson CA, MacGregor GA. Fruit and vegetable consumption and stroke: meta-analysis of cohort studies. *Lancet.* 2006;367(9507):320–26.

13. Zakkar M, Van der Heiden K, Luong LA, et al. Activation of Nrf2 in endothelial cells protects arteries from exhibiting a proinflammatory state. *Arterioscler Thromb Vasc Biol.* 2009;29(11):1851–57. Dwyer JH, Navab M, Dwyer KM, et al. Oxygenated carotenoid lutein and progression of early atherosclerosis: the Los Angeles atherosclerosis study. *Circulation.* 2001;103(24):2922–27.

14. Lopez-Legarrea P, de la Iglesia R, Abete I, et al. The protein type within a hypocaloric diet affects obesity-related inflammation: the RESMENA project. *Nutrition.* 2014;30:424–29.

15. Aune D, Navarro Rosenblatt DA, Chan DS, et al. Dairy products, calcium, and prostate cancer risk: a systematic review and meta-analysis of cohort studies. *Am J Clin Nutr.* 2015;101(1):87–117. Larsson SC, Orsini N, Wolk A. Milk, milk products and lactose intake and ovarian cancer risk: a meta-analysis of epidemiological studies. *Int J Cancer.* 2006;118(2):431–41.

16. U.S. Department of Agriculture and U.S. Department of Health and Human Services. *Dietary Guidelines for Americans, 2010.* 7th ed. Washington, DC: U.S. Government Printing Office, December 2010. Available at health.gov/dietaryguidelines /dga2010/dietaryguidelines2010.pdf.

17. Sacks FM, Svetkey LP, Vollmer WM, et al. DASH-Sodium Collaborative Research Group. Effects on blood pressure of reduced dietary sodium and the Dietary Approaches to Stop Hypertension (DASH) diet. *N Engl J Med.* 2001;344(1):3–10.

18. Dunaief DM, Fuhrman J, Dunaief JL, et al. Glycemic and cardiovascular parameters improved in type 2 diabetes with the high nutrient density (HND) diet. *Open J Prev Med.* 2012;2(3):364–71. Fuhrman J, Singer M. Improved cardiovascular parameter with a nutrient-dense, plant-rich diet-style: a patient survey with illustrative cases. *Amer J Life Med.* October 15, 2015 doi: 10.1177/1559827615611024.

19. Ornish D, Weidner G, Fair WR, et al. Intensive lifestyle changes may affect the progression of prostate cancer. *J Urol.* 2005;174(3):1065–70.

20. Ornish D, Scherwitz LW, Billings JH. Intensive lifestyle changes for reversal of coronary heart disease. *JAMA.* 1998;280(23):2001–7.

21. Grosso G, Yang J, Marventano S, et al. Nut consumption on all-cause, cardiovascular, and cancer mortality risk: a systematic review and meta-analysis of epidemiologic studies. *Am J Clin Nutr.* 2015;101:783–93.

22. Esselstyn CB Jr, Gendy G, Doyle J, et al. A way to reverse CAD? *J Fam Prac.* 2014;63(7):256–64b.

23. Barnard RJ, Guzy P, Rosenberg J, et al. Effects of an intensive exercise and nutrition program on patients with coronary artery disease: a five-year follow-up. *J Cardiac Rehab.* 1983;3:183–90.

24. Beard CM, Barnard RJ, Robbins DC, et al. Effects of diet and exercise on qualitative and quantitative measures of LDL and its susceptibility to oxidation. *Arterioscler Thromb Vasc Biol.* 1996;16:201–7.

25. Rankin P, Morton DP, Diehl HA, et al. Effectiveness of a volunteer-delivered lifestyle modification program for reducing cardiovascular disease risk factors. *Am J of Cardiol*. 2012;109(1):82–6. Morton D, Rankin P, Kent L, Dysinger W. CHIP: History, evaluation and outcomes. *Am J Lifestyle Med*. 2014; DOI:10.1177/1559827614531391.

26. Fuhrman J. Dietary protocols to maximize disease reversal and long term safety. *Am J Lifestyle Med*. 2015 May 4. doi: 10.1177/1559827615580971.

27. Calle-Pascual AL, Saavedra A, Benedi A, et al. Changes in nutritional pattern, insulin sensitivity and glucose tolerance during weight loss in obese patients from a Mediterranean area. *Horm Metab Res*. 1995 Nov;27(11):499–502.

28. Rose GA, Thompson WB, Williams RT. Corn oil treatment of ischaemic heart disease. *Br Med J*. 1965;1(5449):1531–33.

29. Ramsden CE, Zamora D, Leelarthaepin B, et al. Use of dietary linoleic acid for secondary prevention of coronary heart disease and death: evaluation of recovered data from the Sydney Diet Heart Study and updated meta-analysis. *BMJ*. 2013;346:e8707.

Chapter 8: The Nutritarian Plan

1. Bhandarkar SS, Arbiser JL. Curcumin as an inhibitor of angiogenesis. *Adv Exp Med Biol*. 2007;595:185–95. Jurenka JS. Anti-inflammatory properties of curcumin, a major constituent of Curcuma longa: a review of preclinical and clinical research. *Altern Med Rev*. 2009;14:141–53. Noorafshan A, Ashkani-Esfahani S. A review of therapeutic effects of curcumin. *Curr Pharm Des*. 2013;19:2032–45. Goel A, Kunnumakkara AB, Aggarwal BB. Curcumin as "Curecumin": from kitchen to clinic. *Biochen Pharmacol*. 2008;75:787–809.

2. Ali BH, Blunden G, Tanira MO, et al. Some phytochemical pharmacological and toxicological properties of ginger (Zingiber officinale Roscoe): a review of recent research. *Food Chem Toxicol*. 2008;46:409–20. Haniadka R, Saidanha E, Sunita V, et al. A review of the gastroprotective effects of ginger (Zingiber officinale Roscoe). *Food Funct*. 2013;6:845–55. Altman RD, Marcussen KC. Effects of a ginger extract on knee pain in patients with osteoarthritis. *Arthritis Rheum*. 2001;44:2531–38. Rahmani AH, Shabrmi FM, Aly SM. Active ingredients of ginger as potential candidates in the prevention and treatment of diseases via modulation of biological activities. *Int J Physiol Pathophysiol Pharmacol*. 2014;6:125–36.

3. Hiebowicz J, Darwiche G, Bjorgell O, et al. Effect of cinnamon on postprandial blood glucose, gastric emptying, and satiety in healthy subjects. *Am J Clin Nutr*. 2007;85:1552–56. Davis PA, Yokoyama W. Cinnamon intake lowers fasting blood glucose: meta-analysis. *J Med Food*. 2011;14:884–89. Nahas R, Moher M. Complementary and alternative medicine for the treatment of type 2 diabetes. *Can Fam Physician*. 2009;55:591–96.

Chapter 10: Your Questions Answered

1. Grimsmo J, Grundvold I, Maehlum S, et al. High prevalence of atrial fibrillation in long-term endurance cross-country skiers. Echocardiographic findings and

possible predictors. A 28–30 year follow-up study. *Eur J Cardiovasc Prev Rehabil.* 2010;17:100–5.

2. Schnohr P, O'Keefe JH, Marott JL, et al. Dose of jogging and long-term mortality: the Copenhagen City Heart Study. *J Am Coll Cardiol.* 2015;65:411–19.

3. Schnohr P, O'Keefe JH, Marott JL, et al. Dose of jogging and long-term mortality. *J Am Coll Cardiol* 2015; 65:411–419.

4. O'Keefe JH, Patil HR, Lavie CJ, et al. Potential adverse cardiovascular effects from excessive endurance exercise. *Mayo Clin Proc.* 2012;87(6):587–95.

5. Lee DC, Pate RR, Lavie CJ, et al. Leisure-time running reduces all-cause and cardiovascular mortality risk. *J Am Coll Cardiol.* 2014;64(5):472–81.

6. Boutcher SH. High-intensity intermittent exercise and fat loss. *J Obes.* 2011;2011: 868305. doi: 10.1155/2011/868305.

7. Rognmo Ø, Hetland E, Helgerud J, et al. High intensity aerobic interval exercise is superior to moderate intensity exercise for increasing aerobic capacity in patients with coronary artery disease. *Eur J Cardiovasc Prev Rehabil.* 2004 Jun;11(3):216–22.

8. Molmen-Hansen HE, Stolen T, Tjonna AE, et al. Aerobic interval training reduces blood pressure and improves myocardial function in hypertensive patients. *Eur J Prev Cardiol.* 2012;19(2):151–60.

9. Hightower JM, Moore D. Mercury levels in high-end consumers of fish. *Environ Health Perspect.* 2003;11(4):604–8.

10. Mahaffey KR, Clickner RP, Bodurow CC. Blood organic mercury and dietary mercury intake: National Health and Nutrition Examination Survey, 1999 and 2000. *Environ Health Perspect.* 2004;112(5):562–70. Hightower JM, Moore D. Mercury levels in high-end consumers of fish. *Environ Health Perspect.* 2003;111(4):604–8.

11. Dewailly E, Suhas E, Mou Y, et al. High fish consumption in French Polynesia and prenatal exposure to metals and nutrients. *Asia Pac J Clin Nutr.* 2008;17(3):461–70.

12. Diakovich MP, Efimova NV. Assessment of health risks upon exposure to mentholated mercury. *Gig Sanit.* 2001;2:49–51. Masley SC, Masley LV, Gualtieri CT. Effect of mercury levels and seafood intake on cognitive function in middle-aged adults. *J Integr Med.* 2012;11(3):32–40.

13. Foran JA, Carpenter DO, Hamilton MC, et al. Risk-based consumption advice for farmed Atlantic and wild Pacific salmon contaminated with dioxins and dioxin-like compounds. *Environ Health Perspect.* 2005 May;113(5):552–56.

14. Burros, M. Stores say wild salmon, but tests say farm bred. *New York Times.* 2005 Apr 10. Available at http://www.nytimes.com/2005/04/10/dining/stores-say-wild-salmon-but-tests-say-farm-bred.html?_r=0. Salonen JT, Seppänen K, Nyyssönen K, et al. Intake of mercury from fish, lipid peroxidation, and the risk of myocardial infarction and coronary cardiovascular, and any death in eastern Finnish Men. *Circulation.* 1995;91(3):645–55.

15. Hueber, A, Rosentreter A, Severin M. Canthaxanthin retinopathy: long-term observations. *Ophthalmic Res.* 2011;46(2):103–6.

16. Karimi R, Fitzgerald TP, Fisher NS. Stonybrook University seafood mercury database: a quantitative synthesis of mercury in commercial seafood. Supplemental material. 2012.

17. Holmes MV, Dale CE, Zuccolo L, et al. Association between alcohol and cardiovascular disease: Mendelian randomization analysis based on individual participant data. *BMJ*. 2014;349:g4164.

18. Jayasekara H, English DR, Room R, et al. Alcohol consumption over time and risk of death: a systematic review and meta-analysis. *Am J Epidemiol*. 2014;179(9):1049–59.

19. Lim SS, Vos T, Flaxman AD, et al. A comparative risk assessment of burden of disease and injury attributable to 67 risk factors and risk factor clusters in 21 regions, 1990–2010: a systematic analysis for the Global Burden of Disease Study 2010. *Lancet*. 2012;380:2224–60.

20. Rehm J, Baliunas D, Borges GL, et al. The relation between different dimensions of alcohol consumption and burden of disease: an overview. *Addiction*. 2010;105:817–43.

21. Hamajima N, Hirose K, Tajima K, et al. The Collaborative Group on Hormonal Factors in Breast Cancer. Alcohol, tobacco and breast cancer: collaborative reanalysis of individual data from 53 epidemiological studies, including 58,515 women with breast cancer and 95,067 women without the disease. *Br J Cancer*. 2002:87(11):1234–45.

22. Linkins LA, Choi PT, Douketis JD. Clinical impact of bleeding in patients taking oral anticoagulant therapy for venous thromboembolism. *Ann Intern Med*. 2003;139:893–900.

23. Joshipura KJ, Ascherio A, Manson JE, et al. Fruit and vegetable intake in relation to risk of ischemic stroke. *JAMA*. 1999;282(13):1233–39.

24. Sauvaget C, Nagano J, Allen N, et al. Vegetable and fruit intake and stroke mortality in the Hiroshima/Nagasaki Life Span Study. *Stroke*. 2003;34(10):2355–60.

25. Lamas GA, Goertz C, Boineau R, et al. TACT Investigators. Effect of disodium EDTA chelation regimen on cardiovascular events in patients with previous myocardial infarction: the TACT randomized trial. *JAMA*. 2013;309(12):1241–50.

26. Voight BF, Peloso GM, Orho-Melander M, et al. Plasma HDL cholesterol and risk of MI: a Mendelian randomisation study. *Lancet*. 2012;380:572–80.

27. Ridker PM, Genest J, Boekholdt SM, et al. HDL cholesterol and residual risk of first cardiovascular events after treatment with potent statin therapy: an analysis from the JUPITER trial. *Lancet*. 2010;376(9738)333–39. Hausenloy DJ, Opie L, Yellon DM. Dissociating HDL cholesterol from cardiovascular risk. *Lancet*. 2010;376(9738):305–6.

28. Higdon J, Delage B, Williams D, et al. Cruciferous vegetables and human cancer risk: epidemiologic evidence and mechanistic basis. *Pharmacol Res*. 2007;55:224–36. Wu QJ, Yang Y, Vogtmann E, et al. Cruciferous vegetables intake and the risk of colorectal cancer: a meta-analysis of observational studies. *Ann Oncol*. 2013;24(4):1079–87. Liu X, Lv K. Cruciferous vegetables intake is inversely associated with risk of breast cancer: a meta-analysis. *Breast*. 2013;22(3):309–13. Liu B, Mao Q, Cao M, et al. Cruciferous vegetables intake and risk of prostate cancer: a meta-analysis. *Int J Urol*. 2012;19:134–41.

29. Bosetti C, Negri E, Kolonel L, et al. A pooled analysis of case-control studies of thyroid cancer. VII. Cruciferous and other vegetables (International). *Cancer Causes Control*. 2002;13:765–75. Dal Maso L, Bosetti C, La Vecchia C, et al. Risk factors for thyroid cancer: an epidemiological review focused on nutritional factors. *Cancer Causes Control*. 2009;20:75–86.

30. Higdon J, Drake VJ. Cruciferous vegetables. In: *An Evidence-Based Approach to Phytochemicals and Other Dietary Factors*. 2nd ed. New York: Thieme; 2013.

31. Krajcovicova-Kudlackova M, Buckova K, Klimes I, et al. Iodine deficiency in vegetarians and vegans. *Ann Nutr Metab*. 2003;47:183–85. Leung AM, Lamar A, He X, et al. Iodine status and thyroid function of Boston-area vegetarians and vegans. *J Clin Endocrinol Metab*. 2011;96:E1303–7.

32. National Institutes of Health, Office of Dietary Supplements. Dietary supplement fact sheet: iodine. Available at https://ods.od.nih.gov/factsheets/Iodine-Consumer/.

33. McMillan M, Spinks EA, Fenwick GR. Preliminary observations on the effect of dietary brussels sprouts on thyroid function. *Hum Toxicol*. 1986;5:15–19.

34. Chu M, Seltzer TF. Myxedema coma induced by ingestion of raw bok choy. *N Engl J Med*. 2010;362:1945–46.

35. Tonstad S, Nathan E, Oda K, et al. Vegan diets and hypothyroidism. *Nutrients*. 2013;5:4642–52.

36. Leung AM, Lamar A, He X, et al. Iodine status and thyroid function of Boston-area vegetarians and vegans. *J Clin Endocrinol Metab*. 2011;96:E1303–7.

37. Zhang X, Shu XO, Xiang YB, et al. Cruciferous vegetable consumption is associated with a reduced risk of total and cardiovascular disease mortality. *Am J Clin Nutr*. 2011;94:240–46.

38. Barnett JB, Hamer DH, Meydani SN. Zinc: a new risk factor for pneumonia in the elderly? *Nutr Rev*. 2010;68(1):30–37.

39. Bjelakovic G, Nikolova D, Gluud LL, et al. Antioxidant supplements for prevention of mortality in healthy participants and patients with various diseases. *Cochrane Database Syst Rev*. 2008:CD007176.

40. Kim YI. Does a high folate intake increase the risk of breast cancer? *Nutr Rev*. 2006;64(10 Pt 1):468–75. Stolzenberg-Solomon RZ, Chang SC, Leitzmann MI, et al. Folate intake, alcohol use, and postmenopausal breast cancer risk in the Prostate, Lung, Colorectal, and Ovarian Cancer Screening Trial. *Am J Clin Nutr*. 2006;83(4):895–904. Sellers TA, Kushi LH, Cerhan JR, et al. Dietary folate intake, alcohol, and risk of breast cancer in a prospective study of postmenopausal women. *Epidemiology*. 2001;12(4):420–28. Figueiredo JC, Grau MV, Haile RW, et al. Folic acid and risk of prostate cancer: results from a randomized clinical trial. *J Natl Cancer Inst*. 2009;101(6):432–35. Fife J, Raniga S, Hider PN, et al. Folic acid supplementation and colorectal cancer risk: a meta-analysis. *Colorectal Dis*. 2011;13(2):132–37.

41. Oregon State University. Linus Pauling Institute. Micronutrient Information Center. Vitamin K. Available at http://lpi.oregonstate.edu/infocenter/vitamins/vitaminK/.

42. Cockayne S, Adamson J, Lanham-New S, et al. Vitamin K and the prevention of fractures: systematic review and meta-analysis of randomized controlled trials. *Arch Intern Med.* 2006;166:1256–61.

43. Beulens JW, Booth SL, van den Heuvel EG, et al. The role of menaquinones (vitamin K2) in human health. *Br J Nutr.* 2013;110:1357–68. Geleijnse JM, Vermeer C, Grobbee DE, et al. Dietary intake of menaquinone is associated with a reduced risk of coronary heart disease: the Rotterdam Study. *J Nutr.* 2004;134:3100–5. Beulens JW, Bots ML, Atsma F, et al. High dietary menaquinone intake is associated with reduced coronary calcification. *Atherosclerosis.* 2009;203:489–93.

44. Gast GC, de Roos NM, Sluijs I, et al. A high menaquinone intake reduces the incidence of coronary heart disease. *Nutr Metab Cardiovasc Dis.* 2009;19:504–10.

45. Rees K, Guraewal S, Wong YL, et al. Is vitamin K consumption associated with cardio-metabolic disorders? A systematic review. *Maturitas.* 2010;67:121–28.

46. Weingartner O, Bohm M, Laufs U. Controversial role of plant sterol esters in the management of hypercholesterolaemia. *Eur Heart J.* 2009;30:404–9.

47. Berger A, Jones PJ, Abumweis SS. Plant sterols: factors affecting their efficacy and safety as functional food ingredients. *Lipids Health Dis.* 2004;3:5.

48. Woyengo TA, Ramprasath VR, Jones PJ. Anticancer effects of phytosterols. *Eur J Clin Nutr.* 2009;63:813–20. Mendilaharsu M, De Stefani E, Deneo-Pellegrini H, et al. Phytosterols and risk of lung cancer: a case-control study in Uruguay. *Lung Cancer.* 1998;21:37–45. Ronco A, De Stefani E, Boffetta P, et al. Vegetables, fruits, and related nutrients and risk of breast cancer: a case-control study in Uruguay. *Nutr Cancer.* 1999;35:111–19. De Stefani E, Brennan P, Boffetta P, et al. Vegetables, fruits, related dietary antioxidants, and risk of squamous cell carcinoma of the esophagus: a case-control study in Uruguay. *Nutr Cancer.* 2000;38:23–29. De Stefani E, Boffetta P, Ronco AL, et al. Plant sterols and risk of stomach cancer: a case-control study in Uruguay. *Nutr Cancer.* 2000;37:140–44.

49. Klippel KF, Hiltl DM, Schipp B. A multicentric, placebo-controlled, double-blind clinical trial of beta-sitosterol (phytosterol) for the treatment of benign prostatic hyperplasia. German BPH-Phyto Study group. *Br J Urol.* 1997;80:427–32. Berges RR, Kassen A, Senge T. Treatment of symptomatic benign prostatic hyperplasia with beta-sitosterol: an 18-month follow-up. *BJU Int.* 2000;85:842–46.

50. Fuhrman J, Sarter B, Glaser D, et al. Changing perceptions of hunger on a high nutrient density diet. *Nutr J.* 2010;9:51.

Index